Ophthalmology

in Chinese Medicine

(Second Edition)

Project Editor: Zhou Ling

Book Designer: Long Dan-tong   Guo Miao

Typesetter: Bai Ya-ping

International Standard Library of Chinese Medicine

Ophthalmology
in Chinese Medicine

(Second Edition)

Wei Qi-ping (韦企平)

Professor of Ophthalmology,
Beijing University of Chinese Medicine,
Beijing, China

Andy Rosenfarb, ND, L.Ac.

Acupuncture Health Associates,
New Jersey, USA

Liang Li-na (梁丽娜), Ph.D. TCM

Associate Professor of Ophthalmology,
Eye Hospital of China Academy of Chinese Medical Sciences,
Beijing, China

人民卫生出版社
PMPH PEOPLE'S MEDICAL PUBLISHING HOUSE

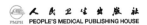
PEOPLE'S MEDICAL PUBLISHING HOUSE

Website: http://www.pmph.com/en

Book Title: International Standard Library of Chinese Medicine: **Ophthalmology in Chinese Medicine** (Second Edition)
国际标准化英文版中医教材：中医眼科学（第 2 版）

Contact address: No. 19, Pan Jia Yuan Nan Li, Chaoyang District, Beijing 100021, P.R. China, phone/fax: 8610 5978 7340, E-mail: pmph@pmph.com/en

For text and trade sales, as well as review copy enquiries, please contact PMPH at pmphsales@gmail.com

Disclaimer
This book is for educational and reference purposes only. In view of the possibility of human error or changes in medical science, the author, editor, publisher and any other party involved in the publication of this work do not guarantee that the information contained herein is in any respect accurate or complete. The medicinal therapies and treatment techniques presented in this book are provided for the purpose of reference only. If readers wish to attempt any of the techniques or utilize any of the medicinal therapies contained in this book, the publisher assumes no responsibility for any such actions. It is the responsibility of the readers to understand and adhere to local laws and regulations concerning the practice of these techniques and methods. The authors, editors and publisher disclaim all responsibility for any liability, loss, injury, or damage incurred as a consequence, directly or indirectly, of the use and application of any of the contents of this book.

First published: 2018
ISBN 978-7-117-27737-2
Cataloguing in Publication Data:
A catalog record for this book is available from the CIP-Database China.
Printed in The People's Republic of China

ISBN 978-7-117-27737-2

9 787117 277372 >

Editorial Board

About the Authors

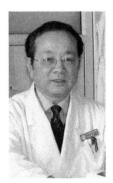

Wei Qi-ping (韦企平)

Professor Wei currently serves as Chief Physician and supervisor of doctoral students at Beijing University of Chinese Medicine. He is the only academic heir of the notable Wei's family Chinese medicine ophthalmology. Dr. Wei is the Chairman of Ophthalmology committee at the National Center for Medical Education Research and Development, vice-chairman of the Ophthalmology Society of China Association of Chinese Medicine, Chairman of the Ophthalmology Society of the Beijing Association of Chinese Medicine, as well as a standing committee member of the Ophthalmology Committee for the World Federation of Chinese Medicine Society. Dr. Wei is an editorial member of the *Chinese Journal of Chinese Ophthalmology, Chinese Journal of Practical Ophthalmology*, and *Chinese Journal of Ophthalmology*. He is also an evaluation expert of the life science department of the National Natural Science Foundation, and a new drug evaluation expert for the State Food and Drug Administration.

He has published over 60 professional articles as first author, and edited 11 professional books as chief editor or editor. Dr. Wei has practiced in the field of ophthalmology for 43 years. He is expert in diagnosis and integrated treatment of ocular surface diseases and difficult eye diseases, particularly specialized in treating all kinds of optic nerve disease and retinal degeneration diseases with Chinese herbs and acupuncture.

In addition to his clinical work, Prof. Wei has hosted and participated in many research programs supported by the Ministry of Health and the State Administration of TCM, and the projects have got many prizes. The project "A Study on Leber's Disease" was awarded the second class of National Scientific Technology Progress Prize. Prof. Wei is currently the principal investigator of two grants from National Nature Science Foundation.

About the Authors

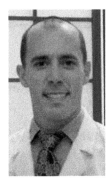

Andy Rosenfarb

Dr. Rosenfarb is a Naturopathic Doctor who has practiced in the field of Chinese medicine since 1994, having received his Master of Traditional Oriental Medicine from Pacific College of Oriental Medicine (Magna Cum Laude). He continued post-graduate work at Zhejiang College of Traditional Chinese Medicine in Hangzhou, China, and is Board Certified in Acupuncture & Chinese Herbal Medicine by the National Certification Commission for Acupuncture & Oriental Medicine (NCCAOM). Dr. Rosenfarb is also the former President of the New Jersey Association of Acupuncture & Oriental Medicine.

Dr. Rosenfarb is the author of *Healing Your Eyes with Chinese Medicine*, published in 2007 by North Atlantic Books, has published many articles on the treatment of ocular diseases with Chinese Medicine, and lectures regularly on TCM Ophthalmology. Dr. Rosenfarb is the Founder and Clinical Director of Acupuncture Health Associates, located in Westfield, New Jersey. He is engaged in ongoing clinical research on the modern applications of Chinese Medicine in the treatment of eye diseases. Dr. Rosenfarb has developed highly effective acupuncture protocols for treating degenerative eye conditions, which has successfully helped hundreds of patients from around the world. Dr. Andy Rosenfarb is the English language editor of this book. (For more information on Dr. Rosenfarb's work, visit www.acupuncture-health.net.)

008

About the Authors

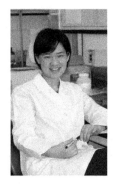

Liang Li-na (梁丽娜)

Dr. Liang has practiced ophthalmology since 1997, having received her Master in Integrative Ophthalmology (Chinese and Western conventional medicine) in 1997, and Doctor of Chinese Medicine in 2003 from the China Academy of Chinese Medical Sciences in Beijing. She continued post-doctoral work in the United States at the University of Alabama at Birmingham and at the Medical College of Wisconsin. Dr. Liang is a committee member of the Ophthalmology Society of Beijing, Association of Chinese Medicine. She is a standing member of the Ophthalmology Committee at the National Center for Medical Education Research and Development.

Dr. Liang is engaged in ongoing clinical research on the modern applications of traditional Chinese medicine in the treatment of eye diseases. She is an expert in the diagnosis and treatment of fundus diseases, and integrates Chinese medicine with Western conventional medicine. Dr. Liang has participated in many research studies supported by the National Nature Science Foundation (China), the Ministry of Science and Technology (China), and National Institutes of Health (USA). She has published many articles on various topics of ophthalmology. Dr. Liang Li-na is the translator of this book.

Author's Preface

Author's Preface

In the 21st century, with the enhancement of the realization of the need for disease prevention and integrative health care, transformation of the conventional medical model, and understanding of the nature of disease, the international community has become more and more interested in natural approaches to health and healing. The increasing popularity of Chinese medicine in Europe and America, and especially in Asia, has brought about a much broader space for the development of Chinese medicine.

Chinese medical ophthalmology is an integral discipline of Chinese medicine with a history of more than 2,000 years. The unique theory and application was formed on the basis of Chinese medicine and has gradually developed and evolved over the years. Concepts of holism, along with principles of pattern differentiation and treatment, form the base of Chinese medicine. Specialized systems like the five-wheel differentiation, external oculopathy differentiation, and fundus differentiation are unique to Chinese medical ophthalmology. As acupuncture (body acupuncture, scalp acupuncture, ear acupuncture) plays an important role in the treatment of eye disease, methods of acupuncture therapy for eye disorders are emphased in this book.

Although Chinese medical ophthalmology is derived from traditional Chinese medicine, it has a close relationship with modern Western medicine. Wide application of equipments such as fluorescence fundus angiography, ophthalmic ultrasonography, and optical coherence tomography not only expands the examination methods of Chinese medical ophthalmology, but also provides objective evaluation for treatment by medicinal and/or acupuncture therapy. At present, there is not a textbook in the English language combing traditional Chinese medical ophthalmology with current examination means of Western ophthalmology, which may be more acceptable and comprehensible to the ophthalmologists and practitioners of Chinese medicine worldwide. Therefore, the publication of this book will fill this gap.

This textbook is written with the intention to highlight the special features of Chinese medicine. It systematically introduces the basic theory of Chinese medical ophthalmology and the diagnose and treatment for eye diseases. The content was selected to meet the practical needs of modern clinicians of Chinese medicine. The authors have strived to make the language concise and accurate, and adapt theoretical expounding to Western

Author's Preface

ways of thinking.

In addition to the etiology, pathogenesis, and diagnostic and treatment procedures for each eye disease, this textbook gives detailed explanations of basic TCM techniques commonly used in the ophthalmic clinic, such as external therapy and acupuncture. There is much information presented on chronic eye diseases and retinal degeneration. These conditions can be effectively treated and/or its progression may be slowed or arrested with medicinal and acupuncture treatment.

The book is composed of two parts – the general introduction to Chinese medical ophthalmology and disease pathology. The general introduction includes five chapters, including a brief introduction to the history of Chinese medical ophthalmology, anatomy and physiology of the eyes, common ophthalmic examination methods, the relationship between the eye and *zang-fu* organs and channels, methods of pattern differentiation, internal and external therapy, commonly used acupoints, and effective acupuncture methods.

The pathology section consists of 10 chapters that introduce 40 eye diseases according to anatomical position (i.e., eyelid, conjunctiva, sclera, cornea, iris, lens, retina, choroids, and optic nerve). Clinically challenging eyes diseases like blepharoptosis, dry eyes, herpes simplex keratitis, ischemic optic neuropathy, retinitis pigmentosa, and optic atrophy, are presented in great detail.

This book is applicable to practitioners of Chinese medicine and integrative medicine in English-speaking countries, especially to the practitioners of Chinese medical ophthalmology. It can also be a reference book for graduate students of TCM and conventional ophthalmologists. However, due to the complexity and variety of clinical medicine, and to the nature of difficult diseases, it is suggested to use this book with flexibility in clinical practice, instead of sticking to a certain medicinal formula or acupoint protocol. A treatment plan should be developed on the basis of pattern differentiation, and suited to the patient's condition, the time of year, and the local climate.

Please see the attached CD for more details on some diseases and manipulation (mainly about acupuncture).

All compilers of the textbook come from notable TCM universities or traditional Chinese medical hospitals in China. They are professors and specialist who have an abundance of scholastic achievement and clinical experience. We anticipate that the publication of this textbook will strengthen the understanding of Chinese medical ophthalmology in clinicians who have a particular interest in treating eye diseases. Our goal is to also

Author's Preface

promote an academic interchange among the doctors of Chinese medicine, integrative medicine, and Western medicine. Our desire is to further promote an international dissemination of Chinese medical ophthalmology so as to benefit eye patients from around the world.

The accompanying DVD-ROM displays the features of Chinese ophthalmology. It introduces the five-wheel theory (the core of Chinese ophthalmology) and the specific acupuncture manipulations in TCM ophthalmology. The disc also introduces the treatment of several diseases with acupuncture.

Special thanks to Dongfang Hospital of Beijing University of Chinese Medicine and Tianjin University of Traditional Chinese Medicine for their support in the making of the DVD-ROM. We are also sincerely grateful to the software production team for their great efforts and all the patients that appear in the videos for their participation.

Wei Qi-ping

Beijing, 2018

Translator's Preface

Translator's Preface

When I was engaged in postdoctoral studies and working in the United States of America, I kept asking the same questions to my Western friends and colleagues: What do you think about traditional Chinese medicine? Do you know many eye diseases can be treated by TCM? The answer to the second question was almost the same as "no". So, I was very excited by the news that PMPH will publish a series of textbooks to introduce Chinese medicine worldwide, and I was invited to be one of the editors-in-chief of this textbook.

The whole textbook has been translated following the PMPH Publication Guidelines. To keep the language characteristics of traditional Chinese medicine as well as facilitate understanding in readers whose mother tongue is English, most of the terms were first translated literally (word-for-word), and then explained with their corresponding Western medical terms. For example, 神水 (*shén shuǐ*) is translated as "spirit water", and its corresponding terms in Western medicine are aqueous humor or tears. However, as the terms yin (阴), yang (阳), and qi (气) have been accepted widely in the English language, they are just given their *pīn yīn* spelling without explanation. In the process of translating classic quotes, I was met with tremendous difficulties. Classical

Chinese, even for a native-Chinese speaker, makes for difficult reading. The classical Chinese text needed to be translated it into modern Chinese first; to do this without distortion of meaning, the translators discussed terminology issues and sought the advice of famous veteran doctors of TCM. I have found that, by patient and careful handling, even the most cumbrous sentences can be rewritten into clear ones.

My personal gratitude goes to the other two editors-in-chief, Dr. Wei Qiping and Dr. Andy Rosenfarb, and the project manager, Ms. Liu Ying, of the People's Medical Publishing House. The translation would not have been finished without their invaluable advice, encouragement, and support.

In a careful final revision of the translation, I have found a number of errors, major and minor; and I fear that others remain undetected. We look forward to receiving any suggestions and criticisms from readers for improving the book for its next edition.

Liang Li-na

Beijing, 2018

Table of Contents

Table of Contents

Part I
Overview

Table of Contents

Part II
Specific Applications

Table of Contents

PART

Overview

I

Chapter 1
A Brief History of Ophthalmology in Chinese Medicine

Ophthalmology in traditional Chinese medicine (TCM) is a clinical discipline gradually formed over time, as a result of the Chinese people struggling with eye diseases over thousands of years. It is a precious part of Chinese culture.

1. Ancient Times - Northern and Southern Dynasties (581 A.D.)

TCM Ophthalmology originated in ancient times and was developed in the Shang, Zhou, Qin, and Han dynasties. After long periods of treating eye diseases with primitive methods, our ancestors began to explore the anatomic structure, physiology, and pathology of the eyes; gaining an understanding of pattern identification of eye diseases. Since the emergence of Chinese characters, the knowledge of eye diseases has been recorded. Among the inscriptions found on the bones or tortoise shells unearthed in Yin Dynasty Ruins in Anyang City, Henan Province, China, there were records about "eye (目)" and " eye diseases (疾目)". In *The Book of Songs* (*Shī Jīng*, 诗经) and *The Book of History* (*Shū Jīng*, 书经, also called *Shàng Shū*, 尚书), the disease of "blindness (目盲)" was recorded. Of the more than 100 different medicinals recorded in *The Classic of Mountains and Seas* (*Shān Hǎi Jīng*, 山海经), written before the Qin Dynasty, seven of them could prevent and treat eye disorders.

According to *Historical Records – Bian Que's Biography* (*Shǐ Jì – Biǎn Què Liè Zhuàn*, 史记·扁鹊列传), Bian Que in the Warring States Period was the first eye doctor (ophthalmologist) in the history of China. *The Yellow Emperor's Inner Classic* (*Huáng Dì Nèi Jīng*, 黄帝内经) had elementarily recorded the anatomy and physiology of the eyes, as well as the etiology, pathology, clinical manifestation, and acupuncture strategies for eye disorders. More than 30 eye diseases were recorded in this book. The relationship between *zang-fu* organs, channels, collaterals and the eyes; the theory of five wheels and eight regions; and the visceral pattern identification of eye diseases were developed from the related content in *The Yellow Emperor's Inner Classic*.

Shen Nong's Classic of Materia Medica (*Shén Nóng Běn Cǎo Jīng*, 神农本草经), compiled in the Qin and Han dynasties, presented 365 kinds of medicinals, around 70 of which could be used to treat diseases of the eyelids, outer and inner cantus, cornea and the fundus, as well as the eye problems caused by general diseases. Quite a few medicinals are still in use today. At the end of the Donghan Dynasty, in the famous medical classic *Treatise on Cold Damage and Miscellaneous Diseases* (*Shāng Hán Zá Bìng Lùn*, 伤寒杂病论), written by Zhang Zhong-jing, more than 20 eye diseases were mentioned when discussing the general diseases of the body.

2. Sui and Tang Dynasties (581 – 907 A.D.)

In the Sui and Tang dynasties, the concentrated records of ophthalmology occurred in some medical and prescription texts including *Treatise on Causes and Manifestations of Various Diseases* (*Zhū Bìng Yuán Hòu Lùn*, 诸病源候论), *Important Prescriptions Worth a Thousand Gold for Emergency* (*Bèi Jí Qiān Jīn Yào Fāng*, 备急千金要方) and *Arcane Essentials from the Imperial Library* (*Wài Tái Mì Yào*, 外台秘要). Famous ophthalmological books of Chinese medicine also occurred such as *Longshu's Treatise on Eye Diseases* (*Lóng Shù Yǎn Lùn*, 龙树眼论) and *Liu Hao's Verse on Eye Diseases* (*Liú Hào Yǎn Lùn Zhǔn Dì Gē*, 刘皓眼论准的歌). In the Sui Dynasty, *Treatise on Causes and Manifestations of Various Diseases*, compiled by Chao Yuan-fang, collected 38 eye diseases of the eyelid, external and internal canthus, conjunctiva, cornea, and fundus. Eyeball protrusion, nearsightedness/myopia, and other eye diseases as they related to general health disorders were also recorded in the book. In the Tang Dynasty, for the first time, the well-known *Important Prescriptions Worth a Thousand Gold for Emergency*, compiled by Sun Si-miao, listed eye diseases in Volume 1 of *Diseases of the Seven Orifices*, and clearly proposed 19 factors that causes eye diseases, several key points in preventing eye diseases, as well as the action of the liver of ox, sheep, and/or goat to brighten the eyes. Other external treatments for eye diseases were also introduced in the book in terms of fumigation, topical application, hooking and cutting, massage, and acupuncture.

Volume 1 of *The Eye Diseases* in *Arcane Essentials from the Imperial Library*, written by Wang Tao, quoted the content of an Indian medical book, *Indian Classics on Eye Diseases* (*Tiān Zhú Jīng Lùn Yǎn*, 天竺经论眼). The book contains the earliest record of the cataractopiesis with the gold needle. *Longshu's Treatise on Eye Diseases* was the first influential ophthalmologic work in China, but the original book was lost. The extant version was collected by the Japanese from the Korean ancient medical book *Categorized Collection of Medical Formulas* (*Yī Fāng Lèi Jù*, 医方类聚). During the reign of Emperor Wuzong of the Tang Dynasty (唐武宗, Li Chan [李瀍], later changed to Li Yan [李炎], 814–846), people were able to construct an artificial eye. China was among the first in recorded history to equip the world with the artificial eye. The Imperial Medical Bureau of the government of the Tang Dynasty was in charge of health care and medical education. Since then, diseases of the five sense organs were separated from the internal and the external medicines; a discipline and specialization of treating the five sense organs in Chinese medicine had been established.

3. Northern Song and Yuan Dynasties (960 – 1368 A.D.)

In the Song and Yuan dynasties, ancient medical books were systematically compiled and sorted out. Literature on TCM ophthalmology was preserved in medicinal prescription books and encyclopedias, such as *Formulas from Benevolent Sages Compiled during the Taiping Era* (*Tài Píng Shèng Huì Fāng*, 太平圣惠方), *Comprehensive Recording of Divine Assistance* (*Shèng Jì Zǒng Lù*, 圣济总录), and *Effective Formulas from Generations of Physicians* (*Shì Yī Dé Xiào Fāng*, 世医得效方). Specific chapters on eye diseases appeared in those books. Monographs of ophthalmology like *Longmu's Ophthalmology Secretly Handed Down* (*Mì Chuán Yǎn Kē Lóng Mù Lùn*, 秘传眼科龙木论) and *Essentials from the Silver Sea* (*Yín Hǎi Jīng Wēi*, 银海精微) were written during this period.

In the 100-volume prescription book *Formulas from Benevolent Sages Compiled during the Taiping Era*, two volumes on eye diseases summarized and developed ophthalmological achievements before the Song Dynasty. 500 prescriptions were classified according to different eye diseases and their patterns, and the pathogenesis of each pattern was briefly stated. The five-wheel theory was applied for the first time, and the relationship between the eyes and the whole body was emphasized. The text stated, "The eyes connect with the five *zang* organs, and qi passes through the five wheels." In addition to numerous records of internal and external treatments for the eye diseases, the book also described an effective acupuncture method used for treating cataracts with a gold needle.

One-hundred years later, the 200-volume *Comprehensive Recording of Divine Assistance*, a medicinal prescription book with discussions was created. The section on eye diseases included 12 volumes based on *Formulas from Benevolent Sages Compiled during the Taiping Era*. The content of the book greatly enriched TCM ophthalmology, and contained 58 kinds of eye diseases, 2 kinds of operations, and more than 750 prescriptions for treating eye diseases.

Over 180 kinds of ophthalmological medicinals were recorded in the officially compiled materia medica, *Revised Classified Materia Medica from Historical Classics for Emergency* (*Chóng Xiū Zhèng Hé Jīng Shǐ Zhèng Lèi Bèi Yòng Běn Cǎo*, 重修政和经史证类备用本草). Some foreign medicinals including myrrh and borneol were also included in the book.

During the Yuan Dynasty, in the book *Effective Formulas from Generations of Physicians*, edited by Wei Yi-lin [危亦林] , one volume was written on eye diseases and discussed the theory of the five wheels and eight regions, and the pattern identification and treatment of 72 different kinds of eye diseases.

The 10-volume *Longmu's Ophthalmology Secretly Handed Down* was a famous monograph of TCM Ophthalmology and was compiled by eye doctors in the Song and Yuan dynasties. Volume 1–6 stated *"The Prescription and Discussion of 72 Eye Diseases (七十二证方论)"*, and the related "Diagnostic Verses (审的歌)" were attached to each disease. Volume 7 recorded the most clinically significant prescriptions of the various famous eye doctors. Volume 8 was based on acupuncture therapy; volume 9-10 discussed the nature of medicinals in the prescriptions. The main content of the book narrated the etiology, symptoms and treatment of 72 kinds of eye diseases according to the classification of internal and external eye diseases. The book also introduced surgical procedures for eye diseases in terms of cataract removal with gold needle, hooking, cutting, knife puncturing and scraping therapy. The content of the book exerted certain influence on the later generations. *Taoist Priest Bao Guang's Discussion on Longmu's Ophthalmology (Bǎo Guāng Dào Rén Yǎn Kē Lóng Mù Jí, 葆光道人眼科龙木集)* was attached to the end of the book. The main content of the book was based on the the "72 *Questions on Eye Diseases* (眼科七十二问)", which was different from *"The Prescription and Discussion of 72 Eye Diseases"*. After the section on the "five-wheel theory", the book described the new principles of the "theory of the eight regions" in detail. Although the theory of the eight regions was not as influential as the theory of the five wheels, it was still clinically applicable.

Essentials from the Silver Sea was written by Sun Si-miao in the Song Dynasty. The book introduced the basic theories of TCM ophthalmology, including the theory of the five wheels and eight regions, and the pattern identification of eye diseases. It also listed the etiology, symptoms and treatment of more than 80 kinds of eye diseases, where simplified illustrations were presented with each eye disease.

In the Song Dynasty, the Imperial Medical Service was in charge of health care and medical education. Since then, TCM ophthalmology became an independent discipline in the medical history of China.

4. Ming and Qing Dynasties (1368 – 1912 A.D.)

Ming and Qing dynasties were the silver age of Chinese medicine, and the ancient medical books that greatly impacted TCM ophthalmology were *Enlightenment of Ophthalmology (Yuán Jī Qǐ Wēi, 原机启微)*, *The Grand Compendium of Materia Medica*

(*Běn Cǎo gāng Mù*, 本草纲目), *Formulas for Universal Relief (Pǔ Jì Fāng*, 普济方), *Standards for Diagnosis and Treatment (Zhèng Zhì Zhǔn Shéng*, 证治准绳), *A Close Examination of the Precious Classic on Ophthalmology (Shěn Shì Yáo Hán*, 审视瑶函), and *The Great Compendium of Classics on Ophthalmology (Mù Jīng Dà Chéng*, 目经大成).

Enlightenment of Ophthalmology was edited by Ni Wei-de [倪维德], a famous eye doctor who lived towards the end of the Yuan Dynasty and into the early Ming Dynasty. In Volume 1, eye diseases were classified into 18 classifications according to the etiologies. In Volume 2, the compatibility of medicinal formulas was discussed where more than 40 prescriptions for eye diseases were attached.

The Grand Compendium of Materia Medica was compiled by Li Shi-zhen [李时珍], who lived in the early Ming Dynasty. The book collected more than 400 kinds of medicinals for eye diseases. *Formulas for Universal Relief*, compiled by Zhu Di [朱棣], was abundant in content. 16 volumes of the text were dedicated to the treatment of eye diseases where a collection of more than 2,300 prescriptions and 300 diseases were named. *Standards for Diagnosis and Treatment*, edited by Wang Ken-tang [王肯堂], recorded more than 170 kinds of eye diseases and was quite helpful to doctors in terms of forming a clear clinical diagnosis.

Forty years later, Fu Ren-yu [傅仁宇] wrote *A Close Examination of the Precious Classic on Ophthalmology* on the basis of the former works on TCM ophthalmology. The front of the book presented numerous case records from many famous traditional eye doctors, including the theory of the five wheels and eight regions and the theory of the five circuits and six qi. Volumes 1–2 discussed the physiology of the eyes and the pattern identification and treatment of the eye diseases. Volumes 3–6 was based on the book *Criterion for Pattern Identification and Treatment*, where Dr. Fu presented his own clinical experiences. He summarized 108 kinds of eye diseases and described in detail the symptoms, diagnosis, and treatment. The book also explained how to treat cataracts with the gold needle, as well as other external therapies. The book was rich in content and, historically, was a very important reference book for the modern practice of TCM ophthalmology.

In the Qing Dynasty, more ophthalmology works were printed and transcribed. Huang Ting-jing [黄庭镜] wrote *The Great Compendium of Classics on Ophthalmology*. In Volume 1, the author discussed the anatomy and physiology of the eyes and the etiology, pattern identification, and internal and external treatment of the eye diseases. In Volume 2, the author investigated 12 kinds of pathogenic factors, 81 kinds of eye diseases, and 8 factors "similar to etiology but not diseases (似因非症)". In Volume 3, over 200 prescriptions were listed with detailed explanations. Huang Ting-jing was a good eye surgeon and thus the description of his operation methods for eye diseases was presented in great detail, including cataractopiesis with the gold needle. The origins of modern cataractopiesis using a gold needle were refined and improved upon over the years. The basic methods presented in the text are the basis for modern day laser cataract surgery.

Other significant ophthalmological works written in the Qing Dynasty were the *Guideline of Opththalmology* (*Yín Hǎi Zhǐ Nán*, 银海指南) by Gu Xi [顾锡], *Compilation of Ophthalmology* (*Yǎn Kē Zuǎn Yào*, 眼科纂要) by Huang Yan (黄岩), *Comprehensive Medicine According to Master Zhang – Section of Seven Orifices* (*Zhāng Shì Yī Tōng – Qī Qiào Mén,* 张氏医通·七窍门) by Zhang Lu [张璐], and *Golden Mirror of the Medical Tradition – Essential Teachings on the Treatment of Eye Diseases* (*Yī Zōng Jīn Jiàn – Yǎn Kē Xīn Fǎ Yào Jué,* 医宗金鉴·眼科心法要诀) by Wu Qian [吴谦]. In the *Complete Records of Ancient and Modern Medical Works of the Grand Compendium of Books* (*Gǔ Jīn Tú Shū Jí Chéng – Yī Bù Quán Lù,* 古今图书集成·医部全录), the section on eye diseases collected ophthalmological works from former dynasties, where brief summaries of respective as well as medicinal prescriptions and other therapeutic modalities were attached. The book was extremely rich in content.

5. Since 1949 (The Foundation of the People's Republic of China)

The Chinese government gave prominence to Chinese medicine and exerted its role in the health care system. Related policies were made, and Chinese medicine began to once again thrive in China.

Research and Educational Institutions:

In 1955, the China Academy of Traditional Chinese Medicine was founded (now called China Academy of Chinese Medical Sciences). A specific institution for Ophthalmology had been established and on October 25, 1986, the Eye Hospital of China Academy of Chinese Medical Sciences was established.

Twenty-five colleges of Chinese medicine were founded since 1956 in cities such as Beijing, Shanghai, Guangzhou, Chengdu, Nanjing, and Changchun. Teaching and research sections of ophthalmology were established, and ophthalmological clinics and hospital wards were opened.

In 1960, five colleges of Chinese medicine edited *Lectures on Ophthalmology in Chinese Medicine* (*Zhōng Yī Yǎn Kē Xué Jiǎng Yì,* 中医眼科学讲义), which became the first version of a universal textbook for institutions of higher education of Chinese medicine. It was revised, enriched, and perfected in 1964, 1975, 1979, and 1983. The fifth edition of *Ophthalmology in Chinese Medicine* (*Zhōng Yī Yǎn Kē Xué*, 中医眼科学) was edited by Chengdu University of Chinese Medicine. In January, 1995, Cooperative Textbook for Institutions of Higher Education of Chinese Medicine, *Ophthalmology in Chinese Medicine* was compiled by Professor Qi Bao-yu [祁宝玉] and published by the People's Medical Publishing House (PMPH). *China's Clinical Complete Book of Integrated Medicine – Ophthalmology* (*Zhōng Guó Zhōng Xī Yī Jié Hé Lín Chuáng Quán Shū – Yǎn Kē Xué*, 中国中西医结合临床全书·眼科学) was compiled by Professor Tang You-zhi [唐由之], Professor Cai Song-nian [蔡松年], and Professor Li Wen-qing [李文清], and was the textbook for the major of Integrated Medicine (integration of Chinese and Western medicine).

In order to adapt to the needs of higher education, the Ministry of Health organized the compilation of the Advanced Reference Book series: *Ophthalmology in Chinese Medicine* (with Li Chuan-ke [李传课] as the chief editor), which became the reference textbook for students of the master's degree program and the teacher's reference book in the colleges and universities of Chinese medicine. Professor Zeng Qing-hua [曾庆华] from Chengdu University of Chinese Medicine compiled the *Ophthalmology in Chinese Medicine* that belonged to the series of textbooks for Institutions of Higher Education of Chinese Medicine. The book was called the seventh version for short and was published by PMPH. The Integration of Traditional Chinese and Western Medical Textbook for Institutions of Higher Education series: *Integration of Traditional Chinese and Western Medical Ophthalmology* (*Zhōng Xī Yī Jié Hé Yǎn Kē Xué*, 中西医结合眼科学) was compiled by Professor Duan Jun-guo [段俊国] from Chengdu University of Chinese Medicine and published by PMPH. All of the above textbooks promoted the development of ophthalmology in Chinese medicine.

Presently, China Academy of Chinese Medical Sciences, Beijing University of CM, Chengdu University of CM, Hunan University of CM, Guangzhou University of CM, and Nanjing University of CM had set up the doctoral programs of Chinese medicine ophthalmology. The universities and colleges of Chinese medicine in different provinces had set up master's degree programs in Chinese medicine ophthalmology. Beijing, Hebei, Guangzhou, Chengdu, and Hunan have conducted training courses for Chinese medicine ophthalmology. Henan Province established the discipline of ophthalmology and otorhinolaryngology in Chinese medicine. The education in TCM ophthalmology is becoming increasingly widespread in the field.

In recent years, the discipline has made great progress in the field of surgery, acupuncture, and medicinal therapy. Some eye diseases that have been difficult to treat were brought into the modern scientific research field, and gained notoriety. Many new Chinese medicinals for treating eye diseases have been approved by The State Food and Drug Administration of China. With the efforts of TCM ophthalmologists, the field of ophthalmology in Chinese medicine is thriving and broadening its horizons.

Since 1949, many works of famous veteran doctors of TCM ophthalmology were published including documented clinical experiences. The works are: *Clinical Notes on Treating Eye Diseases* (*Yǎn Kē Lín Zhèng Bǐ Jì*, 眼科临症笔记) by Lu Ji-ping [路际平], *Wei Wen-gui's Clinical Experiences in Treating Eye Diseases* (*Wéi Wén Guì Yǎn Kē Jīng Yàn Xuǎn*, 韦文贵眼科经验选) by Wei Yu-ying [韦玉英], *Clinical Records of Treating Eye Diseases* (*Yǎn Kē Lín Zhèng Lù*, 眼科临症录) by Lu Nan-shan [陆南山], *Experiences of Syndrome Differentiation and Treatment of Eye Diseases* (*Yǎn Kē Zhèng Zhì Jīng Yàn*, 眼科证治经验) by Yao He-qing [姚和清], *Key Methods of Six Channels in Chinese Medicine Ophthalmology* (*Zhōng Yī Yǎn Kē Liù Jīng Fǎ Yào*, 中医眼科六经法要) by Chen Da-fu [陈达夫], *Clinical Practices of Ophthalmology in Chinese Medicine* (*Zhōng Yī Yǎn Kē Lín Chuáng Shí Jiàn*, 中医眼科临床实践) by Pang Zan-xiang [庞赞襄], *Exploration into Eye Diseases* (*Yǎn Kē Tàn Lí*, 眼科探骊) by Zhang Wang-zhi [张望之], *Chen Xi-nan's Experiences of Treating Eye* Diseases (*Chén Xī Nán Yǎn Kē Jīng Yàn*, 陈溪南眼科经验) by Ma De-xiang [马德祥], and *Zhang Jie-chun's Experiences of Syndrome Differentiation and Treatment of Eye Diseases* (*Zhāng Jiē Chūn Yǎn Kē Zhèng Zhì*, 张皆春眼科证治) by Zhou Feng-jian [周奉建].

The development of modern TCM ophthalmology is embodied by the following works: *Encyclopedia of Medicine - Ophthalmology in Chinese Medicine* (*Yī Xué Bǎi Kē Quán Shū - zhōng Yī Yǎn Kē Fēn Juàn*, 医学百科全书·中医眼科分卷) by Tang You-zhi [唐由之], *Acupuncture and Moxibustion for Eye Diseases* (*Yǎn Kē Zhēn Jiǔ Liáo Fǎ*, 眼科针灸疗法) by Xia Xian-min [夏贤闽], *External Application of Chinese Medicine for Eye Diseases and Clinical Practice* (*Yǎn Kē Wài Yòng Zhōng Yào Yǔ Lín Chuáng*, 眼科外用中药与临床) by Cao Jian-hui [曹建辉], *Ophthalmology in Chinese Medicine Today* (*Jīn Rì Zhōng Yī Yǎn Kē*, 今日中医眼科) by Wang Yong-yan [王永炎] and Zhuang Zeng-yuan [庄曾渊], and *Diagnosis and Treatment for Optic Nerve Diseases with Integration of Traditional Chinese and Western Medicines* (*Shì Shén Jīng Jí Bìng Zhōng Xī Yī Jié Hé Zhěn Zhì*, 视神经疾病中西医结合诊治) by Wei Qi-ping [韦企平] and Wei Shi-hui [魏世辉].

Chapter 2
Anatomy of the Eye

Section 1   The Eyeball

The eyeball is situated in the orbit and surrounded by ocular appendages, muscles, vessels, and orbit fat. The bony orbital cavity houses the eyeball while the soft tissue in-between functions as a cushion. The eyeball has an approximately spherical shape, with the anteroposterior diameter slightly longer than the vertical or horizontal diameter. The average anteroposterior diameter in adults is about 24 mm.[1]

The eyeball consists of three layers. From the exterior to the interior they are the fibrous layer, the uveal tract, and the retina. Within the eyeball, located just behind the iris, is a transparent, crystalline lens whose main function is to focus light rays for vision.

Clinically, the anterior vitreous/hyaloid membrane is used as a landmark to divide the eyeball into two segments: the anterior segment and posterior segment. There are three major chambers in the eye: the anterior, posterior, and vitreous chambers. The former two are in the anterior segment, separated by the lens and iris, but they communicate through the pupil. The latter is in the posterior segment. The anterior and posterior chambers are filled with the aqueous humor and the vitreous chamber is filled with the gelatinous vitreous (Fig. 2-1).

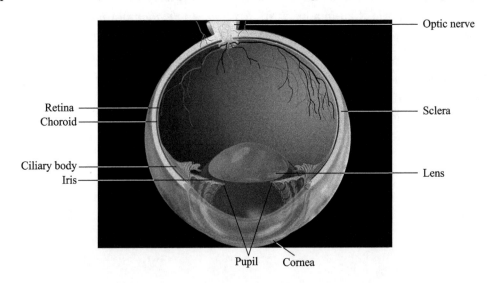

Fig. 2-1   Structure of the human eye

1. The Fibrous Layer

The fibrous layer is composed of the anterior transparent cornea which makes up one-sixth of the structure, and the posterior five-sixths which incluses the opaque sclera. The transitional region between the cornea and sclera is called the limbus. The fibrous layer is very rich in collagen.

■ The Cornea

The transparent cornea convexes and is the most anterior part of the eye. Because its curvature is greater than the sclera, there is a slight circumferential groove, called the scleral sulcus, at the transitional zone. The cornea contributes about 43D to the optical power of the eye.[1] The cornea is slightly elliptical: it is about 10.6 mm in diameter vertically and 11.75 mm in diameter horizontally.[2] The cornea is thinnest at its center and becomes thicker at the periphery. Because the cornea is avascular, its nutrition is supplied by the tear film and the aqueous humor.

Histologically, the cornea has five layers: from the anterior to the posterior, they are the epithelium, Bowman's layer, the stroma, Descemet's membrane, and the endothelium.

The epithelium has five to six layers of cells. The epithelial cells are dynamically shed and replenished with stem cells from the limbus with estimated complete turnover in around 10 to 14 days.[1, 3] Usually, the entire corneal epithelium can be regenerated after an abrasion.

The Bowman's layer is clear and acellular. Scarring will form if this layer is damaged.

The stroma accounts for 90% of the corneal thickness.[4] It is made up of about 200 collagen fibril lamellae.[4] Collagen fibrils within each lamella are parallel. These lamellae stack together so that collagen fibrils in one lamella are orthogonal to those in the adjacent lamella. Corneal stroma is also rich in highly negatively charged glycosaminoglycans and proteoglycans. Because the negative charge attracts water molecules, glycosaminoglycans and proteoglycans exert significant hydration stress to the stroma.[5] This hydration stress can sometimes cause corneal edema and is antagonized by the pump function of the endothelium. Collagen fibrils, together with glycosaminoglycans and proteoglycans, are maintained by keratocytes, which are fibroblast cells residing between collagen lamellae. Lesions of the corneal stroma may lead to scarring and impair corneal transparency.

Descemet's membrane is 10 μm thick[4] and serves as the basement of the endothelium. Under a light microscope, it appears to be a homogenous membrane.

The endothelium consists of a single layer of cells. Corneal endothelial cells are flat and hexagonal and cover the entire posterior corneal surface. When corneal endothelial cells die due to aging, disease, trauma, etc., the adjacent cells enlarge, expand, and finally cover the area left by those dead cells because corneal endothelial cells cannot proliferate. The endothelium is the key component to corneal deturgescence (the mechanism by which the stroma of the cornea remains relatively dehydrated). First, the endothelium forms a physical barrier to the aqueous humor. Second, it functions as a pump; i.e., it actively transports water from the stroma to the anterior chamber. Disruption in the integrity and/or pump function of the endothelium may result in corneal edema and decrease its transparency.

The cornea is rich in fine unmyelinated sensory nerve fibers with unmyelinated ends deriving from the long ciliary nerve — a branch of the ophthalmic division of the trigeminal nerve (V1).

■ **The Sclera**

The sclera is white and opaque. It is enveloped by a fibrous membrane named the Tenon's capsule.

The anterior part of the sclera is continuous with the cornea and is visible as the white of the eye. The posterior region of the sclera is perforated by the optic nerve, forming a sieve-like structure called the lamina cribrosa, where the unmyelinated optic nerve fibers (retinal ganglion cell axons) exit the sclera and become myelinated. The sclera consists of three layers. From the exterior to interior, they are the episclera, the scleral stroma, and the lamina fusca.

The episclera is a layer of loose connective tissue coating the scleral stroma. It is rich in blood vessels but these vessels are not easily discernible. The vessels are branches of the anterior ciliary and short and long posterior arteries.

The scleral stroma is a fibrous tissue with almost no vessels. However, different from the cornea, the collagen fibrils in the sclera are very dense and interwoven irregularly. The irregular arrangement of the collagen fibrils renders the sclera more physical strength but little transparency. The thickness of the sclera is not homogenous: it is the thickest around the optic nerve and the thinnest at the extraocular muscle insertion.

The lamina fusca is the innermost layer. It is brown due to the pigment of melanocytes in this layer. The choroid (a component of the uveal tract) lines the inner surface of the lamina fusca. There is a potential space between the two layers, known as the suprachoroidal space. Fluid accumulation in this space may lead to choroidal detachment.

The sclera is innervated by the ciliary nerves.

■ **The Tenon's Capsule**

The Tenon's capsule is a fibrous layer enveloping the sclera. As mentioned earlier, the eyeball is surrounded by the orbit fat and the Tenon's capsule separates the two structures. The anterior portion of the Tenon's capsule is covered by the bulbar conjunctiva. At the limbus, the Tenon's capsule, the bulbar conjunctiva, and the sclera fuse together.

■ **The Limbus**

The limbus is an important landmark in ophthalmology. In surgery, an incision is usually made here to access the trabecular meshwork or the lens. The limbal stem cells also reside in this region. The limbus is the transitional zone between the transparent cornea and the white opaque sclera. It is about 1.5 to 2.0 mm wide. Exteriorly, it appears as a shallow, circumferential depression, called the external scleral sulcus. A similar groove can be found at the interior surface, named the internal scleral sulcus. If a line is drawn from the termination of Bowman's layer to the termination of Descemet's membrane (Schwalbe's line), it is considered the anterior border of the limbus. The posterior border of the limbus is the line perpendicular to the ocular surface passing the scleral spur, which is a scleral projection at the posterior limit of the internal scleral sulcus.

■ **The Anterior Chamber Angle**

The anterior chamber angle is located at the junction of the peripheral cornea and the root of the iris. Evaluation of this structure bears clinical importance, especially for glaucoma patients, because the majority of the aqueous humor exits the eye through the anterior chamber angle. The anterolateral side of the anterior chamber angle is the limbus, while the posterior side is the anterior part of the ciliary body and root of the iris. Under gonioscopy, the major visible structures in the anterior chamber angle, from anterior to posterior, are Schwalbe's line, the trabecular meshwork, Schlemm's canal, the sclera spur, the ciliary body, and the root of the iris (Fig. 2-2).

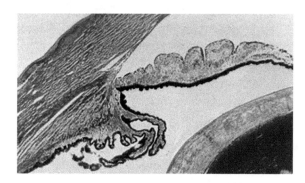

Fig. 2-2   Anterior chamber angle

Schwalbe's line is the termination of Descemet's membrane. Since the cornea has a dome-like shape, Schwalbe's line is actually a ring if considered as a whole; thus, it is also called Schwalbe's ring. It is the anterior limit of the limbus and the trabecular meshwork.

The trabecular meshwork is an avascular spongy, sieve-like structure. Transection of the trabecular meshwork is triangular, with the apex just posterior to the Schwalbe's line and the base pointing the ciliary body. The trabecular meshwork can be further divided into three portions, from the inside out, which are the uveal meshwork, the corneoscleral meshwork, and the juxtacanalicular meshwork (also called the cribiform meshwork). The inner two portions consist of collagen and elastic tissue beams wrapped with trabecular meshwork cells, while the juxtacanalicular meshwork has a dense extracellular matrix embedded with trabecular meshwork cells.[6]

Schlemm's canal is a circumferential channel surrounding the anterior chamber angle. It is situated just anterior to the trabecular meshwork. The lumen of Schlemm's canal is lined with a single layer of endothelium. There are 25–35 collector channels[4] communicating Schlemm's canal with the aqueous vein.

The sclera spur is a projection of the sclera at the posterior limit of the internal scleral sulcus and thus serves as a landmark of the limbus.

The ciliary body and the root of the iris will be described in the subsection on the uveal tract below.

■ **The Aqueous Outflow Pathway**

The anterior segment of the eye is filled with the aqueous humor. The aqueous humor nourishes the avascular ocular structures, including the cornea, the trabecular meshwork, and the lens. It maintains intraocular pressure, which keeps the eye "inflated". A normal intraocular pressure is very important for the eye: too much pressure (ocular hypertension) may damage retinal ganglion cells and their axons (the optic nerve), while too little pressure (ocular hypotension) collapses the eye and leads to atrophy of the eyeball.

The aqueous humor is produced by the nonpigmented ciliary body epithelium and is secreted into the posterior chamber. The majority of the aqueous humor passes the pupil and enters the anterior chamber, where it is filtered through the trabecular meshwork and then transported into Schlemm's canal. Via 25–35 collector channels[4] and aqueous veins, the aqueous humor drains into the episcleral venous system. This outflow pathway is known as the conventional pathway. There also exists a uveoscleral pathway, in which the aqueous humor drains between the ciliary body and the sclera via the suprachoroidal space or through the iris.[7] This pathway contributes a small portion (<10%) to the total outflow.[8]

Intraocular pressure is determined by the production rate of the aqueous humor, outflow resistance, and episcleral vein pressure. Changes in any of the factors may alter intraocular pressure. In glaucoma patients, elevated intraocular pressure is often caused by increased outflow resistance. The endothelial lining of Schlemm's canal and the juxtacanalicular meshwork contribute to the majority of the resistance.[9]

2. The Uveal Tract

The uveal tract is the vascular pigmented layer of the eye. It consists of the iris, the ciliary body, and the choroid. The three components of the uveal tract are continuous. The ciliary body and the choroid lines the inner surface of the sclera with the iris attached to the ciliary body.

■ **The Iris**

The iris is a disc-like tissue with a round aperture, named the pupil in the center (think about the camera diaphragm). It is attached to the ciliary body at the periphery, called the root of the iris. The iris separates the anterior segment into the anterior chamber and the posterior chamber. The anterior surface of the iris (the base of the anterior chamber), which is visible directly, can be divided into the central papillary zone and the peripheral ciliary zone. The collarette, which is a circular ridge on the iris, demarcates the two zones. The anterior surface of the iris shows a lot of crypts, radial streaks, and circular contraction furrows.

The iris has four layers, from anterior to posterior, which are the anterior border, the stroma, the dilator pupillae muscle, and the posterior pigment epithelium. The anterior border is a modified stroma without epithelium lining. The stroma is highly vascularized and consists of loose connective tissue containing fibroblast cells, melanocytes, collagen fibers, and the sphincter pupillae muscle. Depending on the amount of pigment in the iridal stroma, the color of the iris may appear to be brown (more pigment), yellow (intermediate), blue (less pigment), or other colors. The dilator pupillea muscle is a layer of myoepithelial cells. The posterior pigment epithelium has two layers of pigmented cells with the anterior layer continuous with the pigmented epithelial layer of the ciliary body and the posterior layer continuous with the nonpigmented epithelial layer of the ciliary body.

The major function of the iris is to control the amount of light that enters the eye. The size of the pupil is determined by the sphincter pupillae muscle, which contracts the pupil (miosis) and the dilator pupillea muscle, which dilates the pupil (mydriasis). The sphincter pupillae muscle plays a major role in adjusting pupil size (Table 2-1).

Table 2-1　Comparison of Miosis and Mydriasis

	Miosis	Mydriasis
Pupil movement	Constriction	Dilation
Stimuli	Bright light convergence accommodation	Dark condition stress
Muscle	Sphincter pupillae	Dilator pupillea
Innervation	Parasympathetic	Sympathetic

The iris is supplied by the long posterior ciliary arteries and the anterior ciliary arteries. The branches of the long posterior ciliary arteries form the major arterial circle and minor arterial circle. Blood drains through the vortex veins and the anterior ciliary veins.

The iris receives sensory nerve fibers from the long ciliary nerve, which is derived from the nasociliary nerve, a branch of V1. The parasympathetic and sympathetic nerve fibers are from the short ciliary and long ciliary nerves, respectively.

■ The Light Reflex

There are direct and consensual light reflexes. When bright light falls onto the retina, the ipsilateral pupil constricts in order to decrease the amount of light that enters the eye. This is the direct light reflex. Under normal conditions, the contralateral pupil also constricts although there is no direct visual stimulus. This is the consensual light reflex. Light is detected by the retina, and the impulses are carried by the retinal ganglion cell axons and past the optic nerve, optic chiasm, and optic tract. These axons do not enter the lateral geniculate nucleus, but leave the optic tract and synapse on the neurons in the left and right pretectal nuclei, respectively. Some of the axons of the pretectal nuclei project to the ipsilateral Edinger-Westphal nucleus (parasympathetic nucleus), while the others project to the contralateral Edinger-Westphal nucleus. The Edinger-Westphal nucleus sends out axons that join the oculomotor nerve (III) and synapse onto the neurons in the ciliary ganglion. The postganglionic fibers from the ciliary ganglion pass through the short ciliary nerve and innervate the constrictor pupillae muscle.

■ The Ciliary Body

The ciliary body is located between the root of the iris and the choroid. Taken as a whole, it has a ring-like shape. However, on a cross-section, it is roughly triangular. The long side is 6–7 mm wide and is loosely attached to the sclera.[10] The ciliary body extends anteriorly to the scleral spur and continues posteriorly with the choroid. The anterior one-third of the ciliary body is the pars plicata (2 mm in width), which has many radial folds arranged in a circle, known as the ciliary process. The posterior two-thirds of the ciliary body is flat, known as the pars plana (4 mm in width). The junction between the pars plana and the choroid is also the anterior limit of the retina. Because this region looks like saw teeth, it is named the ora serrata.

The ciliary body has the ciliary epithelium, ciliary stroma, and ciliary muscle. The ciliary epithelium is the innermost layer. It has two layers of epithelia: the outer pigmented epithelium and the inner nonpigmented epithelium. The ciliary stroma consists of blood vessels, melanocytes, and fibroblasts. The ciliary muscle has three groups of muscle fibers: the outer longitudinal, the middle radial, and the inner circular muscle fibers.

The functions of the ciliary body include aqueous humor production, maintaining lens zonules, and accommodation. The aqueous humor and the lens zonules are secreted by the nonpigmented epithelium of the ciliary process. Contraction or relaxation of the ciliary muscle regulates accommodation.

The ciliary body has blood and nerve supply as the iris. It receives blood from the long posterior ciliary arteries and anterior ciliary arteries and drains blood into the vortex veins. The ciliary muscle receives parasympathetic and sympathetic nerve fibers from the short ciliary and long ciliary nerves, respectively.

■ The Blood-Aqueous Barrier

The tight junction between the endothelial cells of the iris vessels and that between the nonpigmented ciliary epithelial cells form the blood-aqueous barrier, which prevents blood cells and certain macromolecules from leaking out.[11] This barrier is an important component of the ocular-blood barriers and contributes to ocular immune privilege.[12]

■ The Choroid

The choroid is the most posterior part the uveal tract. It is located between the retina and the sclera. It starts anteriorly from the ora serrata and ends posteriorly at the optic disc. The choroid consists of three layers of blood vessels: large blood vessels (the outer layer), medium blood vessels (the middle layer), and small blood vessels (the inner layer). The small blood vessels in the inner layer are fenestrated capillaries, known as the choroidcapillaris. The junction between the choroid and the sclera is not tight, except at the margin of the optic disc. Thus, there is a potential space between the sclera and choroid, known as the suprachoroidal space. Between the choroid and the underlying retina, there is a layer of membrane named Bruch's membrane. The innermost part of Bruch's membrane serves as the basement of the retinal pigment epithelium. The choroid provides blood supply to the outer layers of the retina.

The choroid is supplied by the posterior and anterior ciliary arteries and drains blood through the vortex veins into the ophthalmic vein. The choroid is innervated by the long ciliary nerves (which carries sensory and sympathetic nerve fibers) and the short ciliary nerves (which carries parasympathetic nerve fibers).

3. The Retina

The retina is a thin, transparent tissue lining the inner surface of the choroid. The anterior limit of the retina is the ora serrata, where the retina is continuous with the choroidal epithelium. Clinically, in the posterior retina, a circular area, which is about 5 to 6 mm in diameter and is temporal to the optic disc, is called the posterior pole. This area is cone-dominated and contains important structures including the macula lutea and the fovea centralis. The macula is about 3 mm in diameter and has a yellowish color due to its xanthophyll (a yellowish pigment) content. In the center of the macula, there is a small depression, which is called the fovea centralis. Under the ophthalmoscope, a reflection from the fovea can be clearly observed. The fovea has only cones and is devoid of rods. About 3 mm nasal to the macula, there is the optic disc, which is a disc-shaped structure of 3.5 mm in diameter.[13] The optic disc has a slightly raised rim and the central depression, known as the optic cup. The optic disc is where the axon of the retinal ganglion cell forms the optic nerve and turns almost 90 degrees posteriorly. Thus, the rim of the optic disc is actually made up of unmyelinated retinal ganglion cell axons. There are also blood vessels passing through the optic cup, including the central retinal arteries and veins. Because there are no photoreceptor cells at the optic disc, this area cannot detect visual signals and thus is the physiological blind spot.

The retina consists of rod and cone photoreceptors, bipolar cells, ganglion cells, horizontal cells, amacrine cells, glial cells (mainly Muller glial cells), and non-neuronal retinal pigment epithelial cells. These cells are organized into ten layers, from inside to outside, which are:

    1) The internal limiting membrane, which is formed by the process of Muller glial cells

    2) The nerve fiber layer, which is formed by retinal ganglion cell axons

    3) The ganglion cell layer, containing the soma (cell body of the neuron) of retinal ganglion cells and a few displaced amacrine cells

    4) The inner plexiform layer, where amacrine cells and bipolar cells form the synaptic

connection (synapse) with ganglion cells

5) The inner nuclear layer, containing the soma of bipolar cells, horizontal cells and amacrine cells, and the cell body of Muller glial cells

6) The outer plexiform layer, where photoreceptor cells synapse on bipolar cells and horizontal cells

7) The outer nuclear layer, containing the nucleus of the photoreceptor

8) The external limiting membrane, which is formed by the junction of Muller glial cells and photoreceptor cells

9) The photoreceptor layer, which contains the outer and inner segments of rods and cones

10) The retinal pigment epithelium, which supports photoreceptors

The retina can be further divided into the non-neuronal retinal pigment epithelium and the neurosensory retina (from the internal limiting membrane to the photoreceptor layer). Developmentally, the retinal pigment epithelium layer originates from the outer layer of the optic cup while the neurosensory retina derives from the inner layer of the optic cup. Thus, the connection between the two layers is not very strong, leaving a potential space. The clinical term, "retinal detachment", refers to detachment of the neurosenory retina from the retinal pigment epithelium at this space.

In the neurosensory retina, photons are first detected by photoreceptors, which then relay the signal to bipolar cells. If this process is initiated by the cone photoreceptor (i.e., in the cone pathway), the signal is directly transduced to ganglion cells via cone bipolar cells, a subgroup of bipolar cells. If it is initiated by the rod photoreceptor (i.e., in the rod pathway), the information is transduced to cone bipolar cells, which relay it to a special group of amacrine cells known as AII amacrine cells. AII amacrine cells then transduce the signal to ganglion cells via cone bipolar cells. The cone pathway is sensitive in the photopic (bright) condition. It is able to differentiate between wavelengths and contributes to color vision. Most of the cones are located in the macula with the highest density in the fovea.[14] Because of this, the fovea provides the best visual acuity. On the contrary, the rod pathway is sensitive in the scotopic (dark) condition but provides achromatic (black and white) vision. Rods are dominant throughout the retina, except in the fovea, where there are no rods, but cones.

Energy consumption is very high in the retina, especially for photoreceptors. Thus, the retina has dual blood supply: the outer five layers are supplied by the choroid capillaries and the inner five layers are supplied by the central retinal artery and its branches. The blood is drained through the central retinal vein (the inner five layers) and the vortex vein (the outer five layers).

The tight junction formed by the nonfenestrated endothelial cells of the retinal blood vessel and by the retinal pigment epithelial cells prevents blood cells and certain macromolecules from leaking out and entering the retina. This barrier also contributes to ocular immune privilege.[12]

4. The Lens

The lens is an avascular, transparent, and biconvex structure. The vertex of the anterior and the posterior surfaces are called the anterior and the posterior poles, respectively. The circumferential region, where the anterior and the posterior surfaces meet, is called the equator. The lens is about 9mm in diameter (at the equator) and 4mm in thickness (between the two poles).[2] The posterior surface of the lens is more curved than the anterior surface. The lens is situated posterior to the iris and the pupil and anterior to the vitreous. It is suspended by the lens suspensory ligament (the zonular fiber or zonule of Zinn). One end of the suspensory ligament is attached to the lens at the equatorial region extending 2 mm anteriorly and 1 mm posteriorly[13] while the other end is attached to the ciliary body.

The lens consists of three parts, which are, from the outside to inside:
1) The lens capsule
2) The lens epithelium
3) The lens fibers

The lens capsule is an acellular elastic basement membrane enclosing the entire lens. It is the structure where the suspensory ligament is attached to the lens. The lens epithelium lies just beneath the lens capsule. However, it is restricted to the anterior lens capsule and the equator, i.e., the posterior lens capsule is devoid of the lens epithelium. Lens epithelial cells undergo continuous proliferation and elongation. The lens fibers are derived from epithelial cells. Epithelial cells at the equator elongate and start to differentiate into lens fibers. They elongate both anteriorly and posteriorly.[13] The old lens fibers are buried in the center and covered by the newly "born" cells. Thus, the structure of the lens fiber is analogous to an onion. The old lens fibers harden with age, forming the nucleus of the lens while the young outer lens fibers form the cortex of the lens. The special arrangement of the lens fibers results in a Y-shaped suture and an inverted Y-shaped suture in the anterior and the posterior regions of the lens, respectively.

■ Accommodation

Accommodation occurs when the eye is directed to a near object. Through accommodation reflex, the ciliary muscle contracts, which leads to decreased tension on the zonules. Then, the slackened zonules allow the elastic lens to become more convex and gain more refractive power, enabling the image of the near object to be properly focused on the retina. When the eye is directed to a far object, the ciliary muscle relaxes, which leads to increased tension on the zonules; the zonules pull the lens and make it less convex to focus the far object.

5. The Vitreous Body

The vitreous body (the vitreous) is an avascular transparent gel occupying the vitreous chamber. The peripheral vitreous is denser, known as the cortex of the vitreous, while the central part is more liquid. Anteriorly, it is attached to the posterior surface of the lens. To accommodate the lens, there is a concave depression in the vitreous called the hyaloid fossa. The rest of its circumference is attached to the ciliary body, the retina, and the optic disc. The strongest attachment is at the pars plana, the fovea, and the optic disc. There is a narrow canal known as the hyaloid canal (Cloquet's canal), extending from the optic disc to the posterior lens. It is the remnant after regression of the hyaloid artery, which supplies the embryonic lens during early development.

The vitreous consists of water (98%), collagens (mainly type II collagens), glycosaminaoglycans/proteoglycans (mainly hyaluronic acid), and other molecules.[13] There is little cellular content in the vitreous except a few hyalocytes, whose major function is to produce hyaluronic acid.

The vitreous is viscoelastic; it buffers impact to the eye and holds the neurosensory retina to the retinal pigment epithelium.

Section 2   The Orbit

The orbit is a bony cavity with a volume of about 30 ml.[2] It is pyramidal-like in shape with the apex pointing posteriorly but slightly medially and the base (opening) directed anteriorly. The orbit consists of seven cranial bones, which are the frontal, the sphenoid, the ethmoid, the palatine, the lacrimal, the maxilla, and the zygomatic bones.

The orbit has four walls (the roof, the floor, and the medial and the lateral walls), one apex, and one base.

The roof (the superior wall) consists primarily of the orbital plate of the frontal bone. The anterolateral part of the roof has a depression, known as the lacrimal fossa, in which the lacrimal gland is located. The posterior part of the roof is composed of the lesser wing of the sphenoid bone, which contains the optic canal, a structure through which the optic nerve exits the orbit.

The floor (the inferior wall) consists of the orbital plate of the maxillary bone, the small orbital process of the sphenoid bone and the orbital surface of the zygomatic bone.

The medial wall consists of the frontal process of the maxillary bone, the lacrimal, the ethmoid, and the sphenoid bone. The anterior part of the medial wall contains the lacrimal groove, in which the lacrimal sac is located.

The lateral wall consists of the greater wing of the sphenoid bone and the zygomatic bone. The lateral wall is separated posteriorly from the roof at the superior orbital fissure and anteriorly from the floor at the inferior orbital fissure. The maxillary nerve (whose name is changed to the infraorbital nerve after entering the infraorbital foramen), the zygomatic nerve, branches of the pterygopalatine ganglion, and the inferior ophthalmic vein pass through the inferior orbital fissure.

Except the lateral wall, which is thick and strong, the other three walls are thin and weak. A blunt trauma may lead to fractures of the thin orbital wall(s), known as blowout fractures.[15] Blowout fractures occur most frequently on the orbital floor and medial wall.[16] In addition, the orbit is very close to the accessory nasal sinuses. The orbit is separated from the frontal sinus by the roof, from the ethmoid sinus and the sphenoid sinus by the medial wall and from the maxillary sinus by the floor. Thus, infection in the sinus may spread to the orbit.

The apex of the orbit is the entrance or exit of the orbit. Vessels and nerves pass through the apex via two structures: the optic canal (which opens at the optic foramen) and the superior orbital fissure.

The optic canal connects the middle cranial fossa with the orbit. The optic nerve, ophthalmic artery, and sympathetic nerve fibers pass through the optic canal.

The superior orbital fissure lies inferolateral to the optic canal. It separates the roof and later walls of the orbit posteriorly. Structures passing through the lateral portion of the superior orbital fissure, from lateral to medial, are the superior ophthalmic vein, the lacrimal nerve, the frontal nerve, and the trochlear nerve. Structures passing through the medial portion, within the annulus of Zinn, are the superior and inferior divisions of the oculomotor nerve, the abducens nerve, and the nasociliary nerve. One branch of the inferior ophthalmic vein passes the medial superior orbital fissure outside the annulus of Zinn.

The annulus of Zinn (the common tendinous ring) is a ring-like fibrous tissue surrounding the optic nerve at the apex. It is the origin of the four rectus muscles. It encircles the structures passing through the optic canal as well as those described above.

The opening of the orbit is anteriorly bounded by a fibrous tissue known as the orbital septum. It separates the orbit from the eyelid. The orbital septum fuses with the orbital periosteum at one end and the tarsal plate at the other end. With age, orbital fat may herniate through the weakened orbital septum. The rim of the orbit is strong, unlike the weak orbit walls (except the lateral wall). At the junction of the medial one-third and the lateral two-thirds of the superior orbital rim, there is the supraorbital notch, through which the supraorbital nerve, supraorbital artery, and supraorbital vein pass. At the junction of the medial one-third and the lateral two-thirds of the inferior orbital rim, there is the opening of the infraorbital canal, known as the infraorbital foramen. Structures passing through the infraorbital foramen are the infraorbital nerve, artery and vein, and the maxillary nerve (The maxillary nerve enters the orbit via the infraorbital fissure; passes forward through the infraorbital groove, the infraorbital groove, and the infraorbital canal; and exits the orbit via the infraorbital foramen.).

Section 3   The Ocular Appendages

The ocular appendages include the eyebrows, the eyelids, the conjunctiva, the lacrimal apparatus, and the extraocular muscles.

1. The Eyebrows

The eyebrows are skin folds covered with hair. They are located anterior to the upper orbital rim.

2. The Eyelids

The eyelids lie anterior to the orbit. Each eye has one upper eyelid and one lower eyelid. The upper eyelid ends at the eyebrow while the lower eyelid blends with the cheek. The space between the upper and lower eyelid margins is the palpebral fissure. When the eyes are open and pointed straight forward, the upper eyelid reaches the limbus. The junctions where the upper and lower eyelids meet are called the external canthus (lateral) and the internal canthus (medial), respectively. The free end of the eyelid is the lid margin. There is a grey line which divides the lid margin into the anterior margin and the posterior margin. The anterior margin is blunt and covered with skin. It has two to three rows of eyelashes, openings of the glands of Zeis (sebaceous glands), and the glands of Moll (sweat glands). The posterior margin is almost at a right angle and in close contact with the eye. It is covered with a layer of mucous membrane, the conjunctiva. Meibomian's glands (tarsal glands) open at this margin. The lacrimal canaliculus also opens at the medial end of this margin. The opening is a small elevation with a central orifice called the lacrimal punctum.

The eyelids consist of five layers, from outer to inner, including:

■ **Skin**

The skin of the eyelid is very thin, loose, and easy to form folds.

■ **Subcutaneous Tissue**

It is composed of loose connective tissue and some adipose tissue.

■ **The Orbicularis Oculi Muscle**

Its striated muscle fibers are circular and roughly parallel to palpebral fissure. It is innervated by the facial nerve (Ⅶ). In the upper eyelid, there is also the levator palpebrae superioris, a striated muscle that lifts the upper eyelid and keeps it open. It is innervated by the oculomotor nerve (Ⅲ). There is a layer of smooth muscle in the levator palpebrae superioris called Muller's muscle, which receives sympathetic nerve fibers.

■ **The Tarsal Plate**

It consists of dense fibrous tissue. The medial and lateral ends of the tarsal plate are attached to the orbital margin by the medial and lateral palpebral ligaments, respectively. Meibomian's glands lie in this layer. These glands are arranged perpendicular to the eyelid margin and have openings on it.

■ **The Palpebral Conjunctiva**

It is the most posterior layer and firmly adherent to the tarsal plate.

The eyelid is supplied by the lateral and medial palpebral arteries. The lateral palpebral artery is a branch of the lacrimal artery, which is derived from the ophthalmic artery. The medial palpebral artery is a branch of the ophthalmic artery. The anastomoses between the lateral and medial palpebral arteries form the marginal arterial arch. The eyelid drains into the ophthalmic vein (then to the cavernous sinus), angular vein, and superficial temporal vein.[4] The ophthalmic division (V1) and maxillary division (V2) of the trigeminal nerve provide sensory nerve fibers to the upper eyelid and lower eyelid, respectively.

3. The Conjunctiva

The conjunctiva is a thin, semitransparent mucous membrane. It can be divided into three portions: the palpebral, the bulbar, and the forniceal conjunctiva. The space enclosed by the three portions is the conjunctival sac, which opens at the palpebral fissure. The palpebral conjunctiva lines and is attached firmly to the posterior surface of the tarsal plate with little mobility. The bulbar conjunctiva covers the anterior sclera. It fuses anteriorly with Tenon's capsule and the sclera at the limbus and ends posteriorly at the fornix. Because the bulbar conjunctiva is easy to fold and is attached loosely to Tenon's capsule, the eyeball is allowed to move freely. There is the semilunar fold, a thickned palpebral conjunctival fold, at the internal canthus. On the medial surface of the semilunar fold, there is a pink, dermatoid nodule known as the lacrimal caruncle. The forniceal conjunctiva is the reflection betwen the palpebral and the bulbar conjunctiva. It forms the superior and inferior limits of the conjunctival sac.

The conjunctiva has secretory function. It contains goblet cells and accessory lacrimal glands (glands of Wolfring and glands of Krause). Goblet cells secrete mucins while accessory lacrimal glands contribute to the aqueous content of the tear.

The conjunctiva is supplied by the anterior ciliary artery and the two palpebral arches from the upper and lower eyelids, respectively. The palpebral arches supply the palpebral and forniceal conjunctivae plus the bulbar conjunctiva 4 mm outside the limbus.[17] The rest of the bulbar conjunctiva (4 mm around the limbus) is supplied by the anterior ciliary artery. The blood is drained into the palpebral veins. The sensory nerve supply of the conjunctiva is primarily from the ophthalmic division of the trigeminal nerve (V1) except the bulbar conjunctiva (from the long ciliary nerve) and the medial portion of the forniceal and palpebral conjunctivae (from the maxillary division V2).

4. The Lacrimal Apparatus

The lacrimal apparatus consists of the lacrimal gland, lacrimal accessory glands, lacrimal puncta, lacrimal canaliculi, lacrimal sac and nasolacrimal duct. The glands produce tears while the other structures drain tears into the nasal cavity.

The lacrimal gland is divided by the lateral horn of the aponeursis of the levator palpebrae superioris into the large orbital portion and small palpebral portion. The orbital portion is situated in the lacrimal fossa, which is in the laterosuperior part of the orbit. The palpebral portion is more superficial and is above the superior conjunctival fornix. The lacrimal gland opens at the conjunctiva fornix via around 10 lacrimal secretory ducts.[2]

The lacrimal accessory glands include the glands of Wolfring and the glands of Krause, both which are located in the conjunctiva.

The lacrimal punctum is a small elevation with a central orifice located in the medial portion of the posterior margin of the eyelid.

The lacrimal canaliculus starts from the lacrimal punctum. The initial part of the canaliculus runs perpendicular to the margin of the eyelid. Then, it turns sharply medially and extends horizontally until it opens at the lacrimal sac. Before the upper and lower lacrimal canaliculi open at the lacrimal sac, sometimes they merge to form a common canaliculus.

The lacrimal sac is situated in the lacrimal fossa formed by the lacrimal bone and frontal bone. The lacrimal canaliculi or the common canaliculus open at the superolateral part of the lacrimal sac. The lacrimal sac is connected to the nasolacrimal duct at the inferior end. Anteriorly, the upper portion of the lacrimal sac is covered by the medial palpebral ligament. Posteriorly, the lacrimal sac is surrounded by the orbicularis oculi muscle. During blinking, movement of the medial palpebral ligament and the orbicularis oculi muscle generates negative pressure in the lacrimal sac.

The nasolacrimal duct is located in the bony nasolacrimal canal, which is formed by the maxillary and the lacrimal bones. It opens at the nasal cavity inferiorly.

Tears form a film (tear film) covering the anterior surface of the eye. The tear film consists of three layers, from anterior to posterior, which are the lipid layer (produced by Meibomian's glands), the aqueous layer (produced by the lacrimal and accessory glands), and the mucus layer (produced by Goblet cells). The tear film lubricates and moistures the ocular surface, maintains the optic power, inhibits microbe growth, and provides nutrition to the ocular surface.

Tears are secreted into the lacrimal sac and are spread over ocular surface during blinking. Blinking also generates negative pressure in the lacrimal sac. Tears are sucked into the lacrimal canaliculi via the lacrimal puncta. They then pass through the lacrimal sac, nasolacrimal duct, and drain into the nasal cavity.

The lacrimal gland is supplied by the lacrimal artery, which is derived from the ophthalmic artery. It drains blood into the ophthalmic vein. The sensory nerve fibers of the lacrimal gland are from the lacrimal nerve, which arises from the ophthalmic division of the trigeminal nerve (V1). The lacrimal nerve also carries sympathetic and parasympathetic postganglionic fibers to innervate the lacrimal gland. These two components control lacrimal secretion (Fig. 2-3).

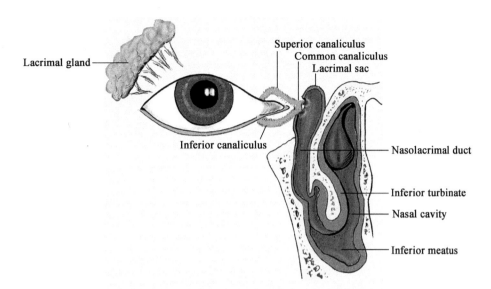

Fig. 2-3   The lacrimal drainage system

5. The Extraocular Muscles

Eye movement is controlled by six extraocular muscles. There are four rectus and two oblique muscles. The extraocular muscles are striated muscle innervated by the cranial nerves (III , IV , and VI) (Fig. 2-4).

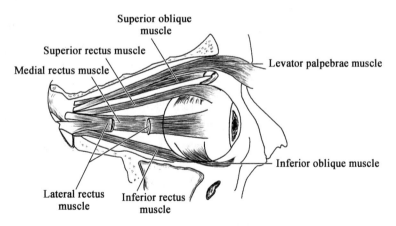

Fig. 2-4   The extraocular muscles

The four rectus muscles are the superior, inferior, lateral, and medial rectus muscles. They originate at the annulus of Zinn (which is located at the orbital apex and encircles the optic nerve) posteriorly and run superiorly, inferiorly, laterally or medially (corresponding to their names). Their tendon inserts into the sclera anterior to the equator (Table 2-2).

Table 2-2   The anatomy and function of the extraocular muscles[17]

Muscle	Origin	Insertion	Anterior or posterior to the equator	Distance between the insertion and limbus	Angle between the visual axis and muscle tendon (degree)	Eye movement	Innervation
Superior rectus	The annulus of Zinn	Superior surface	Anterior	7.7mm	27	Elevation Adduction Intorsion	III
Inferior rectus	The annulus of Zinn	Inferior surface	Anterior	6.5mm	27	Depression Adduction Extorsion	III
Lateral rectus	The annulus of Zinn	Lateral surface	Anterior	6.9mm	0	Adduction	VI
Medial rectus	The annulus of Zinn	Medial surface	Anterior	5.5mm	0	Adduction	III
Superior oblique	The body of the sphenoid bone	Superolateral surface	Posterior		53	Intorsion Depression Adduction	IV
Inferior oblique	The maxillary bone	Inferolateral surface	Posterior		53	Extorsion Elevation Adduction	III

The two oblique muscles are the superior oblique and inferior oblique muscles. The superior oblique originates from the body of the sphenoid bone superomedial to the optic nerve and annulus of Zinn. Its muscle belly runs forward along the orbital wall and its tendon passes through the trochlea, which is on the frontal bone and functions as a pulley. After exiting the trochlea, the superior oblique muscle tendon turns posterolaterally, runs beneath the superior rectus, and inserts into the sclera posterior to the equator. The inferior oblique muscle originates from the anteromedial portion of the orbital floor, very close to the orbital rim and nasolacrimal duct. It runs beneath the inferior rectus and is pointed posteriorly, laterally, and superiorly. Its tendon inserts into the lateral portion of the sclera posterior to the equator.

Each extraocular muscle is supplied by two anterior ciliary arteries except the lateral rectus muscle, which receives blood from the one ciliary artery and the lacrimal artery, and the inferior oblique muscle, which receives additional blood from the infraorbial artery. The seven anterior arteries are derived from the muscular branches of the ophthalmic artery.

Section 4　The Visual Pathway

The visual pathway transmits visual signal from the retina to the primary visual cortex in the brain. It consists of the retina, optic nerve, optic chiasm, optic tract, lateral geniculate body, optic radiation, and primary visual cortex. However, it should be noted that not all the axons follow this pathway. About 10% of the axons project to the pretectal nucleus, superior colliculus, and suprachiasmatic nucleus.[1] These axons are involved in light reflex, saccadic eye movement, and circadian rhythm (Fig. 2-5).

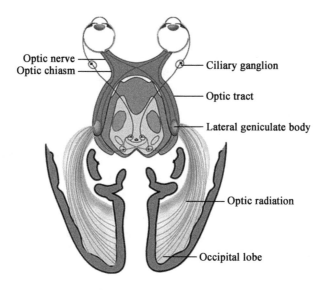

Fig. 2-5　The visual pathway

1. The Optic Nerve

The optic nerve is part of the central nervous system. It is composed of one million axons of retinal ganglion cells.[2] These axons run posteriorly until they form synaptic connections with the neurons in the lateral geniculate bodies. It should be noted that there is no disruption or relay before they enter the lateral geniculate bodies.

The optic nerve starts form the optic disc, runs posteriorly and ends at the optic chiasm. It is often divided into four portions:

■ **The Intraocular Portion**

The intraocular portion starts from the optic disc and ends at the lamina cribrosa and measures about 1 mm.[4] In this portion, the optic nerve is unmyelinated. However, once it exits the lamina cribrosa, the optic nerve becomes myelinated. This portion is supplied by the central retinal arteries and short posterior ciliary arteries.

■ **The Orbital Portion**

The orbital portion is between the lamina cribrosa and the optic canal and measures about 25 mm.[4] It runs in the conical space enclosed by the four extraocular rectus muscles. Starting from this portion, the optic nerve is myelinated and is wrapped with the meninges (the dura mater, arachnoid, and pia mater). The three meningeal membranes are continuous with those in the brain. This portion is supplied by the central retinal arteries and branches of the ophthalmic artery.

■ **The Intracanalicular Portion**

It is the part of the optic nerve within the optic canal and measures about 5 mm.[4] This portion is supplied by the branches of the ophthalmic artery.

■ **The Intracranial Portion**

The intracranial portion starts from where the optic nerve exits the optic canal and ends at the optic chiasm. This portion measures about 10 mm.[17] It is supplied by the branches from the internal carotid artery and the ophthalmic artery.

2. The Optic Chiasm

The left and right optic nerves merge at the optic chiasm, in which optic nerve fibers originating from the nasal retina cross the midline and join the contralateral optic tract. On the contrary, those from the temporal retina do not cross.

The optic chiasm is just above the hypophysis (the pituitary gland). Thus, tumors of the hypophysis may compress the medial portion of the optic chiasm and lead to bitemporal hemianopia.

3. The Optic Tract

The optic tract arises from the optic chiasm. Each optic tract contains the optic nerve fibers corresponding to the temporal retina of the ipsilateral eye and nasal retina of the contralateral eye. The two optic tracts run posteriorly, winds around the cerebral peduncle, and enter the ipsilateral lateral geniculate body.

4. The Lateral Geniculate Body

The lateral geniculate body is an oval structure in the brain. The left and right lateral geniculate bodies receive the ipsilateral optic tract. The neurons in the lateral geniculate body are divided by the white matter into six layers. Most of the axons form synaptic connections with these neurons, which then relay the visual information to the visual cortex. The nerve fibers from the ipsilateral retina terminate at the first, fourth, and sixth layers while those from the contralateral retina terminates at the second, third, and fifth layers.

5. The Optic Radiation

The nerve fibers that exit the lateral geniculate body form the optic radiation and enter the primary visual cortex. The nerve fibers originating from the inferior retina first run anteriorly and then posterolaterally around the inferior horn of the lateral ventricle. After passing the lateral ventricle, these fibers turn posteromedially and enter the primary visual cortex. These fibers are called Meyer's loop. The nerve fibers originating form the superior retina run directly toward the primary visual cortex.

6. The Primary Visual Cortex

The primary visual cortex is in the occipital lobe and specialized for processing visual signal. It is also called the striate cortex, V1 or primary visual cortex.

References

1. Oyster C. *The Human Eye: Structure and Function*. Sunderland, Mass: Sinauer Associates; 1999.

2. Vaughan DA, T; Riordan-Eva, P. *General Ophthalmology*. 14th ed. Stamford, CT: Appleton & Lange; 1999.

3. Hanna C, Bicknell DS, O'Brien JE. Cell turnover in the adult human eye. *Arch Ophthalmol* 1961;65:695-698.

4. Snell RL, MA. *Clinical Anatomy of the Eye*. 2nd ed. Malden, MA: Blackwell Science, Inc; 1998:423.

5. Midelfart A. Swelling pressure in bovine cornea determined by dialysis method. *Acta Ophthalmol (Copenh)* 1987;65:153-158.

6. Llobet A, Gasull X, Gual A. Understanding trabecular meshwork physiology: a key to the control of intraocular pressure? *News Physiol Sci* 2003;18:205-209.

7. Bill A, Hellsing K. Production and drainage of aqueous humor in the cynomolgus monkey (Macaca irus). *Invest Ophthalmol* 1965;4:920-926.

8. Bill A, Phillips CI. Uveoscleral drainage of aqueous humour in human eyes. *Exp Eye Res* 1971;12:275-281.

9. Johnson M. 'What controls aqueous humour outflow resistance?'. *Exp Eye Res* 2006;82:545-557.

10. Moses RA. Detachment of ciliary body—anatomical and physical considerations. *Invest Ophthalmol* 1965;4:935-941.

11. Cunha-Vaz JG. The blood-ocular barriers: past, present, and future. *Doc Ophthalmol* 1997;93:149-157.

12. Streilein JW. Ocular immune privilege: the eye takes a dim but practical view of immunity and inflammation. *J Leukoc Biol* 2003;74:179-185.

13. Forrester JD, AD; McMenamin, PG; Lee, WR. *The eye: basic sciences in practice*. 2nd ed. Edinburgh; New York: W.B. Saunders; 2002:447.

14. Curcio CA, Sloan KR, Jr., Packer O, Hendrickson AE, Kalina RE. Distribution of cones in human and monkey retina: individual variability and radial asymmetry. *Science* 1987;236:579-582.

15. Smith B, Regan WF, Jr. Blow-out fracture of the orbit; mechanism and correction of internal orbital fracture. *Am J Ophthalmol* 1957;44:733-739.

16. Brady SM, McMann MA, Mazzoli RA, Bushley DM, Ainbinder DJ, Carroll RB. The diagnosis and management of orbital blowout fractures: update 2001. *Am J Emerg Med* 2001;19:147-154.

17. Hui Yan-nian. *Ophthalmology*. 5th ed. Beijing, China: People's Medical Publishing House; 2005.

Chapter 3
The Relationship between the Eyes and the *Zang-fu* and Channels

Although the eyes are a local organ, they have a close internal relationship with the whole body, especially *the zang-fu* (visceral and bowels), as well as the channels and collaterals. During the times when *The Yellow Emperor's Inner Classic* was written, there were many descriptions for this relationship; for example, it is said in *The Spiritual Pivot – Great Confusion (Líng Shū – Dà Huò Lùn, 灵枢·大惑论)*: Forms of Disease from Evil Qi in the Bowels and Viscera:

> *"The essential qi of five Zang organs and six Fu organs flow upward into the eyes. The eye is the nest of essence, the essence of the kidney manifests in pupil, the essence of the liver manifests in the black of the eye (cornea), the essence of the heart replenishes in the vessels of the eye, the essence of lung manifests in the white of the eye, the essence of the spleen manifests in the eyelids, together with the essence of bones, muscles, blood and qi combined with collaterals making the eye tie, connecting with the brain and then transfering out from the nape of the neck."* [1]

The above paragraph indicates that the structural development and function of the eyes result from the effect of the essential qi of the five *zang* and six *fu*, and it is the rationale of the five wheels theory.

Section 1   The Eyes and the *Zang-Fu*

1. The Physiological Relationship between the Eyes and the Liver

■ **The liver opens into the eyes, and the eyes reflect the function of the liver.**

In the *Basic Questions - Treatise of the True Doctrine of Golden Coffer (Sù Wèn – Jīn Guì Zhēn Yán Lùn, 素问·金匮真言论)*, it says: "The green color represents the east, and the liver corresponds to the green color. The liver opens into the eyes; the essence of eyes is stored in the liver[2]". This means the eyes are the bridge between the liver and outside world. On one hand, nutrients stored in the liver are transported to the eyes, and so when the eyes are well-nourished, they will function well. On the other hand, if dysfunction arises from the liver, it will reflect in the eyes. It is said in *The Spiritual Pivot – The*

Outward Manifestation and Diseases caused by Five Viscera (Líng Shū – Wǔ Yuè Wǔ Shǐ, 灵枢·五阅五使): "The five sense organs reflect the five *zang* [3]", and among them, "the liver reflects the eyes[4]". This means the five sense organs are the external indicators of the health of the five *zang*, and thus the eyes reflects the liver's function. *The Spiritual Pivot - the Visceral (Líng Shū – Běn Zàng,* 灵枢·本脏) states: "Through observing the reflection of the outside, get the information of the internal organs, thus make a diagnosis of the disease[5]", which means we can know the condition of the internal organs through the survey and evaluation for the information of the external organs. The liver corresponds to the eyes, which establishes the rationale for the theory of "treating eye diseases through treating the liver", reminding us that we should also inspect other sense organs for clues of the health of their associated internal organs.

■ **Liver qi is connected with the eyes, and the harmony of liver qi allows the eyes to see things and distinguish colors.**

The eyes are the sense orifice of the liver, and liver qi can enter the eyes directly, thus the function of liver qi has important effects on visual function. On one hand, the liver can regulate qi circulation, driving qi ascending, descending, exiting and entering in an orderly way, which helps the upward movement of the blood and fluids, nourishing the eyes and enabling them to see. It is stated in *The Spiritual Pivot – Vessel Measurement Standard (Líng Shū – Mài Dù,* 灵枢·脉度): "Liver qi is connected with the eyes, and the harmony of liver qi allows the eyes to see things and distinguish colors[6]". Here, the "harmony of liver qi" means normal flow of qi, neither constrained nor excited. On the other hand, the liver can also regulate the emotions so as to keep the seven modes of emotions at a state of balance, which can not only benefit the overall health of the entire body, but also the health of the eyes, obtaining the goal of "living longer with a sustained vision[7]". It indicates that maintaining emotional health is a very important way of caring for the eyes and preventing eye diseases.

■ **The liver stores the blood; the storage of blood in the liver enables the eyes to see.**

The liver stores blood. In the *Basic Questions - Treatise on the Engenderment of the Five Viscera (Sù Wèn – Wǔ Zàng Shēng Chéng Piān,* 素问·五脏生成篇), it is recorded that "the liver receives blood and there is vision[8]"; Wang Bing's interpretation of this sentence is: "When the body is active, blood is moved to the muscles. When the body is in a state of rest, blood is stored in the liver[9]". The liver's function of storing blood is very helpful to the visual function. Although all the blood and fluids of the five *zang* and six *fu* flow upward into the eyes, the liver is connected with the eyes through a direct channel; thus, among the organs the liver has the biggest effect overall on the visual function. The Chinese medical physicians of later generations called it "true blood"; for example, it is said in *A Close Examination of the Precious Classic on Ophthalmology – Treatise of the Precious Eyes (Shěn Shì Yáo Hán – Mù Wéi Zhì Bǎo Lùn,* 审视瑶函·目为至宝论): "True blood is the clear and lucid blood transformed to the eyes by the liver; it is the blood that nourishes the channels and collaterals of the eyes. The blood is different from the turbid blood flowing in the vessels of muscles; because of its clear and ascendant characteristics, it is called true blood[10]".

■ **The liver governs the tears, and the tears luster the eyes.**

As recorded in *Basic Questions – Treatise Explaining the Five Qi* (*Sù Wèn – Xuān Míng Wǔ Qì Piān*, 素问·宣明五气篇), the five *zang* produce the five fluids and the liver produces the tear[11]. In the *Essentials from the Silver Sea* (*Yín Hǎi Jīng Wēi*, 银海精微) it is clearly pointed out that "tear is the fluid of the liver[12]". Tear has the function of moistening eyes, as it is said in *The Spiritual Pivot – Inquiry About Statement* (*Líng Shū – Kǒu Wèn*, 灵枢·口问): "What is the fluid for? It can enrich essence and moisten the orifices[13]". The production and excretion of tears are related with the liver function. With the normal function of liver qi, the tears will flow orderly without watery eyes (epiphora). When the liver is not functioning well, it can not restrict the tears well, resulting in excessive tearing that is likened to weeping.

2. The Physiological Relationship between the Eyes and the Heart

■ **The heart governs the blood, and the blood nourishes the eyes.**

Basic Questions – Treatise on the Engenderment of the Five Viscera (*Sù Wèn – Wǔ Zàng Shēng Chéng Piān*, 素问·五脏生成篇) states: "All blood belongs to the heart[14]". Under the propelling effect of the heart, the blood flows to the eyes and nourishes the eyes ceaselessly. Meanwhile, the "spirit water" (aqueous humor) originates from the eye blood, which is clear and rich in nourishment, immerses the "spirit jelly" (vitreous body) and the lens, ensuring that the eyes maintain normal visual function. Just as recorded in *A Close Examination of the Precious Classic on Ophthalmology – Treatise of the Precious Eyes*, "The blood produces the spirit water, the spirit water produces the spirit jelly, and the jelly protects the pupil[15]".

■ **The heart is connected with the blood and the vessels, and all the vessels are related to the eyes.**

Basic Questions – Treatise on Regulating the Channels (*Sù Wèn – Tiáo Jīng Lùn*, 素问·调经论) states: "The qi and blood flow in the paths of five *zang*, all of which are branch of channels[16]". The blood must use the channels and vessels as paths to flow up to the eyes. Statements such as "the heart governs the blood and the vessels[17]" (recorded in *Basic Questions – Treatise on Wěi* [*Sù Wèn – Wěi Lùn*, 素问·菱论]) and "the heart is connected with the blood and the vessels[18]" (recorded in *Basic Questions – Treatise on the Engenderment of the Five Viscera*) refer to the notion that the vessels of the whole body are connected with the heart. The vessels in the eyes are the most abundant, so it is said in the in *Basic Questions – Treatise on the Engenderment of the Five Viscera*: "All the vessels are related to the eyes[19]". And, it is pointed out clearly in *The Spiritual Pivot – Inquiry About Statement* (*Líng Shū – Kǒu Wèn*, 灵枢·口问) that "the eye is the confluence point of the channels[20]".

■ **The heart houses the spirit and liveliness, and the eyes are commanded by the heart.**

It is said in *Basic Questions – Treatise of the Arcane Book of the Orchid Chamber of the Spirit Tower* (*Sù Wèn – Líng Lán Mì Diǎn Lùn*, 素问·灵兰秘典论): "The heart holds the office of monarch, whence the spirit light emanates[21]". This means the heart governs the spirit, consciousness, thoughts, and even all life activities. *The Spiritual Pivot – The Spirit* (*Líng Shū – Běn Shén*, 灵枢·本神) says "the organ perceiving and handling stimulus is the heart[22]", which indicates it is the heart that receives stimuli from the outside world and reacts correspondingly, including accepting the stimulus of light and generating the vision. Thus, it is said in *The Spiritual Pivot – Great Confusion* that "the eyes are envoys of the heart, and the heart houses the spirit[23]". The spirit and consciousness are one of the most important factors needed for vision generation, which includes the action of both the heart and the brain. Because the heart is the master of the five *zang* and six *fu* and governs the spirit, all the essential qi of the *zang-fu* aggregate at the heart and then transport to eyes, so either the exuberance and debilitation of *zang-fu* essence or the spirit activities can be reflected at the eyes; therefore, the eyes are the external orifice of the heart, and inspection of the eyes and spirit is of major importance.

3. The Physiological Relationship between the Eyes and the Spleen

■ **The spleen transports essence upward into the eyes.**

The spleen governs the transportation and transformation of the essence of water and grain, and it is the foundation of the acquired constitution. When the spleen is functioning well, it can produce enough nutrients to luster the eyes. When the spleen is not functioning well, the eyes will not function well as a result of lack of nutrients.

Li Dong-yuan, the protagonist of spleen-stomach theory had paid special attention to the relationship between the spleen and the eyes. He pointed out in the *Secrets from the Orchid Chamber – Eye, Ear and Nose Division* (*Lán Shì Mì Cáng – Yǎn Ěr Bí Mén*, 兰室秘藏·眼耳鼻门), "All the essence of the five *zang* and six *fu* first originates from the spleen and is then transported to the eyes…so the deficiency of qi leads to the dysfunction of all the other organs and results in loss of luster in the eyes[24]". This quote highlights the importance of spleen essence to the visual function. Furthermore, the essence of the spleen can also nourish the muscles. With the nourishment of essential qi provided by the spleen, the eyelids are able to open and close, and the eyeballs can move with agility.

■ **The spleen brings clear yang upward to the eyes.**

The eyes are the orifice of clear yang, for it is seated at the superior part of the human body; and the vessel system is tiny that only clear yang can reach it. In *Basic Questions – Great Treatise on the Correspondences and Manifestations of Yin and Yang* (*Sù Wèn – Yīn Yáng Yīng Xiàng Dà Lùn*, 素问·阴阳应象大论), it says: "The clear yang is emitted from the upper orifices[25]". Only when spleen qi ascends can the clear yang be transported to the eyes so that the eyes can see things clearly.

■ **The spleen controls the blood to circulate in the eye vessels.**

The spleen controls the blood. Circulation of the blood in the vessels depends on the control of spleen qi. If there is failure in governing the blood in the vessels, hemorrhaging diseases, especially intraocular hemorrhaging, may develop. The pathomechanism is explained in the *The Complete Works of [Zhang] Jing-yue – Schema of Miscellaneous Patterns (Jǐng Yuè Quán Shū – Zá Zhèng Mó, 景岳全书·杂证谟*): "Since the spleen controls the blood, deficiency of spleen qi makes it fail to keep the blood in the vessels. Since the spleen produces the blood, spleen deficiency leads to failure to transport and transform the essence, which then results in the extravasation of blood[26]". This condition of ocular hemorrhage is commonly seen in diabetics with bleeding diabetic retinaopathies, a clear demonstration of the weak spleen function being the causative factor.

4. The Physiological Relationship between the Eyes and the Lung

■ **The lung is the dominator of qi; the harmony of qi ensures the brightness of the eyes.**

It is said in *Basic Questions – Treatise on the Engenderment of the Five Viscera*: "All qi is ascribed to the lung[27]". It is also pointed out in *Basic Questions – Treatise on the Six Periods and Visceral Manifestation (Sù Wèn – Liù Jié Zàng Xiàng Lùn, 素问·六节脏象论*) that "the lung is the dominator of qi[28]", and "the lung governs qi, the harmony of qi ensures the normal status of *ying-wei* and *zang-fu*[29]". The lung governs qi and controls the breath; it is not only in charge of exchanging air with the nature, but disbursing the essential substance of water and grains to the whole body and warming every organ. If lung qi is abundant, the activity of qi would be harmonious and the clear qi would ascend to the eyes smoothly to ensure sufficient oxygen intake for the eyes. If the lung qi is deficient, the qi of the *zang-fu* would not be sufficient as well and the eyes would lose nourishment and become dim. Just as recorded in *The Spiritual Pivot – Understanding the Qi (Líng Shū – Jué Qì, 灵枢·决气*), "the qi deserts, then the eyes dim[30]". The lung links with all vessels as well as governs the qi; it can promote the dispersion of blood to the whole body. When the lung is functioning well, blood circulates freely to warm and nourish the eyes, protecting the eyes from diseases of vascular obstruction.

■ **The lung governs diffusion and descent, which smooth the ocular collaterals.**

Diffusion means ascent and dispersion, which indicates the lung has the function of dispersing qi, blood, and fluids to the whole body. Descent means depuration and descent, which means the lung has the ability to regulate the waterways and maintain normal fluid metabolism. Diffusion and descent restricts each other, and coordinates and benefits each other, which enable blood to circulate in the vessels freely and make the ocular collateral smooth. On one hand, it enables qi, blood, and fluids to warm and nourish the eyes; on the other hand, it prevents turbid fluid from depositing in the eyes. Moreover, the lung governs the exterior; the orderly ascent and dispersion of lung qi transports *wei* qi and fluids to the body surface, which enables the body exterior and the vessels and collaterals around the eyes to be nourished and warmed, protecting the eyes from damage by external pathogen.

5. The Physiological Relationship between the Eyes and the Kidney

■ **The kidney governs the storage of essence; sufficiency of the essence ensures the brightness of the eyes.**

The Spiritual Pivot – Great Confusion holds that "the eyes are the essence of five *zang* six *fu*[31]", which indicates that the formation of the eyes relies on the essence, and the function of the eyes resorts to the essence. In *Basic Questions – Treatise of Heavenly Truth from Remote Antiquity* (*Sù Wèn – Shàng Gǔ Tiān Zhēn Lùn*, 素问·上古天真论), it says: "The kidney governs water; it receives and stores essence from the five *zang* and six *fu*[32]". Both prenatal and postnatal essence are stored in the kidney. The exuberance or deficiency of kidney essence has a direct effect on the visual function; this is suggested in *Basic Questions – Treatise of the Essential Subtleties of the Pulse* (*Sù Wèn – Mài Yào Jīng Wēi Lùn*, 素问·脉要精微论), which states, "If the essence is abundant, the eyes could see things, distinct color, and judge length. If the essence is deficient, the eyes would see the long as the short, and the white as the black[33]".

■ **The kidney engenders the cerebral marrow, and the eyes are connected with the brain.**

The kidney governs the bone and engenders the cerebral marrow. In the *Basic Questions – Great Treatise on the Correspondences and Manifestations of Yin and Yang*, it says that the kidney genders the bone marrow. All the marrows is ascribed to the brain, as both the brain and the marrow are transformed from kidney essence, so when the kidney essence and marrow are abundant, the vision is sharp. If the kidney essence and marrow are deficient, dizziness and a dim sight would arise.

■ **The kidney governs fluids, and the fluids moisten the eyeball.**

In *Basic Questions– Treatise on Disharmony* (*Sù Wèn – Nì Tiáo Lùn*, 素问·逆调论), it says that "the kidney is a water *zang* organ governing fluid[34]", which indicates clearly the important role of kidney in water metabolism and dispersion. *The Spiritual Pivot – The Five Dribbling Urinary Stoppages and the Differences Between Liquid and Humor* (*Líng Shū – Wǔ Lóng Jīn Yè Bié*, 灵枢·五癃津液别) states that "all the fluids from the five *zang* and six *fu* comes into the eyes[35]". Under the regulation of the kidney, fluids flow into the eyes, ensuring the transport of nutrients to nourish and moisten the eyes. Besides its nourishment function, the fluids play an essential role in maintaining the shape of the eyeball.

■ **The kidney supplies true yin and true yang; and nourishes and supports the function of the pupil.**

The kidney supplies the true yin and true yang, and it is an organ of both water and fire. The water is transformed from the true yin and the fire is transformed from the true yang (thus the root of yin and yang of the whole body). The yang of the five *zang* is produced and ascends from the kidney energy, and the yin of the five *zang* is nourished by the kidney fluids. That the essence produced by the kidney nourishes the eye is supported by *A Close Examination of the Precious Classic on Ophthalmology – Treatise of the Precious Eyes* which says, "The essence of the kidney rises and forms the water wheel[36]". The water wheel is located in the pupil, and the spirit light is stored in the pupil. In *Standards for Diagnosis and Treatment – Miscellaneous Diseases – Section of Seven Orifices* (*Zhèng Zhì Zhǔn Shéng – Zá Bìng – Qī Qiào Mén*, 证治准绳·杂病·七窍门), it says: "The pupil is generated by the prenatal qi and formed by the acquired (postnatal) qi; it is a true wonder of yin and yang, and the essence of water and fire[37]". The quote illustrates that yin and yang is the basis of vision development. Both the nourishment from the kidney essence and the heat energy produced from the life gate fire are requirements for vision.

6. The Physiological Relationship between the Eyes and the Six *fu*

The relationship between the eyes and the six *fu* is dependent on the integrated relationship between the five *zang* and the six *fu*. The *sanjiao* is a solitary *fu* (not correlating to any specific *zang* organ); the other five *fu* organs are paired with their corresponding *zang* in an exterior-interior relationship. The relationships are the small intestine to the heart, the gallbladder to the liver, the stomach to the spleen, the large intestine to the lung, and the bladder to the kidney. Physically, the *zang* moves qi to the *fu*, while the *fu* transports essence to the *zang*. Therefore, the eyes have a close relationship with both the five *zang* and the six *fu* inseparably. Moreover, the main function of the six *fu* organs is to govern reception, control digestion, separate the clear and the turbid, move the waste through the bowels, and transport the essence to the whole body to supply and nourish the organs (including the eyes). It says in *The Spiritual Pivot – the Visceral* that "the six *fu* are the organs in charge of digesting and absorbing the water and grain, and of promoting the circulation of body fluid[38]". Only when the six *fu* organs function optimally, can the eyes have enough nutrients to sustain healthy vision.

Section 2   The Relationships Between the Eyes and the Channels and Collaterals

The channels and collaterals are the places where qi and blood circulate, It can also link up interior and exterior as well as superior and inferior, and connect all the *zang-fu* organs in a complex network. As mentioned earlier, *The Spiritual Pivot – Inquiry About Statement* holds that "the eye is the confluence point of the channels[39]". In another chapter of the same text, *Forms of Disease from Evil Qi in Zang-fu* (*Líng Shū – Xié Qì Zàng Fǔ Bìng Xíng*, 灵枢·邪气脏腑病形), it says that "all the blood and qi of the twelve channels and 365 collaterals run upward to the face and flow into the orifices; the essential yang qi goes into the eyes[40]". The eyes depend on the channels and collaterals for transportation of nutrients, such as qi, blood, and fluids, in order to sustain healthy vision. Therefore, the eyes have a close relationship with the channels and collaterals.

1. The Relationship between the Eyes and the Twelve Channels

The twelve channels are classified into yin channels and yang channels according to the interior or exterior organs with which they are connected. The primary channels link to each other end to end, and divergent channels and collaterals run through the body in a crisscross pattern. The primary channels start from the hand *taiyin* and terminates at the foot *jueyin*; the beginning links up with the end like a circle without end, going around and beginning again, running without stopping. In *The Spiritual Pivot – Treating the Fat and Thin According to Circumstance* (*Líng Shū – Nì Shùn Féi Shòu*, 灵枢·逆顺肥瘦), it is revealed that "the three yang channels of the hand run from the hands to the head, while the three yang channels of the foot go from the head to the feet[41]". So, it can be seen that both the paths of the three yang channels of the hand and the three yang channels of the foot have relationships with the eyes; and although the three yin channels of the hand and the three yin channels of the foot do not go upward to the head and face, some of them correlate with the eyes directly and indirectly. Herein we introduce the channels which have relationships with the eyes according to their stopover at the eyes.

■ **Channels Starting and Ending, Conjoining and Transiting at the Inner Canthus**

➤ The foot *taiyang* bladder channel

The *Spiritual Pivot – Channel Vessels* (*Líng Shū – Jīng Mài*, 灵枢·经脉) states, "The channel of food *taiyang* bladder starts at the internal canthus, goes across the forehead and reach at the top of the head[42]". In detail, the channel starts at BL 1 (*jīng míng*), goes along BL 2 (*cuán zhú*) at the forehead, then across DU 24 (*shén tíng*) and BL 7 (*tōng tiān*), and runs obliquely to meet the *du mai* at DU 20 (*bǎi huì*).

➤ The foot *yangming* stomach channel

The Spiritual Pivot – Channel Vessels: "The foot *yangming* stomach channel starts at the side of the nose...at the forehead." To be more specific, the channel starts at LI 20 (*yíng xiāng*) alongside the nose, passes BL 1 (*jīng míng*) at the inner canthus, and at last connects with the foot *taiyang* bladder channel.

➤ The hand *taiyang* small intestine channel

A branch of the channel travels from the cheek and goes upward to the bottom of the orbit, reaches the side of the nose, and connects with the foot *taiyang* bladder channel.

➢ The hand *yangming* large intestine channel

The two branches of the channel move upward to the head and face, and cross behind the philtrum, then travel along the sides of the nose to LI 20 (*yíng xiāng*), and connect with the foot *yangming* stomach channel, which has a close relationship with the eyes.

■ **Channels Starting and Ending, Conjoining and Transiting at the Outer Canthus**

➢ The foot *shaoyang* gallbladder channel

The channel starts from GB 1 (*tóng zǐ liáo*) at the outer canthus, travels from GB 2 (*tīng huì*) and passes GB 3 (*shàng guān*), goes upward to GB 4 (*hàn yàn*), then moves to the back of the ears, passes GB 20 (*fēng chí*), and then reach the neck. One branch travels from the back of the ear to the inside of the ear, then moves out and up to GB 1 (*tóng zǐ liáo*) at the outer canthus. The other branch moves downward from GB 1 (*tóng zǐ liáo*), passes ST 5 (*dà yíng*) and meets the hand *shaoyang* at the bottom of the orbit.

➢ The hand *shaoyang sanjiao* channel

One branch of the channel travels from the chest to the neck, along SJ 17 (*yì fēng*), moves upward to the superior cornu of the ear and connects with SJ 20 (*jiǎo sūn*), passes GB 14 (*yáng bái*) and LI 19 (*hé liáo*), and then curves and moves downward to the bottom of the orbit. The other branch goes inside of the ear and then moves out and meets the first branch at the cheek and then reaches the outer canthus of the eye, and finally connects with the foot *shaoyang* gallbladder channel. Thereby, the hand *shaoyang sanjiao* channel has relationships with the eyes through two branches.

➢ The hand *taiyang* small intestine channel

One branch of the channel goes upward to the cheek and arrives at the cheek bone, then to the outer canthus, crosses GB 1 (*tóng zǐ liáo*), and moves into the ear.

■ **Channels Connecting with the Eye**

➢ The foot *jueyin* liver channel

The main channel goes along the throat and up to nasopharynx, then passes the outside of ST 5 (*dà yíng*), ST 4 (*dì cāng*), ST 2 (*sì bái*) and GB 14 (*yáng bái*), then connects with the eye directly.

➢ The hand *shaoyin* heart channel

The branch of the channel connects with the eye directly.

➢ The foot *taiyang* bladder channel

One branch of the channel enters the brain through BL 9 (*yù zhěn*, 玉枕), which is also called the "eye branch". BL 9 (*yù zhěn*) is located at the visual area of the scalp, which is commonly used in the treatment of low vision and cortical blindness.

To sum up, all the three yang channels of the foot start from the eye or periorbitally, and all the three yang channels of the hand have one or two branches that stop at the eye or orbit. The foot *jueyin* liver channel, the hand *shaoyin* heart channel, and the foot *taiyang* bladder channel connect with the eye directly. And, as for the foot *jueyin* liver channel, it is the main channel that connects with the eye.

2. The Relationship between the Eyes and the Eight Extraordinary Vessels

The eight extraordinary vessels are different from the twelve regular channels in that they do not pertain to any *zang* and *fu*. However, they cross and run through the twelve channels, enhancing the link between the channels to regulate qi and blood. Among the eight extraordinary vessels, there are five channels have direct relations with the eye at the start, the stop point, or in the pathway, including the *du mai*, the *ren mai*, the *yangqiao mai,* the *yinqiao mai*, and the *yangwei mai*.

■ **Relationship between the Eye and the *Du Mai***

The *du mai* starts from the midpoint inside the pubis. One branch runs upward, winding the buttock, and meets the foot *taiyang* bladder channel at the inner canthus of the eye, then moves upward to the forehead and crosses with each other again at the top of the head, and enters the brain. The other branch starts from the lower abdomen and runs straight up to the belly button, then goes up and crosses the heart, meets the *ren mai* and *chong mai*, then up to the lower mandible and circles around the lips, and then stops below the center of the eye.

■ **Relationship between the Eye and the *Ren Mai***

The *ren mai* is called the "sea of the yin channels", governing all the yin channels of the body. This vessel starts from the perineum, runs up to the pubic hair, goes inside the abdomen, moves out at RN 4 (*guān yuán*), passes through the throat and lower mandible, circles the lips and divides into two branches, and then goes along the cheek and arrives at ST 1 (*chéng qì*) below the eye socket.

■ **Relationship between the Eye and the *Yangqiao Mai***

The foot *taiyang* bladder channel enters the brain at the middle of the neck between two vessels, *yinqiao mai* and *yangwei mai*. The two vessels meet each other at the inner canthus of the eye.

■ **Relationship between the Eye and the *Yinqiao Mai***

The *yinqiao mai* starts from KI 6 (*zhào hǎi*) behind the navicular bone, entersthe chest and crosses ST 12 (*quē pén*), moves out in front of ST 9 (*rén yíng*), arrives at the side of nose, and connects with the inner canthus. Together with the foot *taiyang* bladder channel and the *yangqiao mai,* the *yinqiao mai* nourishes the eye.

■ **Relationship between the Eye and the *Yangwei Mai***

The *yangwei mai* links all the yang channels of the body. It has relations with the eye through GB 14 (*yáng bái*).

Otherwise, although the *yinwei mai, chong mai*, and *dai mai* do not have direct relationships with the eye, the *yinwei mai* links all the yin channels of the body, the *chong mai* is the sea of the blood, and the *dai mai* restrains and connects with all the foot channels; therefore, all of the three vessels have indirect association with the eye.

Endnotes

[1] 五脏六腑之精气,皆上注于目而为之精。精之窠为眼,骨之精为瞳子,筋之精为黑眼,血之精为络,其窠气之精为白眼,肌肉之精为约束,裹撷筋骨血气之精而与脉并为系,上属于脑,后出于项中

[2] 东方青色,入通于肝,开窍于目,藏精于肝

[3] 五官者,五脏之阅也

[4] 目者,肝之官也

[5] 视其外应,以知其内脏,则知所病矣

[6] 肝气通于目,肝和则目能辨五色矣

[7] 长生久视

[8] 肝受血而能视

[9] 人动则血运于诸经,人静则血归于肝藏

[10] 真血者,即肝中升运于目,轻清之血,乃滋目经络之血也。此血非比肌肉间混浊易行之血,因其轻清上升于高而难得,故谓之真也

[11] 五脏化液……肝为泪

[12] 泪乃肝之液

[13] 液者,所以灌精濡空窍者也

[14] 诸血者,皆属于心

[15] 血养水,水养膏,膏护瞳神

[16] 五脏之道,皆出于经隧,以行气血

[17] 心主身之血脉

[18] 心之合脉也

[19] 诸脉者,皆属于目

[20] 目者,宗脉之所聚也,上液之道也

[21] 心者,君主之官,神明出焉

[22] 所以任物者谓之心

[23] 目者,心之使也;心者,神之舍也

[24] 夫五脏六腑之精气皆禀受于脾,上贯于目……故脾虚则五脏之精气皆失所司,不能归明于目矣

[25] 清阳出上窍

[26] 盖脾统血,脾气虚则不能收摄;脾化血,脾气虚则不能运化,是皆血无所主,因而脱陷妄行

[27] 诸气者皆属于肺

[28] 肺者,气之本

[29] 肺主气,气调则营卫脏腑无所不治

[30] 气脱者,目不明

[31] 目者,五脏六腑之精也

[32] 肾者主水，受五脏六腑之精而藏之

[33] 夫精明者，所以视万物、别白黑、审短长；以长为短、以白为黑，如是则精衰矣

[34] 肾者水脏，主津液

[35] 五脏六腑之津液，尽上渗于目

[36] 肾之精腾，结而为水轮

[37] 乃先天之气所生，后天之气所成，阴阳之妙用，水火之精华

[38] 六腑者，所以化水谷而行津液者也

[39] 目者，宗脉之所聚也

[40] 十二经脉，三百六十五络，其血气皆上于面而走空窍，其精阳气上走于目而为睛

[41] 手之三阳，从手走头；足之三阳，从头走足

[42] 膀胱足太阳之脉，起于目内眦，上额交巅

Chapter 4
Diagnostic Essentials

Section 1   Ophthalmologic Examination

This section is to provide an overview of ocular history and complete eye examination as performed by an ophthalmologist.

1. Ocular History

Includes the chief complaint, history of present illness, past medical history and family history.

An understanding of ocular symptomatology is important for performing a proper ophthalmic examination. Ocular symptoms fall into one of the three following categories:

- Visual abnormalities: Loss of vision, blurring, diplopia, visual distortion, flashing, floating, etc.
- Sensational abnormalities: Pain, itching, sensation of foreign body, photophobia, tearing etc.
- Abnormalities of appearance: Redness, secretions, swelling, etc.

2. Ocular Examination

Ocular examinations contain both subjective (which depends on patients' feedback) and objective (which is independent of patients' feedback) exams. The accuracy of the subjective examination relies on patients' cooperation, education, age, mood, etc. Thus, the results from the subjective tests may vary between the exams. Commonly used subjective examinations are visual acuity, Amsler grid, visual field and color vision exams. Commonly used objective exams include slit-lamp examination, ophthalmoscopy, tonometry, fundus fluorescein angiography (FFA), optical coherence tomography (OCT), electrophysiological exams and ultrasonography. In order to examine the posterior ocular structures, the pupil is usually dilated. However, because topical mydriatic drops affects the visual acuity, accommodation, intraocular pressure, anterior chamber angle, these examinations should be performed before pupil dilation. In addition, mydriatic drops may induce acute angle-closure glaucoma in patients with a narrow anterior chamber angle.

■ **Subjective examination**
➤ Visual acuity

Visual acuity, also called spatial visual acuity, is "the finest spatial detail that can be detected, discriminated, or resolved".[1] Visual acuity measures the clearness of central vision, which reflects the "healthiness" of the macula. However, it should be noted that any impairment in the optic or visual pathway, starting from the cornea to the visual cortex, may affect visual acuity. Peripheral vision is often assessed with visual field test.

A Snellen chart is usually used for testing visual acuity at distance (usually 20 feet or 6 meters). The Snellen chart has several rows of black English letters on a white background. It measures the minimum visual angle that the visual system can differentiate at high contrast. Visual acuity is expressed as $V = d/D$.[2] "V" represents visual acuity. "d" represents the distance at which the patient is able to read a certain row of letters. "D" represents the distance at which a person with normal visual acuity is able to read the same row of letters. For example, if a patient can read a row of letters at 20 feet (the commonly used distance for visual acuity test) while a normal person can read the same letters at 40 feet, visual acuity is expressed as 20/40. In some countries, it is also expressed as a decimal number and in this case is 0.5 (20/40=0.5). By convention, visual acuity is tested in the right eye first with the left eye covered. Both uncorrected visual acuity (without glasses or contact lenses) and corrected visual acuity (with glasses or contact lenses, if available) should be tested. If a patient's uncorrected visual acuity is below 1.0 and glasses are not available, a pinhole test can be performed to estimate the patient's corrected visual acuity because small pinholes minimize refractive errors. If a patient can not read the largest letters, ask the patient to move close to the chart until the largest letters can be seen. Record the distance as the numerator. If the patient still cannot read the largest letter at 3 feet (1 meter), extend several fingers and ask the patient to count and record the distance at which the patient can count the number of tester's fingers correctly, e.g. CF (counting fingers) 2ft. If the patient can not count fingers, move the examiner's hand. If the patient can detect hand motion, then record as HM (hand motion). If HM cannot be detected, point a flash light to the patient's eye and ask if he can detect the presence of light. If the patient has light perception (LP), project the light at different directions and ask the patient whether he can identify where the light is. Otherwise, record as NLP (no light perception).

Normal visual acuity is defined as 20/20 or 1.0. Legal blindness is defined as "central visual acuity of 20/200 or less in the better eye with the use of a correcting lens" in ths U.S.

➤ Perimetry

Measurement of the visual field is called perimetry. The visual field can be measured manually or automatically, with or without special instruments (perimeters).

The visual field is "all the space that one eye can see at any given instant".[3] The visual field within the central 30 degree is the central visual field while the visual field outside is the peripheral visual field. The visual field is determined by many factors, e.g. pupil size, stimuli and psychological factors. Generally speaking, the normal visual field extends 60 degrees superiorly, 75 degrees inferiorly, 100 degrees temporally and 60 degrees nasally.[4] The blind spot is temporal to the center of the visual field. Here are the common methods to test peripheral vision.

- The confrontation exam: This method compares patient's visual field with examiner's normal visual field. The patient and examiner sit opposite to each other. When testing the right eye, the patient is asked to fixate the left eye of the examiner, with the patient's left eye and examiner's right eye masked. The examiner places his fingers with equal distance from both the examiner and patient, and moves his fingers from periphery into the patient's visual field in different directions. The patient is asked to report when he first sees the fingers. The confrontation exam is simple but not accurate.

- Amsler charts: The commonly used Amsler chart contains 20×20 squares formed by vertical and horizontal lines. This simple and sensitive test can be used by patients at home to monitor their macular function. The Amsler chart is placed 1 foot (33cm) in front of the patient so that each square corresponds to 1 degree of the visual field.[4] With one eye masked, the patient fixate at the dot in the center. Any scotoma, distortion, wavy or missing lines indicate diseases affecting the central visual field within 10 degrees.

- Goldmann perimetry: The Goldmann perimeter is a manual perimeter. Stimuli with different size and luminance are projected onto a hemispherical screen. The patient is asked to report when he sees the stimuli. The examiner monitors the fixation of the patient during the exam and plots the result. The Goldmann perimeter offers a rapid test for the peripheral visual field.

- Automatic perimetry: Automatic perimeters are computerized perimeters, which are capable of monitoring fixation, performing data analysis, comparing results overtime and have multiple programs for specific diseases. Automatic perimeters offer two strategies: the suprathreshold and threshold exams.[4] The suprathreshold exam uses stimuli that the patient should be able to see. The threshold can be determined by an initial measurement with preset programs. This test is for rapid screening. The threshold test provides accurate results of visual field defects. However, it is time-consuming and may lead to fatigue and distraction, which decrease accuracy and reliability.

➢ Color vision exams

Pseudoisochromatic plates are the most common technique for examine color vision. The patient is asked to report numbers formed by colored dots on a background of other colors. Patients with abnormal color vision can not discern the numbers based on their colors or require prolonged time for the exam. Color vision deficiency is often inherited ("color blindness"). The most common abnormality is red-green color blindness, which is of X-linked recessive inheritance. Color vision deficiency may also be due to acquired retinal or optic nerve diseases.

■ Objective examination

Always start from the healthy eye and check the symmetry of the two eyes. Examine eyelids (check if there is any redness, swelling, tumor, entropion or ectripion, ptosis, etc.), lacrimal apparatus (redness, tendness, discharge, etc.), conjunctiva (redness, papillae, follicles, etc), eye movement and alignment and the orbit first, followed by the cornea (size, curvature, haze, foreign body, neovessels, etc.), sclera (color, congestion, tendness, etc.), anterior chamber (turbidity, hyphema, etc.), pupil (size, circularity, light reflex, etc.) and lens (turbidity, dislocation, etc.).

➢ Slitlamp biomicroscopy

With the help of the slitlamp biomicroscope, most of the ocular structures can be visualized directly. Due to the optic property of the eye, ocular structures including ocular surface, the cornea, anterior chamber, anterior surface of the iris, lens and anterior vitreous are visible under the slitlamp biomicroscope. The anterior chamber angle, posterior vitreous, pars plana of the ciliary body and the retina can also be examined with special lenses (gonioscope, 90D biconvex lens or Goldmann three mirror lens). The slitlamp biomicroscope is equipped with a light source, which projects a slit beam of light onto the ocular structure. The length, width, intensity and angle of projection of the light beam are adjustable. The binocular microscope provides 10× to 16× magnification as well as stereoscopic view. The focus of the light beam and biomicroscope are usually coupled, i.e. at the same focal plane, which provides adequate illumination for visualizing details of the ocular structure. When the light beam is projected to the transparent tissues, e.g. the cornea and lens, an optic cross-section is present. By adjusting focus, the depth and location of abnormalities can be clearly identified. Abnormal content in the aqueous humor is detected with a narrow light beam with minimum length passing the anterior chamber. Normal aqueous humor is optically clear. If there is increased protein concentration and/or presence of cells, the light beam is visible in the aqueous humor, which is called aqueous flare or Tyndall effect. Aqueous flare indicates break of the blood-aqueous humor barrier.

➢ Tonometry

Measurement of intraocular pressure (IOP) is called tonometry. Clinically, IOP is measured by the tonometer. The commonly used tonometers are the indentation tonometer (Schiotz tonometer) and applanation tonometer.[5]

• Indentation tonometry: The indentation tonometer measures corneal depression/

indentation caused by a weight. The measured amount of depression is then converted to pressure readings. The patient is placed supine and topical anesthetics is given to the eyes to be measured. Ask the patient to look straight forward or place his fingers above the non-measured eye as a target for fixation. The examiner holds the indentation tonometer with one hand and opens the eye to be measured by gently retracting the patient's eyelids and hold them against the orbital rim. The indentation tonometer with a 5.5g weight is lowered and placed on the central cornea. The reading (in millimeter) is converted to millimeter mercury (mmHg) according to a conversion chart. If the eye is firm and the reading is less than 3mm, additional weights can be added and repeat IOP measurement.[2]

- Applanation tonometry: Applanation tonometry measures the force required to flatten the cornea to a predetermined level. The amount of the force is converted to IOP. The commonly used applanation tonometers include the Goldmann tonometer, non-contact tonometer, Perkins tonometer and Tono-Pen.[5]

- Goldmann tonometry: Goldmann tonometry is generally accepted as the "golden standard" of IOP measurement. The Goldmann tonometer is attached to a slitlamp. Before measurement, topical anesthetics and fluorescein are given to the patient. In order to visualize fluorescein, a cobalt filter is used with the brightest illumination. The patient is positioned at the slitlamp just like for slitlamp biomicroscopy. The Goldmann tonometer is rotated into place, set at 1, and pre-aligned in front of the cornea from outside the slitlamp biomicroscope. The examiner looks into the slitlamp biomicroscope and moves the tonometer to the patient until the tonometer probe just touches the cornea. Under the slitlamp, two semicircles are present when the cornea is flattened. The force exerted on the cornea is adjusted until the inner edges of the two semicircles are aligned. The reading is multipled by 10 to convert to mmHg.

- Other applanation tonometry: The non-contact tonometer uses air puff to flatten the cornea. Both the amount of cornea applanation and the force of the air puff are detected and calculated.[5] These data are then analyzed and converted to IOP. Although it is not as accurate as the Goldmann tonometer, it does not require topical anesthetics nor fluorescein. This method minimizes the chance of disease transmission and is suitable for rapid IOP screening. The Perkins tonometer is similar to the Goldmann tonometer but it is portable. The Tono-Pen tonometer projects a probe toward and cornea and measures the rate of deceleration when the probe rebounds. Based on the deceleration rate, IOP is calculated. This method requires frequent calibration and is not widely used clinically.

➤ Ophthalmoscopy

Ophthalmoscopes are special optic instruments for examining the vitreous and fundus. There are two types of ophthalmoscopes: direct ophthalmoscope and indirect ophthalmoscope.

- Direct ophthalmoscopy: Direct ophthalmoscopy can be performed with or without pupil dilation. However, a dilated pupil allows visualization of the more peripheral retina. Direct ophthalmoscopy is relatively easy to use because it provides a magnified (usually 15×), upright image. To examine the left eye of the patient, the examiner holds the direct ophthalmoscope with his left hand and uses his left eye. For the patient's right eye, use the right hand and look through the right eye. In order to obtain a wide and clear view, the distance between the patient's eye, ophthalmoscope and examiner's eye should be as short as possible. The refractive error of both the patient and examiner can be compensated by rotating the wheel with series of compensating lenses. Examination of the fundus starts from the optic disc. Ask the patient to fixate on a distant object with both eyes open, turn the ophthalmoscopy slightly to the nasal side and the optic disc should be visible if the optic medium is clear. Shape, color, size, cup-to-disk ratio (C/D ratio, which indicates optic nerve head "cupping"), presence of hemorrhage and symmetry of the optic disc are evaluated and recorded. The size of the optic disc (disk diameters, DD) can also be used as a reference or scale to measure and describe abnormalities in the fundus. After examining the optic disk, the major retinal vessels and the retina are then examined sequentially: from center (optic disc) to periphery and from one quadrant to the adjacent quadrant (either clockwisely or counterclockwisely). To examine the peripheral retina, ask the patient to fixate in the corresponding direction (e.g. to examine the superior peripheral retina, ask the patient to look up). Finally, ask the patient to look at the light source of the ophthalmoscope to examine the macula. A small pinpoint with bright reflection in the center of the macula is the fovea.
- Indirect ophthalmoscopy: Indirect ophthalmoscopy usually requires pupil dilation. The indirect ophthalmoscope is worn on the examiner's head and a condensing lens (usually 20D) is held by the examiner several inches from the patient's eye. By adjusting the distance and orientation of the condensing lens, a magnified (approximately 3×), real image (inverted and reversed) of the patient's fundus is formed in between the examiner and condensing lens. Although indirect ophthalmoscopy is difficult to learn and requires more practice, it has unique advantages over direct ophthalmoscopy: 1) wide field of view; 2) stereoscopic view; 3) less affected by cloudy media (e.g. cataract, vitreous turbidity) and refractive error (e.g. high myopia); 4) Combined with the scleral depressor, the very peripheral retinal region including the ora serrata, and even the pars plana of the ciliary body, are visible.

➢ Fundus fluorescein angiography (FFA)

Fundus fluorescein angiography is an important technique for evaluating retinal vasculature and associated abnormalities. It also provides essential guidance for laser treatment (photocoagulation). Fluorescein is a dye that emits green light when it is excited by light with shorter wavelength. Healthy retinal vessels are impermeable to fluorescein molecules. However, fluorescein molecules diffuse out of the fenestrated choriocapillaris.

Before imaging the fundus, the pupil is dilated to maximize visible retinal area. Fluorescein is injected intravenously, circulates in the body and passes through retinal and choroidal vessels. When fluorescein reaches the fundus, a beam of light is projected to the fundus to excite the dye in the vessels. The green light emitted from the fundus is detected by a fundus camera, through which sequential images are captured.

Fluorescein fills the choroid first, followed by the retinal arteries, capillaries and is drained through the retinal veins. Accordingly, fluorescein angiograms are divided into the choroidal phase, arterial phase, arteriovenous phase, venous phase and late phase.[6] Because the choroidal phase is very short (several seconds) and quickly masked by signals from retinal vessels as well as the "leaky" property of the choroicapillaris, FFA is primarily used for retinal angiography.

Abnormal angiograms are classified into two categories: hyperfluorescence and hypo-fluorescence.[6]

Hyperfluorescence: The intact blood-retinal barrier (non-fenestrated endothelial cells of the retinal vessels and RPE cells) keeps fluorescein from leaking. Any damage to this barrier may lead to fluorescein leakage into the retina (pooling of fluorescein) and staining of the tissue around the leaky vessels, drusen and macular scar tissue. Other disease conditions that may cause hyperfluorescence include lack of pigment (Pigment loss results in visualization of fluorescein in the choroid, which is also called "Window defects"), neovescularization and retinal telangiectasia.

Hypofluorescence: Hypofluorescence is due to either masking or filling defects. Excessive pigment (choroidal nevus, black people, retinal dystrophies) and hemorrhage may mask the fluorescent signal. While occlusion of retinal or choroidal vessels leads to decreased fluorescein circulation in the fudus, causing filling defects.

> Ultrasonography

Ultrasonography uses high frequency sound (ultrasound, >20,000 Hz) to study the ocular and orbital tissue. During ultrasonography, a probe is place against the eye. The probe sends out ultrasound toward the tissue of interest and receives sound waves bounced back (echoes). Signals are transmitted and displayed on an oscilloscope or computer. Two commonly used modes are A-scan and B-scan.

A-scan is an amplitude modulation ("A" means amplitude).[7] In this mode, the sound beam is directed in a straight line. The spikes of sound waves bounced back are displayed according to their temporal order. This mode provides accurate measurement of the intraocular structure, e.g. the axial length.

B-scan is a time-bright modulation ("B" means brightness).[7] In this mode, the linear sound beam sweeps a sector of the eye. The one-dimensional spatial information is summed to construct two-dimensional images. The echoes are displayed as light dots whose brightness varies with their amplitude. Although accurate measure is difficult in

B-scan because differentiation of echo spikes by brightness is not as easy as in A-scan, B-scan provides a direct, anatomical view of intraocular structures and abnormalities.

➢ OCT

OCT is a non-invasive, high resolution (in micrometers) optic biopsy technology in ophthalmology. The first-generation commercial ophthalmic OCT instrument was first introduced in 1996.[8] Currently, third-generation OCT instruments with ultra-high resolution are widely used in ophthalmic care.

The mechanism of OCT is analogous to ultrasonography, except that it uses light wave instead of sound wave to study the retinal structure.[8] Current commercial OCT instruments enable imaging retinal cross sections (2D images, analogous to B-scan) with all the retinal layers clearly visible. The retinal structures shown by OCT images correlate well with histological sections. OCT is particularly helpful in diagnosing, monitoring or measuring retinal diseases and structures e.g. macular holes, macular edema, subretinal fluid accumulation, optic nerve fiber layer.

➢ Electrophysiologic examination

Commonly used electrophyiologic examination includes electro-oculography (EOG), electroretinography (ERG) and visual evoked potential (VEP).

- EOG: EOG measures the resting (without stimuli) corneoretinal potential, which originates from RPE.[9] The recording electrodes are placed at the medial and lateral canthi. Patients are asked to move their eyes horizontally. Time and amplitude of the corneoretinal potential are recorded. This exam is performed in dark and light conditions. EOG abnormalities indicate RPE and photoreceptor dysfunction.

- ERG: ERG measures the electrical responses of the retina to visual stimuli.[9] Different from EOG, the recording electrodes in ERG are placed on the ocular surface (usually on the cornea after administration of topical anesthetics) and the skin close to the eye. In addition, pupil dilation is often required for ERG. Depending on the visual stimulus, ERG is divided into flash ERG and pattern ERG.

- Flash ERG (fEGR): In flash ERG, flashes with various intensities, wavelengths and frequencies are projected to the retina. The recorded electrical responses consist of multiple components. The components of clinical importance are the negative a-wave, positive b-wave and oscillatory potentials (OPs, which are superimposed on the b-wave).[9] These components originate from photoreceptor cells (a-wave), bipolar and Müller glial cells (b-wave) and the inner plexiform layer (OPs). In order to differentiate the function of rods and cones, flash ERG can be performed under light adapted (photopic ERG, for cones) or dark adapted conditions (scotopic ERGs, for rods). Depending on the retinal neurons involved in the retinal disease, ERG components may demonstrate decreased amplitude, abnormal implicit time (time-to-peak), altered b-wave to a-wave ratio etc. Diminished OPs usually indicate retinal ischemia. Because flash ERG represents the summation of electrical responses of the whole retina, it may not be sensitive enough to detect focal retinal abnormalities nor can it specify the location of the diseased retina.

- Pattern ERG: In pattern ERG, alternating/reversing checkboard stimuli are projected to the retina. The recorded electrical responses consist of a positive P50-wave and a negative N95-wave.[9] Pattern ERG abnormalities suggest diseases involving the macula or retinal ganglion cells, Pattern ERG is helpful in detecting ganglion cell damage in the early stage of glaucoma.[10]

- VEP: Similar to ERG, VEP also measures electrical responses of the retina to visual stimuli. However, the recording electrode is placed on the scalp. Thus, it records signals from the visual cortex.[9] In another word, the electrical responses/signals must be transmitted from the retina to the visual cortex via the visual pathway before it can be detected. Thus, any damage in the visual pathway may result in abnormal VEP.[9] Because the projection zone of the macula occupies majority of the visual cortex, VEP primarily reflects the function of both the macula and optic nerve.

References:

1. Norton TT, Corliss DA, Bailey JE. *The psychophysical measurement of visual function.* Wobum, MA: Butterworth-Heinemann; 2002:361.

2. Hui Yan-nian. *Ophthalmology.* 5th ed. Beijing, China: People's Medical Publishing House; 2001:268.

3. Tate GW, Lynn JR. *Principles of quantitative perimetry.* New York, NY: Grune and Stratton; 1977.

4. Henson DB. *Visual fields.* 2nd ed. Boston, MA: Butterworth-Heinemann Ltd.; 2000:159.

5. Riordan-Eva P, Whitcher JP. *Vaughan & Asbury's general ophthalmology.* 16th ed. New York, NY: Lange Medical Books/McGraw Hill Medical Pub. Division; 2004.

6. Chopdar A. *Manual of fundus fluorescein angiography.* Boston, MA: Butterworth-Heinemann Ltd.; 1989:134.

7. Guthoff R, Verlag GT. *Ultrasound in ophthalmologic diagnosis: a practical guide.* New York, NY: Thieme medical publishers, Inc.; 1991:174.

8. Drexler W, Fujimoto JG. State-of-the-art retinal optical coherence tomography. *Prog Retin Eye Res* 2008;27:45-88.

9. Heckenlively JR. *Principles and practice of clinical electrophysiology of vision* St. Louis, MO: Mosby Year Book; 1991:829.

10. O'Donaghue E, Arden GB, O'Sullivan F, et al. The pattern electroretinogram in glaucoma and ocular hypertension. *Br J Ophthalmol* 1992;76:387-394.

Section 2　Common Methods of Pattern Differentiation in Ophthalmology

Based on the concept of holism, pattern differentiation in traditional Chinese medical (TCM) ophthalmology is determined through the analysis and judgement of clinic data collected by the four examinations. Clinical treatment is determined by eight-principle pattern differentiation, cause-of-disease pattern differentiation, visceral pattern differentiation, qi-blood pattern differentiation, etc. TCM ophthalmic pattern differentiation is unique and based on the specific symptoms presented in each case. Therefore, in Chinese medical ophthalmology, local symptoms are the determining factors considered when making pattern differentiation. All symptoms should be considered as well, because most eye diseases are systemic issues and not just localized eye issues, especially in cases of internal, chronic degenerative conditions. Besides the common methods used by general pattern differentiation, a five-wheel pattern differentiation system is a unique method in TCM ophthamology. The traditional eight-stage pattern differentiation is seldom used in the clinic as the primary means of diagnosis when treating ocular conditions; thus, it will not be discussed in this chapter.

1. Five Wheels Pattern Differentiation

■ Theory of Five Wheels

The five wheels theory is a relatively modern theory used in Chinese medicine, and is frequently used in TCM ophthalmology. Derived from the well-known five-phase theory used in TCM ophthalmology, it is based on the "ocular visceral manifestation theory", which traces back to *The Yellow Emperor's Inner Classic. The Spiritual Pivot – Great Confusion* records: "Essential qi of the five *zang* and six *fu* flow upward and changes into ocular essence. The socket of essence is the eye: essence of bone relates to the pupil, essence of sinew relates to the the black of the eye (cornea), essence of blood relates to the vessels, essence of eye socket qi relates to the white of the eye, and essence of ocular muscle relates to the eyelid. All the essence of the sinews, bones, qi, and blood converge into the optic nerve, which connects with vessels that link to the brain and comes out of the nape.

The earliest recordings of the five-wheel theory can be found in *Formulas from Benevolent Sages Compiled during the Taiping Era* (A.D. 922). The five-wheel theory is based on the intimate correlation between the eye and the *zang-fu*; including the eyelid, canthus, white of the eye, the black of the eye (cornea), and the pupil.

The five wheels are divided into the following five categories: flesh wheel, blood wheel, qi wheel, wind wheel, and water wheel, in sequence. This theory illustrates the relationship between the eye structure and the five *zang*, including anatomy, physiology, and pathology.

■ **Anatomy of the Five Wheels and Correspondence with the *Zang-Fu***

➤ The flesh wheel refers to the eyelid, which includes the skin, subcutaneous tissue, muscles, tarsus and palpebral conjunctiva of the eyelid in anatomy. The reason for the eyelid being named as "flesh wheel" is that it is belongs to the spleen, which governs the flesh. The spleen and stomach have an interior-exterior relationship, so diseases of the flesh wheel are always attributed to disorders of the spleen and the stomach.

➤ The blood wheel corresponds to the medial and lateral canthi, including the skin, conjunctiva and vessels of the two canthi, the lacrimal caruncle, the plica semilunaris, and the lacrimal puncta of the inner canthus in anatomy. The reason the two canthi belong to the blood wheel is that they relate to the heart, which governs blood. The heart and small intestine have an interior-exterior relationship, so diseases of the blood wheel are always attributed to disorders of the heart and small intestine.

➤ The qi wheel refers to the white of the eye, including the bulbar conjunctiva and the anterior part of the sclera. The reason why the white of the eye relates to the qi wheel is because it belongs to the lung, which governs qi. The lung and large intestine have an interior-exterior relationship, so diseases of the qi wheel are always attributed to disorders of the lung and large intestine.

➤ The wind wheel refers to the black of the eye, which includes the cornea. The reason the black of the eye relates to the wind wheel is that it belongs to the liver and the liver governs wind. The liver and gallbladder have an interior-exterior relationship, so diseases of the wind wheel are always attributed to disorders of the liver and gallbladder.

➤ The water wheel refers to the pupil spirit (pupil), which means the pupil in a narrow sense, while it also includes the uvea, retina, macula, optic nerve, aqueous humor, lens, and vitreous body in a broad sense. The latter meaning is much more popular and stands for general functions of vision and color-light perception. In the five wheels theory, the reason the pupil is associated with the water wheel is that it belongs to the kidney, which governs water. The kidney and bladder have an interior-exterior relationship, so diseases of the water wheel are always attributed to disorders of the kidney and bladder. However, the pupil spirit is so complicated that its physiology and pathology are not only related to the kidney and bladder but also to other *zang-fu* organs, a notion supported by both ancient and modern conventional doctors (Table 4-1, Fig. 4-1).

Table 4-1　Five-Wheel Correspondence of the *Zang-Fu* and the Eye

Five Wheels	Five Phases	*Zang-Fu*	Eye Structure
Wind wheel	Wood	Liver, gallbladder	Cornea, iris
Blood wheel	Fire	Heart, small intestine	Inner & outter canthus, lacrimal caruncle, plica semilunaris, lacrimal puncta
Flesh wheel	Earth	Spleen, stomach	Eyelid, tarsus, palpebral conjunctiva
Qi wheel	Metal	Lung, large intestine	Bulbar conjunctiva, anterior part of the sclera
Water wheel	Water	Kidney, bladder	Pupil, aqueous humor, lens, vitreous body, choroid, retina, macula, optic nerve, etc.

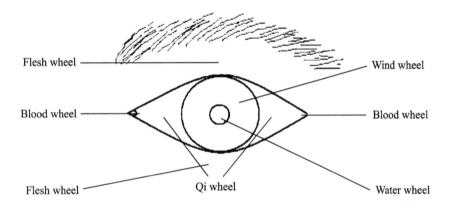

Fig. 4-1　Sketch Map of the Five Wheels (left eye)

■ **Five-Wheel Pattern Differentiation**

In the five-wheel theory, wheels are seen as the branch and the *zang-fu* are the root. Diseases of the wheels are caused by disorders of the organs. In clinical practice, five-wheel pattern differentiation is a method to assess *zang-fu* health based on observing the ocular symptoms. Examining the eyes can give indications about the health of the corresponding organs; similar to how we use tongue and pulse diagnosis. Because the five wheels is just one means of collecting information, we need to consider all other findings, including eight-principle pattern differentiation, disease-cause pattern differentiation, qi-blood pattern differentiation, palpation, etc., to get the most comprehensive and accurate diagnosis.

➤ Pattern Differentiation of the Flesh Wheel

Excess Pattern: Red and swollen eyelids are usually caused by the accumulation of heat in the spleen and stomach. Flushing and erosion of the lid margin is usually caused by damp-heat in the spleen channel. Subcutaneous hardening of the eyelids without pain or hyperemia is due to coagulation of phlegm-dampness. Muco-purulent discharge with papillae in the palpebral conjunctiva is typically caused by damp-heat that has accumulated in the spleen and stomach.

Deficiency Pattern: Blepharoptosis (drooping of the upper eyelid) is due to insufficiency of central qi (spleen qi sinking). A pale-colored palpebral conjunctiva is due to spleen deficiency and blood insufficieny. Puffiness of the eyelids is caused by spleen deficiency and dampness invasion, or can be caused by spleen-kidney yang deficiency. Blepharospasm (spasm of eyelid muscle) is due to blood deficiency engendering wind. Frequent nictation (rapid blinking) is due to spleen deficiency with liver exuberance.

➤ Pattern Differentiation of the Blood Wheel

Excess Pattern: Redness of the canthi is usually caused by the flaring up of heart fire. Dilated blood vessels are due to excess fire in the heart channel. Red pterygium (abnormal tissue growth on the conjunctiva of the inner canthus which obstructs vision) is caused by wind-heat invading the heart and lung. Red swelling and pyorrhea of the lacrimal sac are due to accumulated heat in the heart and spleen.

Deficiency Pattern: Mild conjunctiva hyperemia in both canthi with a dry and uncomfortable sensation is due to the insufficiency of heart yin with ensuing deficiency-fire ascending upward.

➤ Pattern Differentiation of the Qi Wheel

Excess Pattern: Hyperemia of the conjunctiva is due to wind-heat invading the lung channel. Marked redness of the conjunctiva is caused by excess heat in the lung channel. Nodes on the white of the eyes surrounded by a dark-purple vessel are due to stasis of fire-toxin and/or the stagnation of qi and blood. Edema of the white of the eye is due to lung qi failing to disperse qi. Edema with hyperemia is due to lung heat exuberance.

Deficiency Pattern: The carmoisine, small blood streaks in the white of the eye is typically caused by a deficiency-fire of the lung channel. Ultramarine color of the white of the eye is caused by qi deficiency and blood stagnation. Dry sensation with less fluid in the white of the eye is caused by a deficiency of lung yin.

➤ Pattern Differentiation of the Wind Wheel

Excess Pattern: Initial corneal infiltration on the black of the eye (cornea) is caused by the external contraction of wind. A large corneal nebula or corneal ulcer is caused by blazing liver fire. Corneal opacification and/or with filament formation is due to damp-heat in the liver and gallbladder with qi stagnation.

Deficiency Pattern: Long-lasting corneal infiltration or recurrent attacks is due to the deficiency of liver qi or qi-blood deficiency.

➤ Pattern Differentiation of the Water Wheel

Excess Pattern: Contracted pupil (iridocyclitis) with sagging pain of the eyeball that refuses pressure is caused by wind-heat invading the liver channel or excess fire invading the liver and gallbladder. Green glaucoma (acute angle-closure glaucoma) with severe distending pain of the eyeball is due to blazing liver-gallbladder fire.

Deficiency Pattern: Pupillary metamorphosis (posterior synechia) is due to kidney yin deficiency or yin deficiency with effulgent fire. A color change of the pupil spirit is caused by liver-kidney depletion or a heart-spleen deficiency.

Five-wheel pattern differentiation is very popular and has been used in clinical settings for centuries. The five-wheel theory does have its limitations. For example, a yellow color appearing in the white of the eye is a disorder located in the qi wheel, but it is due to the overflow of bile as a result of the steaming of the liver and gallbladder by the damp-heat of the spleen and the stomach, not due to a disorder of the lung. Another example is that diseases of the pupil spirit are not only related to the kidney but also other *zang-fu* organs. Again, we need to not only check the five wheels, but also to perform a complete assessment using all TCM diagnostic tools in order to establish a clear understanding of the pattern presented with each individual patient.

One famous ophthalmology professor of Chinese medicine, Chen Da-fu (陈达夫, now deceased), put forward a six-channel pattern differentiation in TCM ophthalmology in the 1960s. In the book, *Formulas of Six-Channel Pattern Differentiation in Chinese Ophthalmology* (*Zhōng Yī Yǎn Kē Liù Jīng Fǎ Yào*, 中医眼科六经法要), he presented the relationship of the pupil spirit (pupil, aqueous humor, lens, vitreous body, choroid, retina, macula, optic nerve, etc.) to the *zang-fu*. He considered that the choroid belongs to the hand *shaoyin* heart channel; the optic disk, retina, iris, ciliary body, and ciliary zonule belong to the foot *jueyin* liver channel; the retinal macula belongs to the foot *taiyin* spleen channel; the aqueous humor belongs to the foot *shaoyang* gallbladder channel; the vitreous body belongs to the hand *taiyin* lung channel; and all the ocular pigment belongs to the foot *shaoyin* kidney channel. Based on observing the relation of pupil spirit with *zang-fu* and channels, he created the six-channel pattern differentiation in TCM ophthalmology, which has a significant value in clinical practice. The details are presented as follows:

The ocular fundus, the key part of the vision system, includes the vitreous body, optic nerve, retina, choroids, and its vessels. According to TCM theory, the heart governs the blood and vessels, so the vessels of the choroid and retina are ascribed to the heart; therefore, disorders of the choroid and retina refer to the heart. The etiology and pathogenesis are typically heat-fire and qi. The saying that "all fire and heat is ascribed to the heart" basically signifies the clinical presentation of disorders of the vessels in the retina and the choroid. Thus, disorders of the vessels of the retina and choroid have the closest relation with the heart.

Disorders of the vitreous body refers to the lung since they have such a close relationship.

The optic nerve and the nerve fiber layer of the retina are associated with the liver. Anatomically, the nerve fibers of the retina extend from every direction and converge into the optic disk, further condensing into the optic nerve. The optic nerve refers to the "eye connector" in Chinese medicine. This eye connector (optic nerve) belongs to the liver and only the foot *jueyin* liver channel connects to the optic nerve. The foot *jueyin* liver channel distributes to the rib-side (flank), following up to the throat, goes into the nasopharynx, connects with the optic nerve, comes out of the forehead, and assembles with the *du mai* at the top of the head. This shows how the retina and the optic nerve belong to the liver. A pale-colored optic nerve with clear boundary is always due to insufficient nourishment of the optic nerve. The underlying cause of this is due to liver-kidney depletion and liver blood deficiency. Diseases of the optic nerve are usually treated according to the liver. Based on the different disease mechanisms, there are different treatment principles, including soothing the liver and regulating qi, nourishing the liver and extinguishing wind, and clearing the liver and improving vision.

The kidney corresponds to the black color according to TCM theory. As the color of the retinal pigment is black, the retinal pigment epithelium is related to the kidney. Such conditions as retinitis pigmentosa is always differentiated as kidney deficiency, either kidney yang deficiency and/or kidney yin deficiency, in clinical practice, which indicates that kidney deficiency is an essential pathogenesis of retinitis pigmentosa (RP), and disorders of the retinal pigment epithelium (RPE) are treated by improving kidney function.

The macula is the part of the retina which is most sensitive to sight and visual acuity. In traditional Chinese medicine, the color yellow is associated with the spleen. The central direction also belongs to spleen-earth. Therefore, the macula corresponds to the spleen, and in treating any disorder of the macula we need to support the spleen. All vessels belong to the eye, and in order for the eyes to function properly the body must have enough blood for healthy visual function. The spleen governs transportation and transformation of water and grain, and it is the source of qi and blood production. The spleen governs the elevation of the clear (yang) and is responsible for transporting the essence of water and grain into the eyes, bringing clear yang to the upper orifices. Diseases of the macula may influence the vision severely. Macular pathologies include central serous chorioretinopathy, central exudative chorioretinopathy, age-related macular degeneration, myopic macular degeneration, and diabetic macular degeneration. In the clinic, the treatment principle for macular issues is to promote urination, drain dampness, soften hardness, and dissipate masses in the retina (called drusen) by regulating the spleen.

It is important to note that in pattern differentiation and when treating ocular fundus diseases, the practitioner should not limit his/her perspective to the idea that "the pupil spirit belongs to the kidney". We must base our *zang-fu* pattern differentiation on evidence-based clinical findings so as to broaden the diagnosis.

2. Pattern Differentiation of External and Internal Eye Disease

In most ancient Chinese medicine classics, ocular diseases are classified as internal and external oculopathy according to the location of the disease.

■ **External Oculopathy**

Includes diseases of the eyelid, canthi, conjunctiva, sclera, and cornea. These disease processes are always caused by the six external pathogens attacking and/or traumatic injury. Subjective symptoms of external ophthalmic disease may include itching, redness, pain, photophobia, and tearing.

■ **Internal Oculopathy**

Refers to disorders of the pupil spirit (pupil, aqueous humor, lens, vitreous body, choroid, retina, macula, optic nerve, etc.), including disorders of the iris, aqueous humor, lens, vitreous body, retina, and optic nerve. The etiology may include damage to the *zang-fu* organs, deficiency of the qi and blood, imbalance of the seven emotions, qi and blood stasis and traumatic injury of ocular tissues, etc. Symptoms may include impaired vision, distorted shapes or altered colors, floating spots, abnormal visual field, iridization, ophthalmalgia due to eyestrain, and headache.

3. Pattern Differentiation of Common Ocular Conditions

■ **Differentiation of Vision Abnormalities**

➤ Blurred vision with bulbar conjunctiva hyperemia and corneal nebula is caused by the external-contraction of wind-heat or heat-fire blazing in the liver-gallbladder.

➤ Floating spots in front of the eyes, called *yún wù yí jīng* (云雾移睛, vitreous opacity), is caused by turbid qi flooding upward, and/or yin deficiency with effulgent fire, or liver-kidney depletion. Flickering lights that appear when sitting up indicates insufficiency of essence and blood.

➤ Visual decline with normal appearance always indicates insufficiency of the qi and blood, deficiency of the liver and kidney, yin deficiency with effulgent fire, or liver constraint and qi stagnation.

➤ Rapid vision decline with no other symptoms is usually caused by internal wind affecting the head/eyes and phlegm-fire with chaotic movement of hot blood; intemperance of the seven emotions and chaotic counterflow of qi movement with qi stagnation and blood stasis, blood failing to circulate in the vessels; heart deficiency and failure of the spleen to control blood.

➤ Night blindness with contraction of the visual field is always caused by liver-kidney essence deficiency or spleen-kidney yang deficiency.

➤ Myopia is caused by yang deficiency or watching TV, reading or using the computer for extended periods of time. Hyperopia is caused by yin deficiency.

➤ Visual distortion, including seeing straight things as crooked or wavy, seeing large things as small, color-vision abnormalities, and double vision, can be caused by liver-kidney yin deficiency with effulgent fire; suppressed emotional rage impairing the liver and causing qi stagnation and blood stasis; spleen deficiency with damp retention with damp-turbidity floating upwards; deficiency of the heart and kidney; and the consumption of fluid and blood.

■ **Differentiation of Ocular Pain**

Pain is a very common ocular symptom in both internal visual obstruction and external oculopathies.

➢ Differentiation of deficiency and excess syndrome: Acute pain always belongs to excess syndrome and long-lasting pain belongs to deficiency syndrome; continuous pain belongs to excess and intermittent pain that comes and goes belongs to deficiency; and pain with swelling belongs to excess, whereas slight pain without swelling belongs to deficiency. Pain with hyperemia indicates exuberance of a fire pathogen, while vague pain indicates the deficiency of essential qi. Distending eye pain indicates upward reversal of qi and fire with qi stagnation and blood stasis; slight pain and redness in the white of the eye with dryness indicates deficiency of essence and blood.

➢ Differentiation of yin and yang: More pronounced pain presenting from midnight til noon indicates yang exuberance while from noon to midnight indicates yin exuberance. Dry pain, burning pain, and pricking pain in external ophthalmopathy belong to yang excess; ocular distending pain, referred pain, and pain felt in the deep of the eyeball belong to pathogenic yin excess.

➢ Differentiation of heat and cold: Ocular pain with relief by application of cold compresses belong to heat pathology, while relief with heat application belongs to cold pathology; ocular redness, sandy or burning pain and profuse thick exudation belong to external contraction of wind-heat.

➢ Differentiation of meridian tropism: Ocular pain accompanied by pain at the vertex and the back of the neck belongs to *taiyang* channel pathology; pain at the temples and migraine headache correspond to the *shaoyang* channel; pain at the forehead, nose and tooth relates to the *yangming* channel.

■ **Differentiation of Ocular Itch**

The etiology of ocular itch includes wind, fire, and blood deficiency, with wind typically being the most commonly seen in the clinic.

➢ Ocular itch with congestion that is severe when exposed to cold is caused by the external contraction of wind-heat.

➢ Redness and inflammation of the lid-margin with itching or hypertrophic follicle with itching (that feels like a worm crawling) is caused by damp-heat in the spleen and stomach with external wind.

➢ Itching and pain with redness and swelling are caused by exuberance of wind-heat toxin.

➢ Intermittent itching with dryness is caused by blood deficiency engendering wind; the ocular disease has a high probability of occurring because the itching is caused by pathogen. Once the fire pathogen is cleared away and qi and blood are restored, the condition should completely resolve.

■ **Differentiation of Dry Eyes**

Dry eyes is classified into dry and sandy sensations.

> Dry sensation is caused by fluid deficiency and blood deficiency.
> Sandy sensation with redness, itching, pain, photophobia, and tearing is caused by wind-heat invasion, exuberant fire in the lung and liver, or foreign body in the eye.

■ **Differentiation of Redness and Swelling**

Redness with swelling is a common symptom of external ophthalmopathy, and is often seen in the eyelid and the conjunctiva. The differentiation of redness and swelling can be referred to that of the qi wheel and flesh wheel.

■ **Differentiation of Exudation and Tearing**

> Exudation: Pathogenic heat is a very common external pathogen seen in the clinic. Copious hard exudation is caused by excess heat in the lung channel; copious yellow thick pus-like exudation is caused by heat-toxin exuberance; and sticky exudation is caused by damp-heat.
> Tearing: Hot tearing is caused by wind-heat attacking; insufficient tearing with dryness and visual blurring is due to liver-kidney yin deficiency or qi-blood deficiency.

4. Pattern Differentiation of Ocular Nebula and the Ocular Membrane

■ **Differentiation of Ocular Nebula**

An ocular nebula is an opacity of the cornea and/or lens. Opacity of the cornea is called nebula and includes "petaloid nebula" with a sunken center (ulcerative keratitis), "congealed-fat nebula" (purulent keratitis), "frost nebula" (thin nubecula), and "nebulous eye screen" (thick nubecula). Different from the cornea, an opacity of the lens is called a cataract. Various forms of cataracts include the round nebula cataract (senile cataract) and jujube nebula cataract (nuclear cataract). In modern TCM ophthalmology, ocular nebula typically is discussed with regards to keratopathy, so in this chapter we will just expound corneal nebula.

Corneal nebula appears as different shapes, including star, branch, map, worm-eaten shape, and nebulous shape. Names of corneal nebula vary and have been classified by ancient doctors according to the shape, color, and depth of the lesion and presence or absence of ulcerations. Acute nebula and chronic nebula are the two basic classifications.

> Acute nebula: The early stages presents as opacity with a gray color, rough surface, blurry edge, and a developing trend towards the periphery. This is followed by ocular redness, pain, and photophobia. Clustered stars nebula (herpes simplex keratitis), petaloid nebula presenting with a sunken center (ulcerative keratitis), and congealed-fat nebula (purulent keratitis) all belong to this form of nebula which is similar to various keratitis as described in Western conventional medicine. The black of the eye (cornea) corresponds to the liver, so differentiation of the fresh-acute nebula could reveal probems with the liver channel. The etiology may include wind-heat invading the liver channel, liver fire flaring up, damp-heat in the liver channel, or liver-yin deficiency with effulgent fire. Wind-heat-dampness attacking the liver channel and traumatic injury are

the most common forms of corneal nebula.

In the early stages, common symptoms of a corneal nebula may include ciliary flush, and a single or multiple nebula with a light color (which belongs to the category of clustered stars nebula). With the progressive development of the disease, pathogenic qi penetrates inward and/or external pathogenic factors combine with interior pathogens leading to a complex conjunctival congestion. Many corneal nebula present in a linear-patterned flake, or form an ulcer, called petaloid nebula, with a sunken center. If the disease process develops rapidly, the corneal nebula may become thick and large enough to cover the whole cornea in the form of congealed lipids, referred to as the congealed-fat nebula. This kind of the nebula is always combined with an upward rushing of yellow fluid (hypopyon) and easily develops into corneal perforation. The differentiation is intense fire toxin of the *zang-fu*. If the corneal nebula lasts for a long time and has no changes, it is typically caused by deficiency of healthy qi and lingering pathogenic qi, which is differentiated as liver-kidney yin and liver blood deficiency, or qi-blood deficiency.

➢ Chronic nebula: Refers to a glazed corneal nebula with a clear edge, no developing trend and no apparent redness, pain or tearing. This category includes frost nebula, nebulous eye screen, thick nubecula, and speckle-fat nebula or corneal scar in conventional ophthalmology.

According to its thickness and shade, the chronic nebula is divided into four types in modern TCM ophthalmology:

- Nebulas that are very minute and can only be examined under bright light are called "frost nebula" because it is so slight that it resembles cold frost on a glass window (called cloudy nebula in Western medicine).
- Nebula that presents as fine and thin (as the wing of the cicada or a floating cloud) and can be seen in natural light is called a nebulous screen (called macular nebula in Western medicine).
- Nebula that is thick and white (as chinaware) and is easily seen is called a thick nebula (called corneal leukoma in Western medicine).
- Nebula that adheres to the iris and the pupil and is protruding and round is called speckle-fat nebula (adherent leukoma in Western medicine).

Chronic nebula in which there is scarring of the corneal nebula, may be reduced with prompt therapy when the acute corneal nebula is in the process of becoming a chronic nebula; if it already has been chronic for a period of time and the circulation of qi and blood is greatly diminished, as in corneal leukoma, a complete recovery may be unlikely.

■ **Differentiation of Ocular Membrane**

A membrane generating from the white of the eye or the edge of the white and the black of the eye with white or red color, or with flesh-like apophysis, or encroaching on the center of the black of the eye (cornea), is called an ocular membrane. Drooping pannus (trachomatous pannus) and white membrane eye (pterygium) belong to this kind of disease. If the membrane is covered with red silk (vascular engorgement), it is called red membrane; if the membrane is covered with little red silk and the color is white, it is called white membrane. A thin and light membrane that does not cover the pupil is a mild condition; while a thick and red membrane covering part of the pupil is severe; the most severe condition is a thick and large membrane that covers the whole pupil. Membranes of the white and the black parts of the eye (cornea) are caused by blazing lung-liver fire. Thick and red membranes that are rapidly growing belong to excess fire and stagnant heat in the blood level; thin and white membranes without growth belong to qi-yin deficiency.

5. Review & Some Questions for Reflection

■ **What is an internal visual obstruction and what is an external ophthalmopathy?**

Based on the location, ocular diseases are classifed as either internal visual obstructions or external ophthalmopathy in Chinese medicine.

External ophthalmopathy includes diseases of the eyelids, inner and outer canthi, white of the eye, and black of the eye (cornea). External conditions are always caused by one or more of the six pathogenic factors attacking the exterior, or may result from traumatic injury. Subjective symptoms of external ophthalmopathy are usually obvious and may include itching, inflammation, pain, photophobia, weeping exudates, discoloration, and deformities.

Internal visual obstruction refers to disorders of the pupil spirit, which includes the iris, aqueous humor, lens, vitreous body, retina, macula, and optic nerve. The etiology is rooted in an injury to the *zang-fu*, deficiency of qi and blood, imbalance of one or more of the seven emotions, qi and blood stasis, and/or traumatic injury of ocular tissues. Symptoms include progressive visual decline, visual distortion, abnormal color vision, floating spots or "floaters", abnormal visual field, iridization, ophthalmalgia, headache, and eye strain.

■ **What is the basic principle of five-wheel pattern differentiation?**

In the clinic, five-wheel pattern differentiation is a method used to help determine which *zang-fu* organ(s) are dysfunctional and are causing ophthalmic disease. We determine this by observing symptoms in each of the five wheels and relating them to the corresponding organ.

■ **What are the anatomical correlations of the five wheels and its affiliation with *zang-fu* organs?**

The flesh wheel refers to the eyelids, including the skin, subcutaneous tissue, muscles, tarsus, and palpebral conjunctiva of the eyelid. The reason that the eyelid is associated with the flesh wheel is because it correlates to the spleen, which governs the flesh. The spleen and stomach have an interior-exterior relationship and diseases in the flesh wheel are attributed to disorders of the spleen and stomach.

The blood wheel refers to the two canthi (inner and outer), which includes the skin, conjunctiva and vessels of the two canthi, the lacrimal caruncle, the plica semilunaris, and the lacrimal puncta of the inner canthus. The reason the two canthi are referred to as the as blood wheel is because they correspond to the heart, which governs the blood. The heart and small intestine have an interior-exterior relationship, so diseases in the blood wheel are attributed to disorders of the heart and small intestine.

The qi wheel refers to the white of the eye, anatomicaly including the bulbar conjunctiva and anterior part of the sclera. The white of the eye is referred to as the qi wheel because it corresponds to the lung, which governs the qi. The lung and large intestine have an interior-exterior relationship, so diseases in the qi wheel are attributed to disorders of the lung and large intestine.

The wind wheel refers to the black of the eye, which anatomically includes the cornea. The reason that the black of the eye (cornea) is named the wind wheel is because it corresponds to the liver, which governs wind. The liver and gallbladder have an interior-exterior relationship, so diseases in the wind wheel are attributed to disorders of the liver and gallbladder.

The water wheel refers to the pupil spirit, and to the pupil in a narrow sense. Water wheel conditions may include uveitis, retina, macula, optic nerve, aqueous humor, lens, and vitreous body in a broader sense. The latter meaning is much more popular in clinical practice and deals with the main functions of overall vision and color-light perception. In the five wheels theory, the reason for the pupil spirit's affiliation with the water wheel is because it belongs to the kidney, which governs water. The kidney and urinary bladder have an interior-exterior relationship, so diseases of the water wheel are attributed to disorders of the kidney and bladder. The pupil spirit is so complex that its physiology and pathology may not be exclusively related to the kidney and bladder, as proven in clinical practice. Both ancient and modern doctors have agreed that diseases of the pupil spirit may be rooted in other organs besides the kidney and bladder. A detailed intake will allow the practitioner to clarify the existing pattern in each individual case.

Chapter 5
Treatment Essentials

The treatment of eye disorders with TCM includes both internal and external therapy. Internal treatment primarily includes medicinal therapy, while the external treatment includes medicinal and non-medicinal care. The later consists of acupuncture, massage, surgical methods, laser therapy, and other physical therapies. In the external treatment section of this book, only common external therapies are presented. Acupuncture is introduced in a special section of this book. In clinical practice, the recommened treatment plan depends on the patient's condition. The practitioner may choose to utilize one isolated therapy or combine several treatment methods. The main principle is to resolve the condition for the patients as early as possible, using methods with the highest degree of compliance.

Section 1   Internal Treatment

TCM ophthalmology has accumulated a significant amount of information for treating eye disease, forming a complete unique treatment system. Internal treatment is administered through oral consumption of prescribed Chinese medicinals in order to dispel pathogens, regulate *zang-fu* dysfunction, regulate qi and blood, and clear the channels and collaterals in order to resolve eye disease, improve vision, and maintain ocular health. Internal treatment of ophthalmic conditions originated from the traditional Chinese medicinal pharmacy and classic Chinese medicinal formulas. Ophthalmic conditions typically have their own specific patterns as well. Therefore, when using ophthalmic internal treatment in the form of medicinals, we must follow common guidelines for pattern differentiation and treatment and follow the "principles, methods, formulas, and medicinals". We must also comply with the special considerations commonly seen exclusively in ophthalmic pattern differentiation, including five-wheel differentiation, nebula and membrane differentiation, secretion and tearing differentiation.

Basing our strategy on the differences of each individual's constitution, the causes of disease, disease location, and nature of disease will dictate the most appropriate and effective internal (medicinal) treatment method(s). The following are the commonly used methods for treating ophthalmic conditions with Chinese medicinal therapy.

1. Dispelling Wind

The strategy of dispelling wind as a means to treat oculopathy caused by pathogen wind should be done so using Chinese medicinals which have the function of dispelling wind. Pathogenic wind is a common factor that causes eye diseases, including both internal wind and external wind. Because the wind pathogen is the chief pathogen of all disease, and often combines with other pathoigenic influences, the treatment methods usually have a cooperative nature. In addition to dispersing wind, we may scatter wind and clear heat, dispel wind and dissipate cold, dispel wind and unblock the collaterals, dispel wind and relieve itching, and calm the liver to extinguish wind.

■ **Dispersing Wind and Clearing Heat**

For external eye diseases caused by wind-heat pathogen, treat with medicinals which are acrid in flavor and cool-cold in nature. This strategy is applicable to the pattern of wind-heat in the collaterals with symptoms such as redness and swelling of the eyelids, hyperemia of the bulbar conjunctiva, chemosis, inchoate nebula on the black of the eye (cornea), photophobia and tearing; this pattern may also be accompanied by the general signs and symptoms of wind-heat, such as aversion to cold and fever, thin and yellow tongue coating, floating and rapid pulse, or some signs of internal oculopathy, such as contracted pupil (iridocyclitis) or sudden blindness. *Yín Qiào Sǎn* (Lonicera and Forsythia Powder, 银翘散) is a classic representative formula for this pattern.

■ **Dispelling Wind and Dredging the Collaterals**

For eye diseases caused by pathogenic wind striking the channels and collaterals, use this method. Indications of this method include blepharoptosis, twitching eyelids, deviation of the eyes and mouth, double vision, and eye trauma. Select Chinese medicinals which are acrid in flavor and have the effects of penetrating and dredging the collaterals. *Zhèng Róng Tāng* (Face-Restoring Decoction, 正容汤) is one of the classic representative formulas for this pattern.

■ **Dispelling Wind and Arresting Itching**

For itching caused by pathogenic wind, choose medicinals that are acrid in flavor and clear and ascending in nature. According to TCM theory, it is appropriate to treat wind diseases by treating the blood because the wind will disappear naturally once the blood is supplemented, so this method is always used in combination with blood-nourishing medicinals. *Qū Fēng Yī Zì Sǎn* (驱风一字散, Wind-Expelling One-Character Powder) is one of the classic representatives for this pattern.

Most wind-dispelling medicinals are acrid in flavor and dry in nature; in long-term use it may damage yin and fluid. Avoid excessive use and stop taking the formula as soon as the pathogen is removed. For patients with symptoms of yin deficiency and insufficiency of blood, add some enriching and moistening medicinals to the formula in order to protect the yin and blood.

2. Clearing Heat

This method is designed to treat oculopathy marked by inflammation or "heat". Heat pathologies may be caused by a fire or heat pathogen, or maybe be transformed as a result from other syndromes, or caused by other pathogens. The nature of fire and heat is to rise and ascend to the head (and because the eyes are located above the other five sense organs). The heat-clearing method is common in TCM ophthalmology. Medicinal formulas are mostly composed by agents that are cool and cold in nature and have the function of clearing heat. Formulas are modified according to the different organs affected, the invading pathogen, deficiency conditions or excess pathogens, as well as consideration of a patient's individual constitution. The therapeutic method of choice is to clear heat and remove toxins, clear heat and cool blood, clear liver heat and purge the gallbladder, clear lung heat, clear spleen heat, and clear deficiency heat.

Most of the heat-clearing medicinals are bitter and cold, so these must not be used excessively or it will damage the yang and result in impairment of the normal functioning of the spleen and stomach. For the elderly, those who are weak due to chronic disease, and pregnant women, we must be extremely cautious when using these medicinals in formulas to clear heat.

■ **Clearing heat and resolving toxins**

This is a method of treating eye diseases caused by internal heat and fire toxin with fire-draining medicinals that are bitter-cold in nature. It is appropriate to use when there are symptoms of redness, swelling, a burning sensation of the eyelids, severe hyperemia of the bulba conjunctiva, profuse sticky yellow secretion from the eyes, purple-red nodes on the sclera with pain, nebula and ulcerations of the cornea, turbid aqueous, hypopyon (pus in the eye), contracted pupil, hyphema and vitreous hemorrhage, retina exudation, edema or hemorrhage, or severe pain of the head and eyes. Most patients may present with the general symptoms of excess heat pattern, presenting with fever, thirst, yellow urine, dry stool, red tongue with yellow coating, and a surging and rapid pulse. *Wǔ Wèi Xiāo Dú Yǐn* (Five Ingredients Toxin-Removing Beverage, 五味消毒饮) is one of the classic representative formulas for this pattern.

■ **Clearing heat and cooling blood**

Medicinals that clear heat, are cool in nature, and have the action of entering the blood are applicable to eye diseases caused by heat entering *ying*-blood with such symptoms as subconjunctival hemorrhage, hyphema, vitreous hemorrhage, and other intraocular hemorrhage diseases. *Xī Jiǎo Dì Huáng Tāng* (Rhinoceros Horn and Rehmannia Decoction, 犀角地黄汤) is one of the classic representative formulas.

■ **Clearing liver and gallbladder heat**

Treat eye diseases caused by liver-gallbladder constraint-heat with medicinals that clear liver and gallbladder heat. Indications include ciliary congestion, nebula of the cornea, contracted pupil, hypopyon, sudden blindness, green wind glaucoma, and retinal hemorrhage. Besides the symptoms of the eyes, the patients may present with manifestations such as bitter taste in the mouth and dry pharynx, red urine and constipation, a red tongue with yellow coating, and a wiry and rapid pulse. The representative formula *Lóng Dǎn Xiè Gān Tāng* (Gentian Liver-Draining Decoction, 龙胆泻肝汤) is used for this pattern.

■ **Clearing heart heat and draining fire**

Treat the eye diseases caused by fire toxin of the heart channel with medicinals that clear heart heat and drain fire. It is applicable to eye diseases such as marginal blepharitis, canthus pyorrhea, acute dacryocystisis, and pterygium, accompanied by general symptoms such as mouth and tongue sores, dry mouth and vexation, red urine, red tongue tip, and a rapid pulse. The representative formula for this pattern is *Zhú Yè Xiè Jīng Tāng* (Lophatherum Channel-Draining Decoction, 竹叶泻经汤).

■ **Clearing lung fire and draining heat**

Treat eye diseases caused by heat toxin in the lung channel with medicinals that clear and drain excess heat of the lung channel. It is applicable to the symptoms caused by lung heat stagnation such as hyperemia of the bulbar conjunctiva, profuse yellow and white secretion in the eye or profuse secretion and tears, purple-red node on the sclera, and unbearable pain in the eye. The representative formula is *Sāng Bái Pí Tāng* (Mulberry Root Bark Decoction, 桑白皮汤).

3. Dispelling Dampness

Eye diseases caused by dampness are treated with medicinals that transform dampness. Symptoms include edema of the eyelids with skin erosion, fluid discharge, conjunctiva folliculitis with yellow and soft soreness in the palpebral conjunctiva, seasonal eye itching, xanthosis of the conjunctiva, turbid secretion and tearing, rotten dreg-like nebula that is chronic, retinal edema with blurred vision and seeing objects in altered colors and/or shapes. In addition to the ocular symptoms, patients may present with a heavy sensation in the head and weak limbs, a greasy tongue coating, and a soggy pulse. According to the nature and location of the damp pathogen and based on the patient's constitution, the therapeutic strategy may be divided into several possible approaches, which include using aromatic medicinals to remove dampness, bitter-warm medicinals to dry dampness, medicinals that promote urination and percolate dampness, and medicinals that fortify the spleen and remove dampness. A careful pattern differentiation is needed in order to choose the most appropriate herbal strategy. *Sān Rén Tāng* (Three Kernels Decoction, 三仁汤) is one of the representative formulas for this pattern.

Most of the damp-eliminating medicinals are warming and drying, and improper use may damage yin. For damp patterns combining with existing yin deficiency, it is not suitable to use damp-dispelling methods alone, and long-term use should be discouraged.

4. Resolving Phlegm and Softening Hardness

Treat the eye diseases caused by internal accumulation of phlegm-rheum with medicinals that dissolve phlegm, soften hardness, and dissipate masses. It is appropriate for symptoms caused by phlegm-dampness, chronic stubborn phlegm that has gathered to form hard nodules and lumps on the eyelids, distending pain in the eyes, migraine, dark shadow in front of the eyes, seeing things in altered shape, opacities of vitreous, or prolonged exudation. As phlegm can lead to many pathological changes, the method of dissolving phlegm and softening hardness is always used in combination with other methods such as dispelling dampness, moving qi, and dissolving stasis. There are two major considerations when using this method: one is to fortify the spleen in order to resolve the dampness, and the other is to move the qi (because phlegm is easy to disperse when qi is regulated). *Huà Jiān Èr Chén Tāng* (Two Matured Substances Hardness-Resolving Decoction, 化坚二陈汤) is a classic formula used for this pattern.

5. Supplementing the Liver and Kidney

Treat eye diseases caused by deficiency of the liver and kidney by supplementing the liver and kidney. Indications include long-standing cold tearing, dry eyes, late-stage corneal nebula, pupillary metamorphosis, slow-progressive vision loss, clouded vision, opacity of vitreous, cataract, liver deficiency sparrow eye, retinitis pigmentosa, and all kinds of retinal degenerative diseases. The eye symptoms often manifest with general symptoms and signs such as dizziness and tinnitus, limp aching lumbus and knees, spermatorrhea, pale or red tongue, and a deep, weak, thready pulse. Besides the above diseases, the methods can also be used for people with poor vision due to prolonged diseases or senility, and for ocular health care with the premise of right pattern differentiation. *Qǐ Jú Dì Huáng Wán* (Lycium Berry, Chrysanthemum and Rehmannia Pill, 杞菊地黄丸) and *Zuǒ Guī Wán* (Left-Restoring Pill, 左归丸) are the classical representative formulas for liver-kidney yin deficiency, and *Jīn Guì Shèn Qì Wán* (Golden Cabinet's Kidney Qi Pill, 金匮肾气丸) and *Yòu Guī Wán* (Right-Restoring Pill, 右归丸) are the representative formulas for kidney yang deficiency.

6. Enriching Yin and Subduing Fire

This is a treatment method for eye syndromes caused by hyperactivity of fire due to yin deficiency, using medicinals that nourish yin and conduct the fire downward. Indications include dry eyes, chronic conjunctivitis, long-standing corneal nebula, papillary metamorphosis, blurred vision, firefly-like shadow in full visual field, and recurring retinal hemorrhage. Patients may also present with general symptoms and signs such as vexing heat in the five centers (chest, palms, and soles), tidal reddening of the cheeks, night sweating and spermatorrhea, a red tongue with scant coating, and a thready and rapid pulse.

In the case of yin deficiency resulting in vigorous fire, yin deficiency is the root cause of the pattern, and hyperactivity of fire is the branch. Therefore, enriching yin is the primary part of the method with fire-reducing medicinals acting as assistants. Since yin-enriching medicinals have the disadvantage of retaining pathogens, it is not suitable to apply the method alone if there is external pathogen.

7. Calming the Liver and Subduing Yang

Treat eye diseases caused by ascending hyperactivity of liver yang with medicinals that calm the liver, subdue yang, and extinguish wind. Indications include blepharospasm, deviated eyes and mouth, double vision, distending pain of the head and eyes, sudden blindness, mydriasis, green glaucoma, and retinal hemorrhage. In addition to the ocular symptoms, patients often present with red face and ears, dizziness, dysphoria and irascibility, a red tongue, and a wiry or thready-wiry pulse. Generally, the method is always combined with other methods such as dispelling wind, dissolving phlegm, and dredging the collaterals. The primary representative formula for this pattern is *Zhèn Gān Xī Fēng Tāng* (Liver-Sedating and Wind-Extinguishing Decoction, 镇肝熄风汤).

Most of the yang-subduing medicinals are heavy and settling in nature, including minerals and shells. Excess use will damage the stomach and spleen, so one must be very cautious when using these herbs.

8. Supplementing Qi and Nourishing Blood

Treat eye diseases caused by qi and blood deficiency, or qi and blood weakness due to prolonged eye diseases, with medicinals that supplement and nourish qi and blood. This method is applicable for eye diseases presenting with fatigue of the eyelid, clouded vision, chronic vision loss, retinal degenerative diseases, and long-standing ulcerative keratitis with general symptoms and sign such as lethargy, fatigue of the limbs, shortage of qi and a disinclination to talk, a pale or shallow yellow complexion, a pale fat tongue, and a weak pulse. In the clinic, some patients present with a tendency of qi deficiency more than blood deficiency. Others may present with more blood deficiency; therefore, formulas should be prescribed according to the individual's pattern. The classical representative formulas include *Sì Wù Tāng* (Four Substances Decoction, 四物汤), *Sì Jūn Zǐ Tāng* (Four Gentlemen Decoction, 四君子汤), and *Bā Zhēn Tāng* (Eight Gem Decoction, 八珍汤).

Most replenishing medicinals are warm and cloying, so formulas should be combined with herbs that move qi, clear stagnation, and moisten dryness if they are to be used long-term.

9. Soothing the Liver and Rectifying Qi

Treat all internal and external eye diseases caused by liver constraint and qi stagnation with medicinals that soothe the liver, resolve constraint, and rectify qi. Indications include distending pain of the eyes, eyebrow bone pain, mydriasis, green glaucoma, blurred vision, optic atrophy, and sudden blindness, with general symptoms and signs such as oppression in the chest and distending pain of the ribs, depression, signing and belching, rushing, impatience and irascibility, distending pain of the breast, irregular menstruation, and a wiry pulse. The representative formula for this pattern is *Xiāo Yáo Sǎn* (Free Wanderer Powder, 逍遥散).

10. Invigorating Blood and Dissolving Stasis

This treatment method uses medicinals that invigorate blood, dissolve stasis, and unblock the collaterals. It is applicable to eye diseases presenting with stabbing and distending pain of the head and eyes, bleeding, obsolete intraocular hematocele, topical swelling due to ocular trauma, millet sore, chronic conjunctivitis, obstruction of the retinal vessels, hyperblastosis, and scarring in the retina. In clinical practice, this treatment strategy may vary according to the different causes of blood stasis. For example, clearing heat and dissolving stasis is appropriate for cases caused by heat pathogen, warming channels and dissolving stasis for cases caused by cold pathogen, moving qi and dissolving stasis for cases caused by qi stagnation, supplementing qi and dissolving stasis for the cases caused by qi deficiency, supplementing the blood and dissolving stasis for the cases caused by blood deficiency, and nourishing yin and dissolving stasis for cases caused by yin deficiency. The classic representative formulas for this pattern include *Xuè Fǔ Zhú Yū Tāng* (Blood Stasis Expelling Decoction, 血府逐瘀汤) and *Táo Hóng Sì Wù Tāng* (Peach Kernel and Carthamus Four Substances Decoction, 桃红四物汤).

This method should be used with caution because most of the herbs used are acrid-warm and aromatic-drying, which may consume the qi and damage yin; moreover, excessive use may thin the blood and lead to bleeding.

11. Stanching Bleeding

This method is applicable to all kinds of ocular hemorrhage. Indications include retinal hemorrhage, hyphema, subconjunctival hemorrhage, and bleeding due to eye trauma. In clinical practice, several methods may be implemented based on the specific cause of the bleeding. For cases caused by pathogenic heat, blood-quickening medicinals should be combined with medicinals that clear heat and cool the blood. For cases caused by ascending liver fire, one should add medicinals that clear liver heat and drain fire. For cases caused by yin deficiency resulting in vigorous fire, the formula should be combined with herbs that enrich yin and subdue fire. For cases caused by blood stasis, the formula should be combined with herbs that invigorate blood and dissolve stasis. For cases caused by qi deficiency, formulas should be combined with herbs that supplement qi and contain blood. The representative formula for this pattern is *Shí Huī Sǎn* (Ten Charred Substances Powder, 十灰散).

If the bleeding is arrested without recurrence, treatment should be stopped in time to avoid the possibility of inducing blood stasis.

12. Removing Nebula to Improve Vision

This is a unique therapeutic method in TCM ophthalmology that treats corneal nebula with specific nebula-removing medicinals. Treatment is suitable for repairing the corneal nebula by means of decreasing the size or reducing the thickness of the nebula in order to improve the patient's eyesight. According to the theory of TCM, the cornea corresponds to the liver, so most of the medicinals entering the liver channel have the function of removing nebula. The extensional nebula-removing therapies may vary according to the different causes and stages of nebula. At the stage of wind-heat exuberance, the treatment principle is to scatter wind and clear liver heat to remove the nebula. If the patient presents with a blazing liver fire pattern, the treatment principle should be aimed at clearing liver heat and draining fire. For late-stage nebula, all the patterns of coldness, heat, deficiency, and excess are not emphasized. Instead, the treatment should focus on removing nebula by dispelling wind, invigorating blood, dissolving phlegm, softening hardness, nourishing yin, and boosting qi. The representative formula for this condition is a specific formula called *Bō Yún Tuì Yì Wán* (Cloud-Dispelling and Nebula-Removing Pill, 拨云退翳丸).

Unless there is a heat pattern present, do not use medicinals that are excessively cold to remove the nebula, or it may cause qi and blood stagnation and pathogen retention, which will make it more difficult to treat the disease. If the nebula is chronic with a smooth, glossy, porcelain-like appearance, it is very unlikely that the nebula can be treated successfully with medicinal therapy.

Section 2   External Treatment

This is a treatment method of applying Chinese medicinals topically in order to produce an effect on a local area or on the internals through the body surface. Commonly used topical treatments include eye drops, eye ointments, irrigation therapy for the eyes, ophthalmic bath, fumigation therapy for the eyes, and compress therapy. This kind of treatment modality has advantages of working fast and typically being highly effective. The dose is usually small, toxic herbs are seldomly used, and there are few side-effects. It is therefore the preferred external therapy for ocular conditions. According to the patient's specific condition, treatment can be applied alone or with other therapeutic modalities. Generally, external treatment is divided into medicinal external therapy and non-medicinal external therapy.

1. Topical Medicinals

■ Eye Drops

Application of eye drops is the most commonly used ophthalmic therapy. Usually, the method is applied 3 to 5 times a day, or more times in a severe case according to the patient's condition. In case of combined therapy, the eye drops should be administered with an interval of at least 3–5 minutes. When applying eye drops that have toxic properties or adverse effects after systemic absorption, we suggest placing a warm compress over the lacrimal sac for several minutes after administering the eye drops.

■ Eye Ointment

Ointments are applied in the conjunctiva sac (inside the lower eyelid). Because ointments release their content slowly and produce a long-term effect, it is always administered before sleep or after surgery.

■ Eye Powder

Eye powders are applied inside the eyelids. Because there are few powder preparations at present, it is seldom used in the clinic now.

■ Eye Bath

An eye bath is a treatment method where the eye(s) are immersed into a prepared solution or water. This method has the advantage exposing the eyes to the drug solution sufficiently, which makes it more applicable to diseases of the conjunctiva and cornea. The eye-cup and small basin are the common appliances for eye bath therapy. When taking an eye bath, the drug solution must on no account be strong and the temperature should be suitable. For a better effect, it is suggested to open and close the eyes repeatedly while the eyes are under water. The appliance must be well sterilized after use by patients with eye infections.

■ Fumigation-Washing

Fumigation is a treatment method where the eyes are steamed with a boiled decoction, while the washing method is used to bathe the sick eye with the filtrated decoction. The methods can be applied alone or first by fumigating and then by washing the eyes; thus, it is called the fumigation-washing method. In addition to the direct effect of the medicinals, the warmth of the solution can help the medicinals to permeate for a faster result. This method can also improve the local circulation of blood and the absorption of pathogens and toxins. The temperature for fumigation should not be too hot in order to avoid ocular burns. The method is typically administered 2–3 times a day. Patients with new bleeding or corneal ulcer with a tendency for perforation should not use this treatment method.

■ **Compress Therapy**

In this treatment method, medicinals are applied directly on the skin of the eyes (eyelids) according to the patient's condition. This method is most effective for diseases of the eyelids and skin around the eye. The prescribed medicinals are made into fine powder, blended well into pastes with water or tea, green onion or ginger pop, egg white, honey, vinegar, bile, human milk, decoction, etc. Another way is to mash the fresh medicinals and apply directly on the eye, or wrap the mashed medicinals first with gauzes before placing them on the eye. Usually, the method is performed 1–2 times a day. Avoid applying toxic and stimulating medicinals on the eye.

2. Non-medicinal External Treatment

Most of the non-medicinal treatments fall under the category of physical therapies using water, external manipulation, temperature, light, electricity, and radiation.

■ **Thermotherapy (Heat Therapy)**

Thermotherapy creates high temperature on the skin, which promotes vasodilatation, increases blood flow, and reinforces the activities of enzymes, thus alleviating symptoms by improving the absorption of swelling and inflammation, strengthening the immune function of the cells of the eye, relieving pain, and promoting wound healing. It is easy, affordable, and effective. The method is widely used in ophthalmic clinics for such indications as blepharitis, conjunctivitis, keratitis, uveitis, scleritis, visual fatigue, blepharospasm, supraorbital neuralgia, eye trauma, and postsurgical recovery. According to the patient's condition, it can take the form of moist thermotherapy, dry thermotherapy, wax therapy, or many others. Do not use this method at the early stage of bleeding.

Cauterization is a special form of thermotherapy, which can be applied to ophthalmologic surgical hemostasis, treatment for corneal neogenesis pannus, and refractory corneal ulcer.

■ **Cryotherapy (Cold Therapy)**

Cold therapy can be used to stop bleeding in the first 24 hours after an injury. It can also relieve pain, alleviate itching, and astringe lesions (promote wound healing). The applications of this therapy in ophthalmic clinics include swelling, pain and allergy of the eyelid, conjunctiva, and cornea. Moreover, the katogene of hypothermia condensation produced by liquid nitrogen and semiconductor condenser can be used to treat obsolete corneal ulcer, neovascular glaucoma, and retinal holes.

■ **Massage**

Massage is also used in TCM ophthalmology. The main objective is to massage around the eyes; however, local massage can be accompanied by body massage according to pattern differentiation. Common manipulations include pointing, pressing, kneading, pushing, and pinching. Massaging ocular acupoints can dredge the eye collaterals, smooth qi and blood, support healthy qi, dispel pathogens, relax the eyes, and relieve pain. It is usually applied to chronic eye diseases such as blephroptosis, blepharospasm, optic atrophy, adolescent myopia and hyperopia, visual fatigue, ischemic eye diseases, ophthalmoplegia, early- and moderate-stage senile cataract, chronic glaucoma and dry eyes, as well as for eye preventive care.

Specific eyeball massage given after anti-glaucoma surgery can help to keep the new drainage pathway unobstructed and maintain the pressure-reduction effect of the surgery. At the early stage of central retinal artery occlusion, it may help to release the condition through pressing and releasing the eyeball repeatedly to decrease the intraocular pressure.

Patients with acute inflammation and bleeding oculopathy should not use this treatment.

In addition to the therapies mentioned above, there are many other treatment methods such as electrotherapy, iontophoresis, thermal radiation, and galvanic shock therapy. Each has its indications and limitations. In clinical practice, the proper choice of therapy should be determined by the patient's condition.

Section 3　Commonly Used Formulas

Commonly used formulas in TCM ophthalmology have been developed through the experiences of ancient TCM doctors over millennia of past dynasties. We have choosen to suggest some common formulas with reliable and curative clinical effects:

1. *Sāng Jú Yǐn* (Mulberry Leaf and Chrysanthemum Beverage, 桑菊饮)

Systematic Differentiation of Warm Diseases (*Wēn Bìng Tiáo Biàn*, 温病条辨)
【Prescription】

桑叶	*sāng yè*	9 g	Folium Mori
菊花	*jú huā*	9 g	Flos Chrysanthemi
连翘	*lián qiào*	9 g	Fructus Forsythiae
桔梗	*jié gěng*	9 g	Radix Platycodonis
杏仁	*xìng rén*	9 g	Semen Armeniacae Amarum
薄荷	*bò he*	6 g	Herba Menthae
甘草	*gān cǎo*	3 g	Radix et Rhizoma Glycyrrhizae
芦根	*lú gēn*	15 g	Rhizoma Phragmitis

【Actions】
Scatters wind and clears heat

【Indications】

Eye diseases caused by wind-heat, including xerosis conjunctiva, fulminant red eye with acute nebula, conjunctival edema, clustered stars nebula (herpes simplex keratitis), and ulcerative keratitis.

2. *Yín Qiào Sǎn* (Lonicera and Forsythia Powder, 银翘散)

Systematic Differentiation of Warm Diseases (*Wēn Bìng Tiáo Biàn*, 温病条辨)

【Prescription】

金银花	*jīn yín huā*	15 g	Flos Lonicerae Japonicae
连翘	*lián qiào*	12 g	Fructus Forsythiae
桔梗	*jié gěng*	8 g	Radix Platycodonis
薄荷（后下）	*bò he (hòu xià)*	8 g	Herba Menthae (added later)
牛蒡子	*niú bàng zǐ*	8 g	Fructus Arctii
淡豆豉	*dàn dòu chǐ*	6 g	Semen Sojae Praeparatum
甘草	*gān cǎo*	6 g	Herba Schizonepetae
竹叶	*zhú yè*	6 g	Folium Phyllostachydis Henonis
荆芥穗	*jīng jiè suì*	6 g	Spica Schizonepetae
芦根	*lú gēn*	10 g	Rhizoma Phragmitis

【Actions】

Releases the exterior, scatters wind, and clears heat

【Indications】

Eye diseases caused by wind-heat toxic pathogens, including stye, trachoma, dacrocystitis, eyelid myiasis, epidemic red eye, epidemic fulminant red eye with nebula, xerosis conjunctiva, edema of conjunctiva, herpes simplex keratitis, and ulcerative keratitis.

3. *Xǐ Gān Sǎn* (Liver-Washing Powder, 洗肝散)

A Close Examination of the Precious Classic on Ophthalmology (*Shěn Shì Yáo Hán*, 审视瑶函)

【Prescription】

当归	*dāng guī*	9 g	Radix Angelicae Sinensis
川芎	*chuān xiōng*	9 g	Rhizoma Chuanxiong
薄荷	*bò he*	9 g	Herba Menthae
生地	*shēng dì*	9 g	Radix Rehmanniae
羌活	*qiāng huó*	9 g	Radix et Rhizoma Notopterygii

栀子	*zhī zǐ*	9 g	Fructus Gardeniae
大黄	*dà huáng*	9 g	Radix et Rhizoma Rhei
龙胆草	*lóng dǎn cǎo*	9 g	Radix et Rhizoma Gentianae
防风	*fáng fēng*	9 g	Radix Saposhnikoviae
甘草	*gān cǎo*	4.5 g	Radix et Rhizoma Glycyrrhizae

【Actions】

Clears heat and dispels wind, clears liver heat and invigorates blood, eliminates dampness and relieves itching

【Indications】

1. Seasonal itching caused by congestion of wind-heat-damp pathogen
2. Menstrual ophthalmalgia caused by heat in the liver channel

4. *Fáng Fēng Tōng Shèng Sǎn* (Ledebouriella Sage-Inspired Powder, 防风通圣散)

A Close Examination of the Precious Classic on Ophthalmology (*Shěn Shì Yáo Hán*, 审视瑶函)

【Prescription】

防风	*fáng fēng*	6 g	Radix Saposhnikoviae
川芎	*chuān xiōng*	6 g	Rhizoma Chuanxiong
大黄	*dà huáng*	6 g	Radix et Rhizoma Rhei
赤芍	*chì sháo*	6 g	Radix Paeoniae Rubra
连翘	*lián qiào*	6 g	Fructus Forsythiae
麻黄	*má huáng*	6 g	Herba Ephedrae
芒硝	*máng xiāo*	6 g	Natrii Sulfas
薄荷	*bò he*	6 g	Herba Menthae
当归	*dāng guī*	6 g	Radix Angelicae Sinensis
滑石	*huá shí*	6 g	Talcum
炒栀子	*chǎo zhī zǐ*	6 g	Fructus Gardeniae (dry-fried)
白术	*bái zhú*	6 g	Rhizoma Atractylodis Macrocephalae
桔梗	*jié gěng*	6 g	Radix Platycodonis
石膏	*shí gāo*	6 g	Gypsum Fibrosum
荆芥穗	*jīng jiè suì*	6 g	Spica Schizonepetae
黄芩	*huáng qín*	6 g	Radix Scutellariae
甘草	*gān cǎo*	6 g	Radix et Rhizoma Glycyrrhizae

【Actions】
Scatters wind and clears heat, cools and invigorates the blood
【Indications】
Marginal blepharitis caused by wind-heat pathogen

5. *Chái Hú Qīng Gān Sǎn* (Bupleurum Liver-Clearing Powder, 柴胡清肝散)

A Close Examination of the Precious Classic on Ophthalmology (*Shěn Shì Yáo Hán*, 审视瑶函)
【Prescription】

柴胡	*chái hú*	10 g	Radix Bupleuri
黄芩	*huáng qín*	8 g	Radix Scutellariae
人参	*rén shēn*	8 g	Radix et Rhizoma Ginseng
川芎	*chuān xiōng*	8 g	Rhizoma Chuanxiong
炒栀子	*chǎo zhī zǐ*	8 g	Fructus Gardeniae (dry-fried)
连翘	*lián qiào*	5 g	Fructus Forsythiae
甘草	*gān cǎo*	5 g	Radix et Rhizoma Glycyrrhizae
桔梗	*jié gěng*	6 g	Radix Platycodonis

【Actions】
Dispels wind and clears heat
【Indications】
Frequent nictitation (rapid blinking or winking) caused by wind-heat in the liver and gallbladder.

6. *Qiāng Huó Shèng Fēng Tāng* (Notopterygium Wind-Dispelling Decoction, 羌活胜风汤)

Enlightenment of Ophthalmology (*Yuán Jī Qǐ Wēi*, 原机启微)
【Prescription】

柴胡	*chái hú*	10 g	Radix Bupleuri
黄芩	*huáng qín*	9 g	Radix Scutellariae
白术	*bái zhú*	9 g	Rhizoma Atractylodis Macrocephalae
荆芥	*jīng jiè*	8 g	Herba Schizonepetae
枳壳	*zhǐ qiào*	8 g	Fructus Aurantii
川芎	*chuān xiōng*	8 g	Rhizoma Chuanxiong
白芷	*bái zhǐ*	8 g	Radix Angelicae Dahuricae
羌活	*qiāng huó*	8 g	Radix et Rhizoma Notopterygii

防风	*fáng fēng*	8 g	Radix Saposhnikoviae
独活	*dú huó*	8 g	Radix Angelicae Pubescentis
前胡	*qián hú*	8 g	Radix Peucedani
薄荷	*bò he*	8 g	Herba Menthae
桔梗	*jié gěng*	6 g	Radix Platycodonis
甘草	*gān cǎo*	6 g	Radix et Rhizoma Glycyrrhizae

【 Actions 】
Dispels wind and clears heat
【 Indications 】
Eyelid dermatitis with fulminant wind and invading fire caused by a prevalent wind pathogen

7. *Qiān Zhèng Sǎn* (Symmetry-Correcting Powder, 牵正散)

Secret Formulas of the Yang Family (*Yáng Shì Jiā Cáng Fāng,* 杨氏家藏方)
【 Prescription 】

白附子	*bái fù zǐ*	10 g	Rhizoma Typhonii
僵蚕	*jiāng cán*	10 g	Bombyx Batryticatus
全蝎	*quán xiē*	10 g	Scorpio

【 Actions 】
Dispels wind and dissolves phlegm, unblocks the collaterals
【 Indications 】
Dry mouth and eyes; squinting caused by wind-phlegm obstructing the channels of the head and eyes

8. *Zhèng Róng Tāng* (Face-Restoring Decoction, 正容汤)

A Close Examination of the Precious Classic on Ophthalmology (*Shěn Shì Yáo Hán,* 审视瑶函)
【 Prescription 】

羌活	*qiāng huó*	9 g	Radix et Rhizoma Notopterygii
白附子	*bái fù zǐ*	9 g	Rhizoma Typhonii
防风	*fáng fēng*	9 g	Radix Saposhnikoviae
秦艽	*qín jiāo*	9 g	Radix Gentianae Macrophyllae
胆南星	*dǎn nán xīng*	9 g	Arisaema cum Bile
白僵蚕	*bái jiāng cán*	9 g	Bombyx Batryticatus

姜半夏	*jiāng bàn xià*	9 g	Rhizoma Pinelliae Praeparatum
木瓜	*mù guā*	9 g	Fructus Chaenomelis
黄松节 （抱木茯神）	*huáng sōng jié* *(bào mù fú shén)*	9 g	Lignum Pini Nodi; Sclerotium Poriae Pararadicis
炙甘草	*zhì gān cǎo*	6 g	Radix et Rhizoma Glycyrrhizae Praeparata cum Melle
生姜	*shēng jiāng*	3 sheets	Rhizoma Zingiberis Recens

【Actions】

Dispels wind and unblocks the collaterals, dissolves phlegm and stops spasm

【Indications】

Eye diseases caused by wind-phlegm-dampness obstructing the collaterals, including blephar numbness, drooping of the upper eyelid, squinting, wry eyes and mouth, seeing upright objects inclined, seeing still objects moving, seeing large objects as small, mydriasis, "backward turning spirit ball" (paralytic strabismus), "backward turned pupil spirit" (paralytic strabismus), infantile convergent strabismus, and downward turned pupil.

9. *Wàn Yìng Chán Huā Sǎn* (Myriad Application Cordyceps Cicadae Powder, 万应蝉花散)

Enlightenment of Ophthalmology (Yuán Jī Qǐ Wēi, 原机启微)

【Prescription】

石决明	*shí jué míng*	15 g	Concha Haliotidis
蝉蜕	*chán tuì*	5 g	Periostracum Cicadae
当归身	*dāng guī shēn*	10 g	Radix Angelicae Sinensis (body)
甘草	*gān cǎo*	10 g	Herba Schizonepetae
川芎	*chuān xiōng*	10 g	Rhizoma Chuanxiong
防风	*fáng fēng*	10 g	Radix Saposhnikoviae
茯苓	*fú líng*	10 g	Poria
羌活	*qiāng huó*	10 g	Radix et Rhizoma Notopterygii
苍术	*cāng zhú*	18 g	Rhizoma Atractylodis
蛇蜕	*shé tuì*	9 g	Periostracum Serpentis
赤芍	*chì sháo*	15 g	Radix Paeoniae Rubra

【Actions】

Dispels wind and clears heat, eliminates dampness and relieves itching

【Indications】
Extreme itching caused by complex wind-heat-damp pathogen

10. *Gōu Téng Yǐn Zǐ* (Uncaria Beverage, 钩藤饮子)

A Close Examination of the Precious Classic on Ophthalmology (Shěn Shì Yáo Hán, 审视瑶函)
【Prescription】

钩藤	*gōu téng*	6 g	Ramulus Uncariae Cum Uncis
麻黄	*má huáng*	5 g	Herba Ephedrae
甘草	*gān cǎo*	5 g	Radix et Rhizoma Glycyrrhizae
天麻	*tiān má*	12 g	Rhizoma Gastrodiae
川芎	*chuān xiōng*	12 g	Rhizoma Chuanxiong
防风	*fáng fēng*	12 g	Radix Saposhnikoviae
人参	*rén shēn*	12 g	Radix et Rhizoma Ginseng
僵蚕	*jiāng cán*	18 g	Bombyx Batryticatus
全蝎	*quán xiē*	15 g	Scorpio

【Actions】
Dispels wind and unblocks the collaterals
【Indications】
Nystagmus caused by wind pathogen

11. *Pái Fēng Sǎn* (Wind-Expelling powder, 排风散)

Longmu's Ophthalmology Secretly Handed Down (Mì Chuán Yǎn Kē Lóng Mù Lùn, 秘传眼科龙木论)
【Prescription】

天麻	*tiān má*	9 g	Rhizoma Gastrodiae
桔梗	*jié gěng*	9 g	Radix Platycodonis
防风	*fáng fēng*	9 g	Radix Saposhnikoviae
乌梢蛇	*wū shāo shé*	3 g	Zaocys
五味子	*wǔ wèi zǐ*	6 g	Fructus Schisandrae Chinensis
细辛	*xì xīn*	3 g	Radix et Rhizoma Asari
芍药	*sháo yào*	6 g	Radix Paeoniae Alba; Radix Paeoniae Rubra
全蝎	*quán xiē*	3 g	Scorpio

【Actions】
Dispels wind, unblocks the collaterals and stops spasms

【Indications】
Paralytic strabismus caused by the internal stirring of liver wind

12. *Jú Huā Sǎn* (chrysanthemum powder, 菊花散)

Formulas from the Imperial Pharmacy (*Hé Jì Jú Fāng*, 和剂局方)
【Prescription】

蝉蜕	*chán tuì*	3 g	Periostracum Cicadae
木贼	*mù zéi*	3 g	Herba Equiseti Hiemalis
白蒺藜	*bái jí lí*	9 g	Fructus Tribuli
羌活	*qiāng huó*	9 g	Radix et Rhizoma Notopterygii
菊花	*jú huā*	12 g	Flos Chrysanthemi
荆芥	*jīng jiè*	6 g	Herba Schizonepetae
甘草	*gān cǎo*	6 g	Radix et Rhizoma Glycyrrhizae

【Actions】
Scatters wind, clears heat, relieves itching
【Indications】
Extreme itching caused by wind-heat

13. *Qū Fēng Yī Zì Sǎn* (Wind-Expelling One-Character Powder, 驱风一字散)

Standards for Diagnosis and Treatment (*Zhèng Zhì Zhǔn Shéng*, 证治准绳)
【Prescription】

川乌	*chuān wū*	15 g	Radix Aconiti
川芎	*chuān xiōng*	15 g	Rhizoma Chuanxiong
荆芥	*jīng jiè*	15 g	Herba Schizonepetae
羌活	*qiāng huó*	7.5 g	Radix et Rhizoma Notopterygii
防风	*fǎng fēng*	7.5 g	Radix Saposhnikoviae

【Actions】
Dispels wind and relieves itching
【Indications】
Extremely itching caused by wind pathogen

14. *Chuān Xiōng Chá Tiáo Sǎn* (Tea-Mix and Chuanxiong Powder, 川芎茶调散)

Formulas from the Imperial Pharmacy (*Hé Jì Jú Fāng*, 和剂局方)

【Prescription】

羌活	qiāng huó	6 g	Radix et Rhizoma Notopterygii
防风	fáng fēng	6 g	Radix Saposhnikoviae
白芷	bái zhǐ	6 g	Radix Angelicae Dahuricae
甘草	gān cǎo	6 g	Radix et Rhizoma Glycyrrhizae
川芎	chuān xiōng	12 g	Rhizoma Chuanxiong
荆芥	jīng jiè	12 g	Herba Schizonepetae
细辛	xì xīn	3 g	Radix et Rhizoma Asari
薄荷	bò he	3 g	Herba Menthae

【Actions】

Dispels wind and pathogens, relieves itching

【Indications】

Marginal blepharitis caused by wind pathogen

15. *Chú Fēng Qīng Pí Yǐn* (Wind-Eliminating Spleen-Clearing Beverage, 除风清脾饮)

A Close Examination of the Precious Classic on Ophthalmology (*Shěn Shì Yáo Hán,* 审视瑶函)

【Prescription】

陈皮	chén pí	9 g	Pericarpium Citri Reticulatae
连翘	lián qiào	9 g	Fructus Forsythiae
防风	fáng fēng	9 g	Radix Saposhnikoviae
知母	zhī mǔ	9 g	Rhizoma Anemarrhenae
玄明粉	xuán míng fěn	9 g	Natrii Sulfas Exsiccatus
黄芩	huáng qín	9 g	Radix Scutellariae
玄参	xuán shēn	9 g	Radix Scrophulariae
黄连	huáng lián	9 g	Rhizoma Coptidis
荆芥穗	jīng jiè suì	9 g	Spica Schizonepetae
大黄	dà huáng	9 g	Radix et Rhizoma Rhei
桔梗	jié gěng	9 g	Radix Platycodonis
生地	shēng dì	9 g	Radix Rehmanniae

【Actions】

Dispels wind and pathogens, clears heat and dredges the bowels

【Indications】

Conjunctival folliculitis, trachoma, and trichiasis caused by wind-heat pathogen

16. *Dāng Guī Huó Xuè Yǐn* (Chinese Angelica Blood-Invigorating Beverage, 当归活血饮)

A Close Examination of the Precious Classic on Ophthalmology (Shěn Shì Yáo Hán, 审视瑶函)

【Prescription】

当归	*dāng guī*	15 g	Radix Angelicae Sinensis
白芍	*bái sháo*	12 g	Radix Paeoniae Alba
川芎	*chuān xiōng*	9 g	Rhizoma Chuanxiong
苍术	*cāng zhú*	6 g	Rhizoma Atractylodis
薄荷	*bò he*	6 g	Herba Menthae
黄芪	*huáng qí*	9 g	Radix Astragali
熟地黄	*shú dì huáng*	9 g	Radix Rehmanniae Praeparata
防风	*fáng fēng*	9 g	Radix Saposhnikoviae
羌活	*qiāng huó*	9 g	Radix et Rhizoma Notopterygii
甘草	*gān cǎo*	4.5 g	Radix et Rhizoma Glycyrrhizae

【Actions】
Nourishes the blood and dispels wind
【Indications】
Blepharospasm caused by blood deficiency engendering wind

17. *Zhèn Gān Xī Fēng Tāng* (Liver-Sedating and Wind-Extinguishing Decoction, 镇肝熄风汤)

Records of Chinese Medicine with Reference to Western Medicine (Yī Xué Zhōng Zhōng Cān Xī Lù, 医学衷中参西录)

【Prescription】

怀牛膝	*huái niú xī*	30 g	Radix Achyranthis Bidentatae
代赭石	*dài zhě shí*	30 g	Haematitum
龙骨	*lóng gǔ*	15 g	Os Draconis; Fossilia Ossis Mastodi
牡蛎	*mǔ lì*	15 g	Concha Ostreae
龟板	*guī bǎn*	15 g	Plastrum Testudinis
白芍	*bái sháo*	15 g	Radix Paeoniae Alba

玄参	xuán shēn	15 g	Radix Scrophulariae
天冬	tiān dōng	15 g	Radix Asparagi
川楝子	chuān liàn zǐ	6 g	Fructus Toosendan
麦芽	mài yá	6 g	Fructus Hordei Germinatus
茵陈	yīn chén	6 g	Herba Artemisiae Scopariae
甘草	gān cǎo	4.5 g	Radix et Rhizoma Glycyrrhizae

【Actions】
Tranquilizes the liver and extinguishes internal wind
【Indications】
Strabismus and deviated eyes and mouth caused by liver wind disturbing upward

18. *Bàn Xià Bái Zhú Tiān Má Tāng* (Pinellia, Atractylodes Macrocephala and Gastr odia Decoction, 半夏白术天麻汤)

Medical Revelations (*Yī Xué Xīn Wù*, 医学心悟)
【Prescription】

制半夏	zhì bàn xià	12 g	Rhizoma Pinelliae (prepared)
陈皮	chén pí	10 g	Pericarpium Citri Reticulatae
茯苓	fú líng	15 g	Poria
甘草	gān cǎo	3 g	Radix et Rhizoma Glycyrrhizae
白术	bái zhú	12 g	Rhizoma Atractylodis Macrocephalae
天麻	tiān má	10 g	Rhizoma Gastrodiae

【Actions】
Dissolves phlegm and extinguishs internal wind, fortifies the spleen and removes dampness
【Indications】
Reversed vision caused by wind phlegm

19. *Xiān Fāng Huó Mìng Yǐn* (Immortal Formula Life-Giving Beverage, 仙方活命饮)

Elaboration on External Medicine (*Wài Kē Fā Huī*, 外科发挥)

【Prescription】

陈皮	chén pí	9 g	Pericarpium Citri Reticulatae
金银花	jīn yín huā	9 g	Flos Lonicerae Japonicae
穿山甲	chuān shān jiǎ	3 g	Squama Manitis
天花粉	tiān huā fěn	3 g	Radix Trichosanthis
甘草节	gān cǎo jié	3 g	Radix Tenuis Glycyrrhizae
乳香	rǔ xiāng	3 g	Olibanum
没药	mò yào	3 g	Myrrha
赤芍	chì sháo	3 g	Radix Paeoniae Rubra
当归尾	dāng guī wěi	3 g	Radix Angelicae Sinensis (extremities)
皂角刺	zào jiǎo cì	3 g	Spina Gleditsiae
白芷	bái zhǐ	3 g	Radix Angelicae Dahuricae
贝母	bèi mǔ	3 g	Bulbus Fritillaria
防风	fáng fēng	3 g	Radix Saposhnikoviae

【Actions】

Clears heat and resolves toxins, moves qi and invigorates blood, disperses swelling and softens hardness

【Indications】

Stye, eyelid effusion, inflammatory swelling of the eyelid, and ocular polyp caused by an accumulation of heat toxins

20. *Wǔ Wèi Xiāo Dú Yǐn* (Five Ingredients Toxin-Removing Beverage, 五味消毒饮)

Golden Mirror of the Medical Tradition (Yī Zōng Jīn Jiàn, 医宗金鉴)

【Prescription】

金银花	jīn yín huā	12 g	Flos Lonicerae Japonicae
野菊花	yě jú huā	30 g	Flos Chrysanthemi Indici
蒲公英	pú gōng yīng	30 g	Herba Taraxaci
紫花地丁	zǐ huā dì dīng	30 g	Herba Violae
紫背天葵	zǐ bèi tiān kuí	15 g	Herba Gynurae Bicoloris

【Actions】

Clears heat and resolves toxins

【Indications】
1. Stye and eye carbuncles caused by wind-heat toxin
2. Eyelid myiasis presenting with hyperemia and edema of conjunctiva, hypopyon, and ocular polyp
3. Signs of inflammation and purulence after ocular trauma

21. *Pǔ Jì Xiāo Dú Yǐn* (Universal Relief Toxin-Removing Beverage, 普济消毒饮)

Medical Formulas Collected and Analyzed (*Yī Fāng Jí Jiě*, 医方集解)
【Prescription】

黄连	*huáng lián*	15 g	Rhizoma Coptidis
黄芩	*huáng qín*	15 g	Radix Scutellariae
陈皮	*chén pí*	6 g	Pericarpium Citri Reticulatae
甘草	*gān cǎo*	6 g	Radix et Rhizoma Glycyrrhizae
玄参	*xuán shēn*	6 g	Radix Scrophulariae
柴胡	*chái hú*	6 g	Radix Bupleuri
桔梗	*jié gěng*	6 g	Radix Platycodonis
连翘	*lián qiào*	3 g	Fructus Forsythiae
板蓝根	*bǎn lán gēn*	3 g	Radix Isatidis
马勃	*mǎ bó*	3 g	Lasiosphaera seu Calvatia
牛蒡子	*niú bàng zǐ*	3 g	Fructus Arctii
薄荷	*bò he*	3 g	Herba Menthae
僵蚕	*jiāng cán*	2 g	Bombyx Batryticatus
升麻	*shēng má*	2 g	Rhizoma Cimicifugae

【Actions】
Clears heat and resolves toxins, scatters and dissipates wind
【Indications】
Acute dacryocystitis and acute contagious conjunctivitis caused by intense heat pathogen

22. *Xiè Gān Sǎn* (Liver-Draining Powder, 泻肝散)

Essentials from the Silver Sea (*Yín Hǎi Jīng Wēi*, 银海精微)

【Prescription】

当归尾	dāng guī wěi	12 g	Radix Angelicae Sinensis
大黄	dà huáng	6 g	Radix et Rhizoma Rhei
黄芩	huáng qín	6 g	Radix Scutellariae
知母	zhī mǔ	6 g	Rhizoma Anemarrhenae
桔梗	jié gěng	6 g	Radix Platycodonis
茺蔚子	chōng wèi zǐ	6 g	Fructus Leonuri
芒硝	máng xiāo	6 g	Natrii Sulfas
车前子	chē qián zǐ	6 g	Semen Plantaginis
防风	fáng fēng	6 g	Radix Saposhnikoviae
赤芍	chì sháo	6 g	Radix Paeoniae Rubra
栀子	zhī zǐ	6 g	Fructus Gardeniae
连翘	lián qiào	6 g	Fructus Forsythiae
薄荷	bò he	6 g	Herba Menthae

【Actions】

Clears heat and resolves toxins, drains fire and unblocks the bowels, dispels wind and invigorates the blood

【Indications】

1. Ulcerative keratitis caused by fire-heat pathogen and traumatic external oculopathy

2. Thunder head wind cataract accompanied with constipation caused by intense wind-fire pathogen

3. Iridocyclitis and pupillary metamorphosis caused by residual fire pathogen in the liver and gallbladder

23. Sì Shùn Qīng Liáng Yǐn Zi (Four Favorable Cool Beverage, 四顺清凉饮子)

A Close Examination of the Precious Classic on Ophthalmology (Shěn Shì Yáo Hán, 审视瑶函)

【Prescription】

当归身	dāng guī shēn	12 g	Radix Angelicae Sinensis (body)
龙胆草	lóng dǎn cǎo	12 g	Radix et Rhizoma Gentianae
黄芩	huáng qín	12 g	Radix Scutellariae
桑白皮	sāng bái pí	12 g	Cortex Mori
车前子	chē qián zǐ	12 g	Semen Plantaginis

生地	*shēng dì*	12 g	Radix Rehmanniae
赤芍	*chì sháo*	12 g	Radix Paeoniae Rubra
枳壳	*zhǐ qiào*	12 g	Fructus Aurantii
熟大黄	*shú dà huáng*	9 g	Radix et Rhizoma Rhei
川芎	*chuān xiōng*	9 g	Rhizoma Chuanxiong
防风	*fáng fēng*	9 g	Radix Saposhnikoviae
黄连	*huáng lián*	9 g	Rhizoma Coptidis
木贼草	*mù zéi cǎo*	9 g	Herba Equiseti Hiemalis
羌活	*qiāng huó*	9 g	Radix et Rhizoma Notopterygii
柴胡	*chái hú*	9 g	Radix Bupleuri
炙甘草	*zhì gān cǎo*	5 g	Radix et Rhizoma Glycyrrhizae Praeparata cum Melle

【Actions】
Drains fire and resolves toxin, scatters wind and clears heat
【Indications】
1. Purulent keratitis caused by wind-heat in the liver channel
2. Scleritis caused by blood heat during the menstrual period

24. *Huán Yīn Jiù Kǔ Tāng* (Yin-Returning Bitterness-Returning Decoction, 还阴救苦汤)

Enlightenment of Ophthalmology (*Yuán Jī Qǐ Wēi*, 原机启微)
【Prescription】

当归尾	*dāng guī wěi*	10 g	Radix Angelicae Sinensis (extremities)
川芎	*chuān xiōng*	15 g	Rhizoma Chuanxiong
升麻	*shēng má*	8 g	Rhizoma Cimicifugae
苍术	*cāng zhú*	8 g	Rhizoma Atractylodis
炙甘草	*zhì gān cǎo*	8 g	Radix et Rhizoma Glycyrrhizae Praeparata cum Melle
柴胡	*chái hú*	8 g	Radix Bupleuri
防风	*fáng fēng*	8 g	Radix Saposhnikoviae
桔梗	*jié gěng*	8 g	Radix Platycodonis
黄连	*huáng lián*	8 g	Rhizoma Coptidis

黄芩	huáng qín	8 g	Radix Scutellariae
黄柏	huáng bǎi	8 g	Cortex Phellodendri Chinensis
知母	zhī mǔ	8 g	Rhizoma Anemarrhenae
连翘	lián qiào	8 g	Fructus Forsythiae
生地	shēng dì	8 g	Radix Rehmanniae
羌活	qiāng huó	8 g	Radix et Rhizoma Notopterygii
龙胆草	lóng dǎn cǎo	5 g	Radix et Rhizoma Gentianae
藁本	gāo běn	6 g	Rhizoma Ligustici
红花	hóng huā	3 g	Flos Carthami
细辛	xì xīn	1 g	Radix et Rhizoma Asari

【Actions】
Clears heat and resolves toxin, invigorates blood and dissolves stasis
【Indications】
Late-stage scleratitis caused by heat toxin accumulation

25. *Xīn Zhì Chái Lián Tāng* (New Bupleurum and Coptis Decoction, 新制柴连汤)

Compilation of Ophthalmology (*Yǎn Kē Zuǎn Yào*, 眼科纂要)
【Prescription】

柴胡	chái hú	9 g	Radix Bupleuri
黄连	huáng lián	12 g	Rhizoma Coptidis
黄芩	huáng qín	9 g	Radix Scutellariae
赤芍	chì sháo	12 g	Radix Paeoniae Rubra
蔓荆子	màn jīng zǐ	9 g	Fructus Viticis
山栀	shān zhī	9 g	Fructus Gardeniae
龙胆草	lóng dǎn cǎo	15 g	Radix et Rhizoma Gentianae
木通	mù tōng	9 g	Caulis Akebiae
荆芥	jīng jiè	6 g	Herba Schizonepetae
防风	fáng fēng	6 g	Radix Saposhnikoviae
甘草	gān cǎo	3 g	Radix et Rhizoma Glycyrrhizae

【Actions】
Drains fire and resolves toxin, scatters wind and dissipates heat

【Indications】

Purulent keratitis caused by wind-heat congestion; iridocyclitis caused by excess heat in the liver and gallbladder

26. *Xī Jiǎo Dì Huáng Tāng* (Rhinoceros Horn and Rehmannia Decoction, 犀角地黄汤)

Important Formulas Worth a Thousand Gold Pieces for Emergency (Bèi Jí Qiān Jīn Yào Fāng, 备急千金要方)

【Prescription】

犀角	*xī jiǎo*	1.5–3 g	Cornu Rhinocerotis
生地	*shēng dì*	30 g	Radix Rehmanniae
芍药	*sháo yào*	12 g	Radix Paeoniae Alba
牡丹皮	*mǔ dān pí*	9 g	Cortex Moutan

【Actions】

Clears the *ying* level and cools the blood, resolves toxins

【Indications】

1. Hyphema and vitreous hemorrhage caused by heat entering *ying*-blood and causing frenetic movement of blood

2. Eye carbuncle and hypopyon caused by intense heat toxin

3. Signs of purulence after ruptured wound of the eyeball and chemical ophthalmic injury

27. *Qīng Yíng Tāng* (*Ying* Level Clearing Decoction, 清营汤)

Systematic Differentiation of Warm Diseases (Wēn Bìng Tiáo Biàn, 温病条辨)

【Prescription】

犀角	*xī jiǎo*	1.5–3 g	Cornu Rhinocerotis
生地	*shēng dì*	15 g	Radix Rehmanniae
玄参	*xuán shēn*	9 g	Radix Scrophulariae
竹叶心	*zhú yè xīn*	6 g	Folium Pleioblasti
麦冬	*mài dōng*	9 g	Radix Ophiopogonis
丹参	*dān shēn*	9 g	Radix et Rhizoma Salviae Miltiorrhizae
黄连	*huáng lián*	6 g	Rhizoma Coptidis
金银花	*jīn yín huā*	15 g	Flos Lonicerae Japonicae
连翘	*lián qiào*	9 g	Fructus Forsythiae

【Actions】

Clears the *ying* level and resolves toxins, clears heat and nourishes yin

【Indications】

1. Hypopyon and iridocyclitis caused by intense fire toxin

2. Suddern blindness, hyphema and vitreous hemorrhage caused by heat entering the *ying*-blood

28. *Lóng Dǎn Xiè Gān Tāng* (Gentian Liver-Draining Decoction, 龙胆泻肝汤)

Golden Mirror of the Medical Tradition (*Yī Zōng Jīn Jiàn*, 医宗金鉴)

【Prescription】

龙胆草	*lóng dǎn cǎo*	12 g	Radix et Rhizoma Gentianae
生地	*shēng dì*	18 g	Radix Rehmanniae
当归	*dāng guī*	6 g	Radix Angelicae Sinensis
柴胡	*chái hú*	6 g	Radix Bupleuri
木通	*mù tōng*	6 g	Caulis Akebiae
泽泻	*zé xiè*	9 g	Rhizoma Alismatis
车前子	*chē qián zǐ*	9 g	Semen Plantaginis
栀子	*zhī zǐ*	9 g	Fructus Gardeniae
黄芩	*huáng qín*	9 g	Radix Scutellariae
甘草	*gān cǎo*	3 g	Radix et Rhizoma Glycyrrhizae

【Actions】

Clears liver and drains fire, clears damp-heat in the lower *jiao*

【Indications】

All kinds of eye diseases causd by excess heat in the liver and gallbladder or damp-heat pathogen

29. *Liáng Gān Sǎn* (Liver-Cooling Powder, 凉肝散)

Essentials from the Silver Sea (*Yín Hǎi Jīng Wēi*, 银海精微)

【Prescription】

草决明	*cǎo jué míng*	3 g	Semen Cassiae
天花粉	*tiān huā fěn*	9 g	Radix Trichosanthis
赤芍	*chì sháo*	9 g	Radix Paeoniae Rubra
绿豆衣	*lǜ dòu yī*	6 g	Testa Glycinis
谷精草	*gǔ jīng cǎo*	6 g	Flos Eriocauli
甘草	*gān cǎo*	3 g	Radix et Rhizoma Glycyrrhizae

【Actions】

Clears heat and calms the liver

【Indications】

The initial stage of smallpox invading the eyes

30. *Dǎo Chì Sǎn* (Red Guiding Powder, 导赤散)

Essentials from the Silver Sea (Yín Hǎi Jīng Wēi, 银海精微)

【Prescription】

生地	*shēng dì*	18 g	Radix Rehmanniae
木通	*mù tōng*	9 g	Caulis Akebiae
淡竹叶	*dàn zhú yè*	12 g	Herba Lophatheri
栀子	*zhī zǐ*	12 g	Fructus Gardeniae
黄柏	*huáng bǎi*	9 g	Cortex Phellodendri Chinensis
知母	*zhī mǔ*	9 g	Rhizoma Anemarrhenae
灯心草	*dēng xīn cǎo*	6 g	Medulla Junci
甘草	*gān cǎo*	6 g	Radix et Rhizoma Glycyrrhizae

【Actions】

Clear heart heat and drain fire; promotes urination

【Indications】

Chronic conjunctivitis and marginal blepharitis caused by heat fire

31. *Xiè Xīn Tāng* (Heart-Draining Decoction, 泻心汤)

Essentials from the Silver Sea (Yín Hǎi Jīng Wēi, 银海精微)

【Prescription】

黄连	*huáng lián*	9 g	Rhizoma Coptidis
黄芩	*huáng qín*	9 g	Radix Scutellariae
大黄	*dà huáng*	9 g	Radix et Rhizoma Rhei
连翘	*lián qiào*	9 g	Fructus Forsythiae
车前子	*chē qián zǐ*	9 g	Semen Plantaginis
薄荷	*bò he*	9 g	Herba Menthae
菊花	*jú huā*	9 g	Flos Chrysanthemi
赤芍	*chì sháo*	9 g	Radix Paeoniae Rubra

【Actions】

Clears heart fire, eliminates damp-heat, and dispels wind

【Indications】
Chronic conjunctivitis, cornea pannus, marginal blepharitis, corneal perforation, and iridocyclitis caused by heart fire or wind-heat-damp pathogen

32. *Xiè Bái Sǎn* (White-Draining Powder, 泻白散)

Key to Diagnosis and Treatment of Children's Diseases (Xiǎo Ér Yào Zhèng Zhí Jué, 小儿药证直诀)

【Prescription】

地骨皮	*dì gǔ pí*	12 g	Cortex Lycii
桑白皮	*sāng bái pí*	15 g	Cortex Mori
甘草	*gān cǎo*	3 g	Radix et Rhizoma Glycyrrhizae
粳米	*jīng mǐ*	9 g	Semen Oryzae Sativae

【Actions】
Clears and drains lung heat
【Indications】
Follicular conjunctivitis, conjunctiva edma, pseudopterygium, and measles infecting the eyes caused by lung heat

33. *Sāng Bái Pí Tāng* (Mulberry Root Bark Decoction, 桑白皮汤)

A Close Examination of the Precious Classic on Ophthalmology (Shěn Shì Yáo Hán, 审视瑶函)

【Prescription】

桑白皮	*sāng bái pí*	12 g	Cortex Mori
泽泻	*zé xiè*	5 g	Rhizoma Alismatis
玄参	*xuán shēn*	5 g	Radix Scrophulariae
甘草	*gān cǎo*	3 g	Radix et Rhizoma Glycyrrhizae
麦冬	*mài dōng*	6 g	Radix Ophiopogonis
黄芩	*huáng qín*	6 g	Radix Scutellariae
旋覆花	*xuán fù huā*	6 g	Flos Inulae
菊花	*jú huā*	5 g	Flos Chrysanthemi
地骨皮	*dì gǔ pí*	6 g	Cortex Lycii
桔梗	*jié gěng*	6 g	Radix Platycodonis
茯苓	*fú líng*	6 g	Poria

【Actions】
Clears and drains lung heat, nourishes yin to brighten the eyes
【Indications】
　1. Severe conjunctival edema caused by lung-stomach heat congestion
　2. Acute contagious conjunctivitis, follicular conjunctivitis, and dry eyes caused by lung heat

34. *Xiè Fèi Yǐn* (Lung-Draining Beverage, 泻肺饮)

Compilation of Ophthalmology (*Yǎn Kē Zuǎn Yào*, 眼科纂要)
【Prescription】

石膏	*shí gāo*	9 g	Gypsum Fibrosum
赤芍	*chì sháo*	9 g	Radix Paeoniae Rubra
黄芩	*huáng qín*	9 g	Radix Scutellariae
桑白皮	*sāng bái pí*	9 g	Cortex Mori
枳壳	*zhǐ qiào*	9 g	Fructus Aurantii
木通	*mù tōng*	9 g	Caulis Akebiae
连翘	*lián qiào*	9 g	Fructus Forsythiae
荆芥	*jīng jiè*	9 g	Herba Schizonepetae
防风	*fáng fēng*	9 g	Radix Saposhnikoviae
栀子	*zhī zǐ*	9 g	Fructus Arctii
白芷	*bái zhǐ*	9 g	Radix Angelicae Dahuricae
羌活	*qiāng huó*	6 g	Rhizoma et Radix Notopterygii
甘草	*gān cǎo*	3 g	Radix et Rhizoma Glycyrrhizae

【Actions】
Clears and drains lung heat, dispels wind and pathogens
【Indications】
Fulminant wind and invading heat and fulminant red eye with nebula (epidemic keratoconjunctivitis) caused by wind-heat pathogen

35. *Tōng Pí Xiè Wèi Tāng* (Spleen-Freeing and Stomach-Draining Decoction, 通脾泻胃汤)

Golden Mirror of the Medical Tradition (*Yī Zōng Jīn Jiàn*, 医宗金鉴)
【Prescription】

知母	*zhī mǔ*	6 g	Rhizoma Anemarrhenae
大黄	*dà huáng*	6–12 g	Radix et Rhizoma Rhei

黄芩	*huáng qín*	9 g	Radix Scutellariae
芫蔚子	*chōng wèi zǐ*	6 g	Fructus Leonuri
石膏	*shí gāo*	12 g	Gypsum Fibrosum
栀子	*zhī zǐ*	6 g	Fructus Arctii
黑参	*hēi shēn*	6 g	Radix Scrophulariae
防风	*fáng fēng*	6 g	Radix Saposhnikoviae

【Actions】
Clears stomach heat, resolves toxins

【Indications】
Stye and eye carbuncle caused by accumulation of heat in the spleen and stomach; hypopyon and trachomatous pannus caused by spleen-stomach damp-heat ascending upward to the eyes.

36. *Sān Huáng Tāng* (Three Yellow Decoction, 三黄汤)

Essentials from the Silver Sea (*Yín Hǎi Jīng Wēi*, 银海精微)

【Prescription】

黄芩	*huáng qín*	30 g	Radix Scutellariae
黄连	*huáng lián*	30 g	Rhizoma Coptidis
大黄	*dà huáng*	30 g	Radix et Rhizoma Rhei

【Actions】
Clears accumulation of heat in the spleen and stomach

【Indications】
Pterygium caused by accumulated heat in the spleen and stomach

37. *Xiāo Yáo Sǎn* (Free Wanderer Powder, 逍遥散)

Formulas from the Imperial Pharmacy (*Hé Jì Jú Fāng*, 和剂局方)

【Prescription】

当归	*dāng guī*	9 g	Radix Angelicae Sinensis
白术	*bái zhú*	9 g	Rhizoma Atractylodis Macrocephalae
茯苓	*fú líng*	9 g	Poria
白芍	*bái sháo*	9 g	Radix Paeoniae Alba
柴胡	*chái hú*	9 g	Radix Bupleuri
甘草	*gān cǎo*	3 g	Radix et Rhizoma Glycyrrhizae Praeparata cum Melle

【Actions】

Soothes the liver and resolves constraint, fortifies the spleen and nourishes the blood

【Indications】

Eye diseases caused by liver constraint, such as frequent nictation, Pulley eye (nystagmus), bluish blindness (optic atrophy), seeing straight objects as crooked, and seeing objects in altered colors

38. *Dān Zhī Xiāo Yáo Sǎn* (Peony Bark and Gardenia Free Wanderer Powder, 丹栀逍遥散)

Summary of Internal Medicine (*Nèi Kē Zhāi Yào*, 内科摘要)

【Prescription】

丹皮	*dān pí*	12 g	Cortex Moutan
栀子	*zhī zǐ*	9 g	Fructus Gardeniae
当归	*dāng guī*	9 g	Radix Angelicae Sinensis
白术	*bái zhú*	9 g	Rhizoma Atractylodis Macrocephalae
茯苓	*fú líng*	15 g	Poria
白芍	*bái sháo*	15 g	Radix Paeoniae Alba
柴胡	*chái hú*	9 g	Radix Bupleuri
煨姜	*wèi jiāng*	3 g	Rhizoma Zingiberis Rosc.
薄荷	*bò he*	3 g	Herba Menthae
甘草	*gān cǎo*	3 g	Radix et Rhizoma Glycyrrhizae

【Actions】

Soothes the liver and resolves constraint, fortifies the spleen and nourishes the blood, clears heat and invigorates the blood

【Indications】

Eye diseases caused by liver constraint, including tinted vision, blurred vision, "green-wind" glaucoma, "blue wind" glaucoma (acute angle-closure glaucoma), "black wind" glaucoma (acute angle-closure glaucoma), postpartum eye disease, and sudden blindness

39. *Chái Hú Shū Gān Sǎn* (Bupleurum Liver-Soothing Powder, 柴胡疏肝散)

The Complete Works of [Zhang] Jing-yue (*Jǐng Yuè Quán Shū*, 景岳全书)

【Prescription】

柴胡	*chái hú*	6 g	Radix Bupleuri
白芍	*bái sháo*	9 g	Radix Paeoniae Alba
枳壳	*zhǐ qiào*	4.5 g	Fructus Aurantii
陈皮	*chén pí*	6 g	Pericarpium Citri Reticulatae
川芎	*chuān xiōng*	6 g	Rhizoma Chuanxiong
香附	*xiāng fù*	6 g	Rhizoma Cyperi
甘草	*gān cǎo*	3 g	Radix et Rhizoma Glycyrrhizae

【Actions】

Soothes the liver and resolves constraint, moves qi and invigorates the blood

【Indications】

Tinted vision (seeing objects in altered colors) and "black wind glaucoma" caused by liver constraint and qi stagnation.

40. *Gān Lù Xiāo Dú Dān* (Sweet Dew Toxin-Removing Elixir, 甘露消毒丹)

Warp and Woof of Warm-Heat Diseases (*Wēn Rè Jīng Wěi*, 温热经纬)

【Prescription】

滑石	*huá shí*	25 g	Talcum
茵陈	*yīn chén*	18 g	Herba Artemisiae Scopariae
黄芩	*huáng qín*	15 g	Radix Scutellariae
石菖蒲	*shí chāng pú*	9 g	Rhizoma Acori Tatarinowii
川贝母	*chuān bèi mǔ*	8 g	Bulbus Fritillariae Cirrhosae
木通	*mù tōng*	8 g	Caulis Akebiae
藿香	*huò xiāng*	6 g	Herba Agastachis
射干	*shè gān*	6 g	Rhizoma Belamcandae
连翘	*lián qiào*	6 g	Fructus Forsythiae
薄荷	*bò he*	6 g	Herba Menthae
豆蔻	*dòu kòu*	6 g	Fructus Amomi Rotundus

【Actions】

Clears heat and drains dampness; removes turbidity with aromatic medicinals

【Indications】

Blurred vision and screen vision caused by damp-heat pathogenic factors

41. *Sān Rén Tāng* (Three Kernels Decoction, 三仁汤)

【Prescription】

杏仁	*xìng rén*	15 g	Semen Armeniacae Amarum
滑石	*huá shí*	18 g	Talcum
白通草	*bái tōng cǎo*	6 g	Medulla Tetrapanacis
白豆蔻	*bái dòu kòu*	6 g	Fructus Amomi Kravanh
竹叶	*zhú yè*	6 g	Folium Phyllostachydis Henonis
厚朴	*hòu pò*	6 g	Cortex Magnoliae Officinalis
薏苡仁	*yì yǐ rén*	18 g	Semen Coicis
半夏	*bàn xià*	15 g	Rhizoma Pinelliae

【Actions】
Clears and drains heat-damp, diffuses and harmonizes qi
【Indications】
Eye diseases caused by damp-heat pathogens: chronic dacrocystitis, scleritis, herpes simplex keratitis, screen vision, white membrane invading eye, iridocyclitis, vitreous opacity, tinted vision, seeing straight objects appear as crooked

42. *Qiāng Huó Chú Shī Tāng* (Notopterygium Dampness-Dispelling Decoction, 羌活除湿汤)

Direct Records of Ophthalmology (*Yǎn Kē Jié Jìng,* 眼科捷径)
【Prescription】

柴胡	*chái hú*	3 g	Radix Bupleuri
羌活	*qiāng huó*	9 g	Radix et Rhizoma Notopterygii
防风	*fáng fēng*	6 g	Radix Saposhnikoviae
苍术	*cāng zhú*	12 g	Rhizoma Atractylodis
藁本	*gāo běn*	9 g	Rhizoma Ligustici
升麻	*shēng má*	3 g	Rhizoma Cimicifugae

【Actions】
Dispels wind, resolves dampness, and clears heat
【Indications】
Phlyctenular kerato-conjunctivitis caused by complex wind-heat-damp pathogen

43. *Yì Yáng Jiŭ Lián Săn* (Inhibiting Excessive Yang Rhizoma Coptidis Powder, 抑阳酒连散)

Enlightenment of Ophthalmology (*Yuán Jī Qǐ Wēi*, 原机启微)
【Prescription】

独活	*dú huó*	12 g	Radix Angelicae Pubescentis
生地	*shēng dì*	12 g	Radix Rehmanniae
黄柏	*huáng bǎi*	9 g	Cortex Phellodendri Chinensis
汉防己	*hàn fáng jǐ*	9 g	Radix Stephaniae Tetrandrae
知母	*zhī mǔ*	9 g	Rhizoma Anemarrhenae
蔓荆子	*màn jīng zǐ*	12 g	Fructus Viticis
前胡	*qián hú*	12 g	Radix Peucedani
羌活	*qiāng huó*	12 g	Radix et Rhizoma Notopterygii
防风	*fáng fēng*	12 g	Radix Saposhnikoviae
白芷	*bái zhǐ*	12 g	Radix Angelicae Dahuricae
甘草	*gān cǎo*	12 g	Radix et Rhizoma Glycyrrhizae
山栀	*shān zhī*	15 g	Fructus Gardeniae
黄芩	*huáng qín*	15 g	Radix Scutellariae
寒水石	*hán shuǐ shí*	15 g	Glauberitum
黄连	*huáng lián*	15 g	Rhizoma Coptidis

【Actions】
Dispels wind, eliminates dampness, and clears heat
【Indications】
Iridocyclitis caused by complex wind-heat-damp pathogen

44. *Èr Chén Tāng* (Two Matured Substances Decoction, 二陈汤)

Formulas from the Imperial Pharmacy (*Hé Jì Jú Fāng*, 和剂局方)
【Prescription】

半夏	*bàn xià*	9 g	Rhizoma Pinelliae
橘红	*jú hóng*	9 g	Exocarpium Citri Rubrum
茯苓	*fú líng*	9 g	Poria
甘草	*gān cǎo*	3 g	Radix et Rhizoma Glycyrrhizae

【Actions】
Dries dampness and dissolves phlegm, moves qi and relieves edema

【Indications】

　1. Conjunctival edema caused by phlegm-damp

　2. Treat blepharospasm caused by phlegm-damp in combination with *Bǔ Zhōng Yì Qì Tāng* (补中益气汤, Center-Supplementing and Qi-Boosting Decoction)

45. *Liù Jūn Zǐ Tāng* (Six Gentlemen Decoction, 六君子汤)

Fine Formulas for Women (*Fù Rén Liáng Fāng,* 妇人良方)

半夏	*bàn xià*	9 g	Rhizoma Pinelliae
陈皮	*chén pí*	6 g	Pericarpium Citri Reticulatae
茯苓	*fú líng*	9 g	Poria
甘草	*gān cǎo*	6 g	Radix et Rhizoma Glycyrrhizae
人参	*rén shēn*	9 g	Radix et Rhizoma Ginseng
白术	*bái zhú*	9 g	Rhizoma Atractylodis Macrocephalae
生姜	*shēng jiāng*	3 pieces	Rhizoma Zingiberis Recens
大枣	*dà zǎo*	5 pieces	Fructus Jujubae

【Actions】
Dissolves phlegm and unblocks the collaterals; fortifies the spleen and boosts qi
【Indications】
Paralytic strabismus caused by phlegm-damp

46. *Huà Jiān Èr Chén Wán* (Hardness-Removing Two Matured Substances Pill, 化坚二陈丸)

Golden Mirror of the Medical Tradition (*Yī Zōng Jīn Jiàn,* 医宗金鉴)
【Prescription】

半夏	*bàn xià*	10 g	Rhizoma Pinelliae
陈皮	*chén pí*	10 g	Pericarpium Citri Reticulatae
茯苓	*fú líng*	15 g	Poria
甘草	*gān cǎo*	3 g	Radix et Rhizoma Glycyrrhizae
白僵蚕	*bái jiāng cán*	20 g	Bombyx Batryticatus
黄连	*huáng lián*	3 g	Rhizoma Coptidis

【Actions】
Dissolves phlegm and dissipates masses
【Indications】
Chalazion caused by phlegm-damp

47. *Dǎo Tán Tāng* (Phlegm-Expelling Decoction, 导痰汤)

Formulas to Aid the Living (Jì Shēng Fāng, 济生方)
【 Prescription 】

半夏	*bàn xià*	9 g	Rhizoma Pinelliae
陈皮	*chén pí*	9 g	Pericarpium Citri Reticulatae
茯苓	*fú líng*	9 g	Poria
甘草	*gān cǎo*	3 g	Radix et Rhizoma Glycyrrhizae
枳壳	*zhǐ qiào*	9 g	Fructus Aurantii
胆南星	*dǎn nán xīng*	12 g	Arisaema cum Bile
生姜	*shēng jiāng*	9 g	Rhizoma Zingiberis Recens

【 Actions 】
Dispels wind and clears up phlegm, moves qi and resolves constraint
【 Indications 】
Seeing still objects that appear to be moving and/or sudden blindness caused by wind-phlegm

48. *Shēng Pǔ huáng Tāng* (Raw Typha Decoction, 生蒲黄汤)

Essential Teachings of the Six Channel on TCM Ophthalmology (Zhōng Yī Yǎn Kē Liù Jīng Fǎ Yào, 中医眼科六经法要)
【 Prescription 】

生蒲黄	*shēng pú huáng*	24 g	Pollen Typhae
旱莲草	*hàn lián cǎo*	24 g	Herba Ecliptae
丹参	*dān shēn*	15 g	Radix et Rhizoma Salviae Miltiorrhizae
荆芥炭	*jīng jiè tàn*	12 g	Herba Schizonepetae Carbonisatum
郁金	*yù jīn*	15 g	Radix Curcumae
生地	*shēng dì*	12 g	Radix Rehmanniae
川芎	*chuān xiōng*	6 g	Rhizoma Chuanxiong
牡丹皮	*mǔ dān pí*	12 g	Cortex Moutan

【 Actions 】
Stanches bleeding and invigorates the blood, cools the blood and dissolves stasis
【 Indications 】
1. Hyphema, vitreous hemorrhage and retinal hemorrhage

2. Eye bleeding caused by ocular trauma

49. *Níng Xuě Tāng* (Blood-Quieting Decoction, 宁血汤)

Ophthalmology of Chinese medicine (*Zhōng Yī Yǎn Kē Xué*, 中医眼科学)

【Prescription】

仙鹤草	*xiān hè cǎo*	30 g	Herba Agrimoniae
旱莲草	*hàn lián cǎo*	12 g	Herba Ecliptae
生地	*shēng dì*	15 g	Radix Rehmanniae
栀子炭	*zhī zǐ tàn*	15 g	Fructus Gardeniae (carbonized)
白芍	*bái sháo*	9 g	Radix Paeoniae Alba
白蔹	*bái liǎn*	9 g	Radix Ampelopsis
白茅根	*bái máo gēn*	30 g	Rhizoma Imperatae
侧柏叶	*cè bǎi yè*	18 g	Cacumen Platycladi
阿胶	*ē jiāo*	9 g	Colla Corii Asini

【Actions】
Cools the blood and stanches bleeding
【Indications】
Hyphema and intraocular bleeding

50. *Táo Hóng Sì Wù Tāng* (Peach Kernel and Carthamus Four Substances Decoction, 桃红四物汤)

Golden Mirror of the Medical Tradition (*Yī Zōng Jīn Jiàn*, 医宗金鉴)

【Prescription】

熟地黄	*shú dì huáng*	12 g	Radix Rehmanniae Praeparata
川芎	*chuān xiōng*	6 g	Rhizoma Chuanxiong
赤芍	*chì sháo*	9 g	Radix Paeoniae Rubra
当归	*dāng guī*	9 g	Radix Angelicae Sinensis
桃仁	*táo rén*	12 g	Semen Persicae
红花	*hóng huā*	9 g	Flos Carthami

【Actions】
Nourishes the blood and cools the blood, invigorates the blood and dissolves stasis
【Indications】
1. Conjunctival diseases such as subconjunctival hemorrhage, chronic conjunctivitis,

and severe conjunctival edema

2. Hyphema, intraocular bleeding, vitreous opacity, optic atrophy, and sudden blindness caused by blood stasis

51. *Tōng Qiào Huó Xuè Tāng* (Orifice-Freeing Blood-Quickening Decoction, 通窍活血汤)

Correction of Errors in Medical Works (*Yī Lín Gǎi Cuò*, 医林改错)
【Prescription】

赤芍	*chì sháo*	9 g	Radix Paeoniae Rubra
川芎	*chuān xiōng*	9 g	Rhizoma Chuanxiong
桃仁	*táo rén*	9 g	Semen Persicae
红花	*hóng huā*	9 g	Flos Carthami
大枣	*dà zǎo*	9 g	Fructus Jujubae
生姜	*shēng jiāng*	9 g	Rhizoma Zingiberis Recens
老葱	*lǎo cōng*	3 g	Bulbus Allii Fistulosi
麝香	*shè xiāng*	0.3 g	Moschus

【Actions】
Invigorates the blood and unblock the orifices
【Indications】
Sudden blindness

52. *Xuè Fǔ Zhú Yū Tāng* (Blood Stasis Expelling Decoction, 血府逐瘀汤)

Correction of Errors in Medical Works (*Yī Lín Gǎi Cuò*, 医林改错)
【Prescription】

桃仁	*táo rén*	12 g	Semen Persicae
红花	*hóng huā*	9 g	Flos Carthami
生地	*shēng dì*	9 g	Radix Rehmanniae
川芎	*chuān xiōng*	4.5 g	Rhizoma Chuanxiong
赤芍	*chì sháo*	6 g	Radix Paeoniae Rubra
当归	*dāng guī*	6 g	Radix Angelicae Sinensis
牛膝	*niú xī*	9 g	Radix Achyranthis Bidentatae
桔梗	*jié gěng*	4.5 g	Radix Platycodonis
柴胡	*chái hú*	3 g	Radix Bupleuri
枳壳	*zhǐ qiào*	6 g	Fructus Aurantii
甘草	*gān cǎo*	6 g	Radix et Rhizoma Glycyrrhizae

【Actions】

Invigorates blood and dissolves stasis

【Indications】

Conjunctival hyperemia and edema, hyphema, intraocular bleeding, and vitreous opcity caused by blood stasis

53. *Bŭ Yáng Huán Wŭ Tāng* (Yang-Supplementing and Five-Returning Decoction, 补阳还五汤)

Correction of Errors in Medical Works (*Yī Lín Găi Cuò*, 医林改错)

【Prescription】

黄芪	*huáng qí*	60 – 120 g	Radix Astragali
当归	*dāng guī*	9 g	Radix Angelicae Sinensis
桃仁	*táo rén*	9 g	Semen Persicae
红花	*hóng huā*	9 g	Flos Carthami
地龙	*dì lóng*	9 g	Pheretima
川芎	*chuān xiōng*	9 g	Rhizoma Chuanxiong
赤芍	*chì sháo*	9 g	Radix Paeoniae Rubra

【Actions】

Invigorates blood and unblocks the collaterals, resolves spasm and relaxes tension

【Indications】

Infantile convergent strabismus caused by residual heat pathogen

54. *Chú Fēng Yì Sŭn Tāng* (Wind-Eliminating Boosting Decoction, 除风益损汤)

Enlightenment of Ophthalmology (*Yuán Jī Qĭ Wēi*, 原机启微)

熟地黄	*shú dì huáng*	9 g	Radix Rehmanniae Praeparata
川芎	*chuān xiōng*	9 g	Rhizoma Chuanxiong
赤芍	*chì sháo*	9 g	Radix Paeoniae Rubra
当归	*dāng guī*	9 g	Radix Angelicae Sinensis
藁本	*gāo běn*	6 g	Rhizoma Ligustici
前胡	*qián hú*	6 g	Radix Peucedani
防风	*fáng fēng*	6 g	Radix Saposhnikoviae

【Actions】

Nourishes and invigorates the blood, eliminates wind and supplements deficiency

【Indications】

Hyphema and intraocular bleeding, traumatic cataract, wry mouth and eyes caused by trauma

55. *Sì Jūn Zǐ Tāng* (Four Gentlemen Decoction, 四君子汤)

Formulas from the Imperial Pharmacy (*Hé Jì Jú Fāng*, 和剂局方)

【Prescription】

人参	*rén shēn*	9 g	Radix et Rhizoma Ginseng
白术	*bái zhú*	9 g	Rhizoma Atractylodis Macrocephalae
茯苓	*fú líng*	9 g	Poria
甘草	*gān cǎo*	6 g	Radix et Rhizoma Glycyrrhizae

【Actions】

Supplements the center and boosts qi, reinforces healthy qi and dispels pathogen

【Indications】

Fascicular keratitis, corneal fistular, seeing big things as small, patients with weak constitutions. This formula is always given in combination with other medicinals to enhance the effectiveness.

56. *Shēn Líng Bái Zhú Sǎn* (Ginseng, Poria and Atractylodes Macrocephalae Powder, 参苓白术散)

Formulas from the Imperial Pharmacy (*Hé Jì Jú Fāng*, 和剂局方)

【Prescription】

人参	*rén shēn*	10 g	Radix et Rhizoma Ginseng
白术	*bái zhú*	10 g	Rhizoma Atractylodis Macrocephalae
茯苓	*fú líng*	10 g	Poria
甘草	*gān cǎo*	10 g	Radix et Rhizoma Glycyrrhizae
山药	*shān yào*	10 g	Rhizoma Dioscoreae
白扁豆	*bái biǎn dòu*	7.5 g	Semen Lablab Album
莲子肉	*lián zǐ ròu*	5 g	Semen Nelumbinis
薏苡仁	*yì yǐ rén*	5 g	Semen Coicis
砂仁	*shā rén*	5 g	Fructus Amomi
桔梗	*jié gěng*	5 g	Radix Platycodonis

【Actions】
Fortifies the spleen and boosts qi
【Indications】
Frequent nictation, dry eyes, malnutrition involving the eyes, tinted vision caused by spleen-stomach qi deficiency

57. *Dìng Zhì Wán* (Mind-Calming Pill, 定志丸)

Important Prescriptions Worth a Thousand Gold for Emergency (*Bèi Jí Qiān Jīn Yào Fāng*, 备急千金要方)
【Prescription】

远志	*yuǎn zhì*	10 g	Radix Polygalae
石菖蒲	*shí chāng pú*	10 g	Rhizoma Acori Tatarinowii
人参	*rén shēn*	5 g	Radix et Rhizoma Ginseng
茯苓	*fú líng*	5 g	Poria

【Actions】
Boosts qi and brightens the eyes
【Indications】
Myopia

58. *Shēng Mài Sǎn* (Pulse-Engendering Powder, 生脉散)

Important Prescriptions Worth a Thousand Gold for Emergency (*Bèi Jí Qiān Jīn Yào Fāng*, 备急千金要方)
【Prescription】

人参	*rén shēn*	3–9 g	Radix et Rhizoma Ginseng
麦冬	*mài dōng*	12 g	Radix Ophiopogonis
五味子	*wǔ wèi zǐ*	6 g	Fructus Schisandrae Chinensis

【Actions】
Boosts qi and promotes fluid production
【Indications】
In the oculopathy treatment, this formula is always prescribed in combination with other formulas, such as with *Liù Wèi Dì Huáng Wán* (Six Ingredients Rehmannia Pill, 六味地黄丸) to treat vitreous opacity caused by liver and kidney deficiency, *Zhù Jǐng Wán* (Long Vistas Pill, 驻景丸) to treat sudden blindness caused by retina detachment, with *Sì Jūn Zǐ Tāng* (Four Gentlemen Decoction) to treat corneal fistula caused by qi and yin deficiency.

59. *Fù Míng Tāng* (Light-Restoring Decoction, 复明汤)

A Close Examination of the Precious Classic on Ophthalmology (*Shěn Shì Yáo Hán*, 审视瑶函)

【Prescription】

黄芪	*huáng qí*	18 g	Radix Astragali
当归	*dāng guī*	18 g	Radix Angelicae Sinensis
柴胡	*chái hú*	18 g	Radix Bupleuri
连翘	*lián qiào*	18 g	Fructus Forsythiae
甘草	*gān cǎo*	18 g	Radix et Rhizoma Glycyrrhizae
生地	*shēng dì*	18 g	Radix Rehmanniae
黄柏	*huáng bǎi*	5 g	Cortex Phellodendri Chinensis
川芎	*chuān xiōng*	6 g	Rhizoma Chuanxiong
苍术	*cāng zhú*	6 g	Rhizoma Atractylodis
广陈皮	*guǎng chén pí*	6 g	Pericarpium Citri Reticulatae

【Actions】
Boosts qi and nourishes the blood, harmonizes the liver to brighten the eyes
【Indications】
Tinted vision (altered color vision).

60. *Yì Qì Cōng Míng Tāng* (Qi-Boosting Intelligence Decoction, 益气聪明汤)

Treatise on the Spleen and Stomach (*Pí Wèi Lùn*, 脾胃论)
【Prescription】

蔓荆子	*màn jīng zǐ*	16 g	Fructus Viticis
黄芪	*huáng qí*	6 g	Radix Astragali
人参	*rén shēn*	6 g	Radix et Rhizoma Ginseng
黄柏	*huáng bǎi*	12 g	Cortex Phellodendri Chinensis
白芍	*bái sháo*	12 g	Radix Paeoniae Alba
炙甘草	*zhì gān cǎo*	4 g	Radix et Rhizoma Glycyrrhizae Praeparata cum Melle
升麻	*shēng má*	4 g	Rhizoma Cimicifugae
葛根	*gé gēn*	4 g	Radix Puerariae Lobatae

【Actions】
Boosts qi and brightens the eyes
【Indications】
Altered color vison

61. *Sì Wù Tāng* (Four Substances Decoction, 四物汤)

Formulas from the Imperial Pharmacy (*Hé Jì Jú Fāng*, 和剂局方)

当归	*dāng guī*	9 g	Radix Angelicae Sinensis
川芎	*chuān xiōng*	6 g	Rhizoma Chuanxiong
白芍	*bái sháo*	9 g	Radix Paeoniae Alba
熟地黄	*shú dì huáng*	12 g	Radix Rehmanniae Praeparata

【Actions】
Supplements and regulates the blood
【Indications】
1. Conjunctival edema and frequent nictation caused by blood deficiency
2. Night blindness after measles

62. *Bā Zhēn Tāng* (Eight Gem Decoction, 八珍汤)

Categorized Synopsis of the Whole (*Zhèng Tǐ Lèi Yào*, 正体类要)
【Prescription】

人参	*rén shēn*	9 g	Radix et Rhizoma Ginseng
白术	*bái zhú*	9 g	Rhizoma Atractylodis Macrocephalae
茯苓	*fú líng*	9 g	Poria
甘草	*gān cǎo*	6 g	Radix et Rhizoma Glycyrrhizae
当归	*dāng guī*	9 g	Radix Angelicae Sinensis
川芎	*chuān xiōng*	9 g	Rhizoma Chuanxiong
白芍	*bái sháo*	9 g	Radix Paeoniae Alba
熟地黄	*shú dì huáng*	9 g	Radix Rehmanniae Praeparata
生姜	*shēng jiāng*	3 pieces	Rhizoma Zingiberis Recens
大枣	*dà zǎo*	3 pieces	Fructus Jujubae

【Actions】
Supplements qi and blood
【Indications】
Dry eyes, night blindness, malnutrition involving the eyes, and halovision caused by qi

and blood deficiency.

63. *Guī Pí Tāng* (Spleen-Restoring Decoction, 归脾汤)

Formulas to Aid the Living (*Jì Shēng Fāng*, 济生方)

【Prescription】

白术	*bái zhú*	9 g	Rhizoma Atractylodis Macrocephalae
黄芪	*huáng qí*	9 g	Radix Astragali
茯神	*fú shén*	9 g	Sclerotium Poriae Pararadicis
党参	*dǎng shēn*	9 g	Radix Codonopsis
甘草	*gān cǎo*	6 g	Radix et Rhizoma Glycyrrhizae
木香	*mù xiāng*	6 g	Radix Aucklandiae
远志	*yuǎn zhì*	9 g	Radix Polygalae
枣仁	*zǎo rén*	9 g	Semen Ziziphi Spinoae
龙眼肉	*lóng yǎn ròu*	9 g	Arillus Longan
当归	*dāng guī*	9 g	Radix Angelicae Sinensis
生姜	*shēng jiāng*	2 pieces	Rhizoma Zingiberis Recens
大枣	*dà zǎo*	3 pieces	Fructus Jujubae

【Actions】
Boosts qi and supplements blood, fortifies the spleen and nourishes the heart
【Indications】
Hyphema and intraocular bleeding caused by deficiency of both the heart and spleen, and spleen failing to control the blood.

64. *Bǔ Zhōng Yì Qì Tāng* (Center-Supplementing and Qi-Boosting Decoction, 补中益气汤)

Treatise on the Spleen and Stomach (*Pí Wèi Lùn*, 脾胃论)

【Prescription】

黄芪	*huáng qí*	15 g	Radix Astragali
人参	*rén shēn*	5 g	Radix et Rhizoma Ginseng
炙甘草	*zhì gān cǎo*	8 g	Radix et Rhizoma Glycyrrhizae Praeparata cum Melle
当归	*dāng guī*	5 g	Radix Angelicae Sinensis
橘皮	*jú pí*	5 g	Pericarpium Citri Reticulatae
升麻	*shēng má*	5 g	Rhizoma Cimicifugae

| 柴胡 | *chái hú* | 5 g | Radix Bupleuri |
| 白术 | *bái zhú* | 5 g | Rhizoma Atractylodis Macrocephalae |

【Actions】
Boosts qi and fortifies the spleen, supplements qi and raises yang

【Indications】
Eye diseases caused by qi and blood deficiency, such as conjunctival edema, unopenable eye, blepharopotosis, blepha numbness, blepharospasm, retinitis pigmentosa, and senile cataract.

65. *Liù Wèi Dì Huáng Wán* (Six Ingredients Rehmannia Pill, 六味地黄丸)

Key to Diagnosis and Treatment of Children's Diseases (*Xiǎo Ér Yào Zhèng Zhí Jué*, 小儿药证直诀)

【Prescription】

熟地黄	*shú dì huáng*	12 g	Radix Rehmanniae Praeparata
山茱萸	*shān zhū yú*	6 g	Fructus Corni
干山药	*gān shān yào*	6 g	Rhizoma Dioscoreae
泽泻	*zé xiè*	5 g	Rhizoma Alismatis
茯苓	*fú líng*	5 g	Poria
牡丹皮	*mǔ dān pí*	5 g	Cortex Moutan

【Actions】
Nourishes water to moisten wood, supplements the kidney to improve vision

【Indications】
Eye diseases caused by yin-essence deficiency, such as pterygium, seasonal eye diseases, parenchymatous dryness of the conjunctiva, vitreous opacity, measles involving the eyes, frequent nictaition, and black eyelid (dark circles).

66. *Zhī Bǎi Dì Huáng Wán* (Anemarrhena, Phellodendron and Rehmannia Pill, 知柏地黄丸)

Golden Mirror of the Medical Tradition (*Yī Zōng Jīn Jiàn*, 医宗金鉴)

【Prescription】

熟地黄	*shú dì huáng*	12 g	Radix Rehmanniae Praeparata
山茱萸	*shān zhū yú*	6 g	Fructus Corni
干山药	*gān shān yào*	6 g	Rhizoma Dioscoreae
泽泻	*zé xiè*	5 g	Rhizoma Alismatis

茯苓	*fú líng*	5 g	Poria
牡丹皮	*mǔ dān pí*	5 g	Cortex Moutan
知母	*zhī mǔ*	5 g	Rhizoma Anemarrhenae
黄柏	*huáng bǎi*	5 g	Cortex Phellodendri Chinensis

【Actions】

Enriches yin and subdues fire, improves vision

【Indications】

Eye diseases caused by yin deficiency and effulgent fire, such as chronic conjunctivitis, subconjunctival hemorrhage, stromal keratitis, herpes simplex keratitis, ulcerative keratitis, iridocyclitis, hyphema and intraocular bleeding, glaucoma, blurred vision, tinted vision, sudden blindness, seeing still objects as moving.

67. *Qǐ Jú Dì Huáng Wán* (Lycium Berry, Chrysanthemum and Rehmannia Pill, 杞菊地黄丸)

The Advancement of Medicine (*Yī Jí*, 医级)

【Prescription】

熟地黄	*shú dì huáng*	12 g	Radix Rehmanniae Praeparata
山茱萸	*shān zhū yú*	6 g	Fructus Corni
干山药	*gān shān yào*	6 g	Rhizoma Dioscoreae
泽泻	*zé xiè*	5 g	Rhizoma Alismatis
茯苓	*fú líng*	5 g	Poria
牡丹皮	*mǔ dān pí*	5 g	Cortex Moutan
枸杞子	*gǒu qǐ zǐ*	8 g	Fructus Lycii
菊花	*jú huā*	5 g	Flos Chrysanthemi

【Actions】

Nourishes the liver and kidney, removes nebula to improves vision

【Indications】

Eye diseases caused by yin defiecency of the liver and kidney, such as cold tearing, dry eyes, parenchymatous dryness of the conjunctiva, iridocyclitis, senile cataract, retinitis pigmentosa, sudden blindness, and glaucoma.

68. *Míng Mù Dì Huáng Wán* (Eye Brightener Rehmannia Pill, 明目地黄丸)

A Close Examination of the Precious Classic on Ophthalmology (*Shěn Shì Yáo Hán*, 审视瑶函)

【Prescription】

熟地黄	shú dì huáng	12 g	Radix Rehmanniae Praeparata
山茱萸	shān zhū yú	6 g	Fructus Corni
干山药	gān shān yào	6 g	Rhizoma Dioscoreae
泽泻	zé xiè	5 g	Rhizoma Alismatis
茯神	fú shén	5 g	Sclerotium Poriae Pararadicis
牡丹皮	mǔ dān pí	5 g	Cortex Moutan
当归	dāng guī	5 g	Radix Angelicae Sinensis
柴胡	chái hú	3 g	Radix Bupleuri
五味子	wǔ wèi zǐ	6 g	Fructus Schisandrae Chinensis

【Actions】
Supplements the liver and kidney, benefits essence and improves vision
【Indications】
Optic atrophy and sudden blindness caused by liver and kidney yin deficiency

69. *Zuǒ Guī Wán* (Left-Restoring Pill, 左归丸)

The Complete Works of [Zhang] Jing-yue (*Jǐng Yuè Quán Shū*, 景岳全书)
【Prescription】

熟地黄	shú dì huáng	12 g	Radix Rehmanniae Praeparata
山茱萸	shān zhū yú	6 g	Fructus Corni
山药	shān yào	6 g	Rhizoma Dioscoreae
枸杞子	gǒu qǐ zǐ	6 g	Fructus Lycii
川牛膝	chuān niú xī	5 g	Radix Cyathulae
菟丝子	tù sī zǐ	6 g	Semen Cuscutae
鹿角胶	lù jiǎo jiāo	6 g	Colla Cornus Cervi
龟板胶	guī bǎn jiāo	6 g	Colla Testudinis Plastri

【Actions】
Nourishes yin and supplements the kidney
【Indications】
Eye diseases caused by liver and kidney deficiency leaning more to the kidney yin deficiency, including parenchymatous dryness of the conjunctiva, optic neuropathy, retinitis pigmentosa, seeing straight objects as inclined, reversed vision.

70. *Zēng Yè Tāng* (Humor-Increasing Decoction, 增液汤)

Systematic Differentiation of Warm Diseases (*Wēn Bìng Tiáo Biàn*, 温病条辨)

【Prescription】

玄参	*xuán shēn*	30 g	Radix Scrophulariae
麦冬	*mài dōng*	24 g	Radix Ophiopogonis
生地	*shēng dì*	24 g	Radix Rehmanniae

【Actions】
Increases fluids to moisten dryness

【Indications】
Combined with *Gān Lù Yǐn* (Sweet Dew Beverage, 甘露饮) to treat parenchymatous dryness of the conjunctiva caused by yin deficiency and dryness-heat.

71. *Dì Zhī Wán* (Rehmannia Root Pill, 地芝丸)

Ten Treatises of Li Dong-yuan (Dōng Yuán Shí Shū, 东垣十书)

【Prescription】

生地	*shēng dì*	20 g	Radix Rehmanniae
枳壳	*zhǐ qiào*	10 g	Fructus Aurantii
天门冬	*tiān mén dōng*	20 g	Radix Asparagi
菊花	*jú huā*	10 g	Flos Chrysanthemi

【Actions】
Nourishes yin to improves vision

【Indicatons】
Hyperopia

72. *Yòu Guī Wán* (Right-Restoring Pill, 右归丸)

The Complete Works of [Zhang] Jing-yue (Jǐng Yuè Quán Shū, 景岳全书)

【Ingredients】

熟地黄	*shú dì huáng*	12 g	Radix Rehmanniae Praeparata
山茱萸	*shān zhū yú*	5 g	Fructus Corni
山药	*shān yào*	6 g	Rhizoma Dioscoreae
枸杞子	*gǒu qǐ zǐ*	6 g	Fructus Lycii
鹿角胶	*lù jiǎo jiāo*	6 g	Colla Cornus Cervi
菟丝子	*tù sī zǐ*	6 g	Semen Cuscutae
杜仲	*dù zhòng*	6 g	Cortex Eucommiae
当归	*dāng guī*	5 g	Radix Angelicae Sinensis
肉桂	*ròu guì*	3 g	Cortex Cinnamomi
制附子	*zhì fù zǐ*	3 g	Radix Aconiti Lateralis Praeparata

【Actions】
Warms the kidney and supplements essence
【Indications】
Eye diseases caused by liver and kidney deficiency leaning more to the kidney yang deficiency, such as optic neuropathy and retinitis pigmentosa.

73. Zhù Jǐng Wán Jiā Jiǎn Fāng (Modified Long vistas pill, 驻景丸加减方)

Key Methods of Six Channels in Ophthalmology of Chinese Medicine (Zhōng Yī Yǎn Kē Liù Jīng Fǎ Yào, 中医眼科六经法要)

菟丝子	tù sī zǐ	15 g	Semen Cuscutae
楮实子	chǔ shí zǐ	15 g	Fructus Broussonetiae
茺蔚子	chōng wèi zǐ	12 g	Fructus Leonuri
枸杞子	gǒu qǐ zǐ	4 g	Fructus Lycii
车前子	chē qián zǐ	4 g	Semen Plantaginis
木瓜	mù guā	4 g	Fructus Chaenomelis
寒水石	hán shuǐ shí	6 g	Glauberitum
三七粉	sān qī fěn	1 g	Radix et Rhizoma Notoginseng
紫河车粉	zǐ hé chē fěn	6 g	Placenta Hominis (powder)
五味子	wǔ wèi zǐ	4 g	Fructus Schisandrae Chinensis

【Actions】
Supplements the liver and kidney, benefits essence and improves vision
【Indications】
Eye diseases caused by liver and kidney deficiency, including extenal oculopathy like dry eyes and parenchymatous dryness of the conjunctiva; internal oculopathy like tinted vision, blurred vision, vitreous opacity, senile cataract, optic atrophy, blindness, retinitis blindness, seeing straight objects as crooked, double vision, and late stage of gestational eye diseases.

74. Jú Jīng Wán (Chrysanthemum Eye Pill, 菊睛丸)

Formulas for Universal Relief (Pǔ Jì Fāng, 普济方)
【Prescription】

巴戟天	bā jǐ tiān	5 g	Radix Morindae Officinalis
五味子	wǔ wèi zǐ	15 g	Fructus Schisandrae Chinensis
枸杞子	gǒu qǐ zǐ	20 g	Fructus Lycii

| 肉苁蓉 | ròu cōng róng | 10 g | Herba Cistanches |
| 菊花 | jú huā | 25 g | Flos Chrysanthemi |

【Actions】
Enriches and nourishes the liver and kidney, stops tearing
【Indications】
Cold tearing caused by liver-kidney deficiency

75. *Shí Hú Yè Guāng Wán* (Dendrobium Night Vision Pill, 石斛夜光丸)

Enlightenment of Ophthalmology (*Yuán Jī Qǐ Wēi*, 原机启微)
【Prescription】

天门冬	tiān mén dōng	15 g	Radix Asparagi
麦冬	mài dōng	15 g	Radix Ophiopogonis
人参	rén shēn	15 g	Radix et Rhizoma Ginseng
茯苓	fú líng	15 g	Poria
熟地黄	shú dì huáng	15 g	Radix Rehmanniae Praeparata
生地	shēng dì	15 g	Radix Rehmanniae
牛膝	niú xī	10 g	Radix Achyranthis Bidentatae
杏仁	xìng rén	10 g	Semen Armeniacae Amarum
枸杞子	gǒu qǐ zǐ	10 g	Fructus Lycii
草决明	cǎo jué míng	12 g	Semen Cassiae
川芎	chuān xiōng	8 g	Rhizoma Chuanxiong
犀角	xī jiǎo	1.5–3 g	Cornu Rhinocerotis
白蒺藜	bái jí lí	8 g	Fructus Tribuli
羚羊角	líng yáng jiǎo	8 g	Cornu Saigae Tataricae
枳壳	zhǐ qiào	8 g	Fructus Aurantii
石斛	shí hú	8 g	Caulis Dendrobii
五味子	wǔ wèi zǐ	8 g	Fructus Schisandrae Chinensis
青葙子	qīng xiāng zǐ	8 g	Semen Celosiae
甘草	gān cǎo	8 g	Radix et Rhizoma Glycyrrhizae
防风	fáng fēng	8 g	Radix Saposhnikoviae
肉苁蓉	ròu cōng róng	8 g	Herba Cistanches
黄连	huáng lián	8 g	Rhizoma Coptidis
菊花	jú huā	10 g	Flos Chrysanthemi
菟丝子	tù sī zǐ	10 g	Semen Cuscutae
山药	shān yào	10 g	Rhizoma Dioscoreae

【Actions】

Enriches and nourishes the liver and kidney, supplements qi and blood, dispels wind and clears heat, dissipates stagnation and improves vision

【Indications】

Optic atrophy, sudden blindness, and blurred vision

76. *Zhēn Wŭ Tāng* (True Warrior Decoction, 真武汤)

Treatise on Cold Damage and Miscellaneous Diseases (*Shāng Hán Zá Bìng Lùn*, 伤寒杂病论)

【Prescription】

茯苓	*fú líng*	9 g	Poria
芍药	*sháo yào*	9 g	Radix Paeoniae Alba; Radix Paeoniae Rubra
生姜	*shēng jiāng*	9 g	Rhizoma Zingiberis Recens
白术	*bái zhú*	9 g	Rhizoma Atractylodis Macrocephalae
附子	*fù zĭ*	9–12 g	Radix Aconiti Lateralis Praeparata

【Actions】

Warm yang and promote urination

【Indications】

Sudden blindness caused by kidney yang deficency

77. *Sì Wèi Féi Ér Wán* (Four Ingredients Childhood-Malnutrition Rectifying Pill, 四味肥儿丸)

Standards for Diagnosis and Treatment (*Zhèng Zhì Zhŭn Shéng*, 证治准绳)

【Prescription】

芜荑	*wú yí*	6 g	Fructus Ulmi Macrocarpae Praeparata
神曲	*shén qū*	6 g	Massa Medicata Fermentata
麦芽	*mài yá*	6 g	Fructus Hordei Germinatus
黄连	*huáng lián*	6 g	Rhizoma Coptidis

【Actions】

Expels worms, disperses infantile malnutrition with accumulation (*gān*, 疳), and clears heat

【Indications】

Night blindness caused by worm accumulation

78. *Tuì Yì Sǎn* (Nebula-Removing Powder, 退翳散)

Ophthalmology Secretly Handed Down (*Yǎn Kē Mì Chuán*, 眼科秘传)
【Prescription】

当归	*dāng guī*	9 g	Radix Angelicae Sinensis
大黄	*dà huáng*	6 g	Radix et Rhizoma Rhei
防风	*fáng fēng*	6 g	Radix Saposhnikoviae
白芷	*bái zhǐ*	6 g	Radix Angelicae Dahuricae
木通	*mù tōng*	9 g	Caulis Akebiae
菊花	*jú huā*	9 g	Flos Chrysanthemi
蝉蜕	*chán tuì*	6 g	Periostracum Cicadae
蒺藜	*jí lí*	12 g	Fructus Tribuli
连翘	*lián qiào*	9 g	Fructus Forsythiae
甘草	*gān cǎo*	6 g	Herba Schizonepetae
桔梗	*jié gěng*	6 g	Radix Platycodonis
薄荷	*bò he*	4.5 g	Herba Menthae
石决明	*shí jué míng*	15 g	Concha Haliotidis

【Actions】
Dispels wind and clears heat, improves vision and removes nebula
【Indications】
Keratic pannus caused by wind-heat of the lung and the liver

Instructions for the Preparation and Intake of Medicinal Formulas:
1. Place the dried and crushed medicinals in a cooking pot.
2. Pour in water to cover the medicinals.
3. Cover with a lid and allow medicinals to steep for 30 to 45 minutes.
4. Bring to a boil, reduce heat, and simmer for 20–30 minutes.
5. Remove from the heat, filter out the dregs and allow the decoction cool to room temperature.
6. Drink in two divided doses per batch, per day.

Section 4　Acupuncture

Acupuncture and moxibustion are effective and safe, which is why they are widely used in the clinic. Because moxibustion is seldom used in ophthalmology, only acupuncture methods are introduced here. Many kinds of eye diseases may get better faster with a combined approach of medicinal therapy and acupuncture rather than just using Chinese medicinals alone. Moreover, for some stubborn eye diseases, especially for chronic and degenerative eye diseases, acupuncture can improve visual acuity, enlarge the visual field, and improve symptoms. It has been proven by many recent studies that acupuncture can stimulate blood circulation to the eye, regulate the function of ocular muscles, promote secretion of tears, regulate intraocular pressure, strengthen the function of the retina and optic nerve, protect visual function under ocular hypertension, improve visual acuity, and relieve pain. Acupuncture is also a good method for general visual care.

1. Commonly used Acupoints in Ophthalmology

■ **Acupoints around the eyes (12 points)**

1) **ST 1** (***chéng qì***): Between the infraorbital ridge and the eyeball, 0.7 *cun* directly below the pupil when the eyes are looking straight ahead. Puncture perpendicularly 0.5 – 1.5 *cun* along the infraorbital ridge. Do not lift and thrust the needle at this acupoint. Indications include sore red swollen eyes, tearing, night blindness, optic atrophy, wry eyes and mouth, frequent eyelid nictation, and many other internal oculopathies.

2) **BL 1** (***jīng míng***): 1 *fēn* superior to the inner canthus. When puncturing, ask patients to close the eyes, and then push the eyeball outward gently, puncture slowly in the depression between the eyeball and nasal bone to a depth of 0.5–1 *cun*. It is not advisable to lift and thrust. Indications include tearing on exposure to wind, itching and pain of the canthus, sore red swollen eyes, eye screen, pterygium, myopia, night blindness, color blindness, malnutrition involving the eyes and many other internal oculopathies.

3) ***Shàng jīng míng*** (上睛明; "above BL 1"): Several *fen* superior to BL 1 (*jīng míng*), the indication is almost the same as that of BL 1. Because there is less bleeding and pain when puncturing at this point, it can take the place of BL 1 or be used alternatively.

4) **BL 2** (*cuán zhú*): In the depression over the medial end of the eyebrow. Oblique puncture downward to a depth of 0.3–0.5 *cun*. Indications include pain of supraorbital bone, drooping of the eyelid, tearing on exposure to wind, red eye, dizziness, pain of the eyeball, blurred vision, and myopia.

5) *Yú yāo* (鱼腰): At the midpoint of the eyebrow, directly above the pupil. Horizontally puncture towards medial or lateral side for 0.5 *cun*. Indications include pain of supraorbital eyebrow, frequent eyelid nictation, drooping of the eyelid, squinting, wry eyes and mouth, sore red swollen eyes, and herpes simplex keratitis.

6) *Qiú hòu* (球后): At the junction of lateral 1/4 and medial 3/4 of the inferior border of the orbit. Puncture slowly along the infraorbital border. Indications include retinitis pigmentosa, optic atrophy, and other internal oculopathies.

7) **GB 14** (*yáng bái*): 1 *cun* above the middle of the eyebrow. Subcutaneously puncture to a depth of 0.4–0.8 *cun*. Indications include blepharospasm, drooping of the upper eyelid, weakness of the eyelid to open, pain in the external canthus, profuse discharge, night blindness.

8) **SJ 23** (*sī zhú kōng*): In the depression over the tip of the eyebrow. Horizontally puncture to 0.3–0.5 *cun*. Indications include frequent eyelid nictation, trichiasis, dizziness and headache, blurred vision.

9) **ST 2** (*sì bái*): 1 *cun* directly below the pupil, in the depression over the infraorbital foramen. Perpendicularly puncture for 0.2–0.3 *cun*. Indications include conjunctival congestion, eye itching and eye pain, keratitis, wry eyes and mouth, frequent eyelid nictation, headache and dizziness, myopia, and visual fatigue.

10) **GB 1** (*tóng zǐ liáo*): 0.5 *cun* lateral to the external canthus, in the depression over the extraorbital ridge. Puncture horizontally toward the back of the head or obliquely to a depth of 0.3–0.5 *cun*. Indications include red eye, eye pain, eye itching, tearing on exposure to wind, profuse discharge, eye nebula, optic atrophy, myopia.

11) *Tài yáng* (太阳): In the depression about 1 *cun* behind the midpoint between the lateral end of the eyebrow and the outer canthus. Perpendicularly or obliquely puncture for 0.3–0.5 *cun*. Indications include paralytic strabismus, wry eyes and mouth, red sore swollen eye, dry eye, optic atrophy, and night blindness.

12) **SI 18** (*quán liáo*): Directly below the external canthus, in the depression over the lower bonder of the zygomatic bone. Perpendicularly puncture to 0.3–0.5 *cun*. Indications include wry eyes and mouth, blepharospasm, and tearing on exposure to wind.

■ **Relative body acupoints (44 acupoints)**

1) **ST 3** (*jù liáo*): Directly below the middle of the eye, at the level of the inferior border of nasal ala. Perpendicularly puncture to a depth of 0.5–0.8 *cun*. Indications include bleparospasm, wry eyes and mouth, optic atrophy, myopia.

2) **ST 4** (*dì cāng*): About 0.4 *cun* from the angle of the mouth. Perpendicularly puncture to a depth of 0.2 *cùn* or horizontally puncture towards ST 6 (*jiá chē*) to 0.5–0.8 *cun*. Indications include night blindness, bleparospasm, wry eyes and mouth.

3) **ST 6** (*jiá chē*): Anterior and inferior to the ear lobe, at the prominent point of the masseter when biting the teeth tightly, or one finger-breadth anterior and superior to

the angle of the mandible, in the depression when opening mouth. Perpendicularly puncture to a depth of 0.3–0.4 *cun* or obliquely puncture towards ST 4 (*dì cāng*) to 0.7–0.9 *cun*. Indications include bleparospasm and wry eyes and mouth.

4) **LI 20 (*yíng xiāng*)**: In the nasolabial groove, at the level of the midpoint of the lateral border of ala nasi. Perpendicularly puncture to a depth of 0.1–0.2 *cun* or obliquely puncture to a depth of 0.3–0.5 *cun*. Indications include wry eyes and mouth, conjunctival congestion, photophobia, nasal obstruction, and tearing.

5) **GB 2 (*tīng huì*)**: Anterior to the intertragic notch, at the posterior border of the condyloid process of the mandible; the point is located with the mouth wide open. Perpendicularly puncture to a depth of 0.5 *cun*. Indications include bleparospasm and wry eyes and mouth, tearing and dizziness, blurred vision.

6) **SJ 20 (*jiǎo sūn*)**: In the depression over the superior angle of the ear conch. Horizontally puncture to a depth of 0.3–0.5 *cun*; moxibustion is also applicable. Indications include redness and swelling of the eyelids and conjunctiva, nebulous eye screen, dry eyes, clouded vision, double vision.

7) **SJ 17 (*yì fēng*)**: Behind the lobule of the auricle, in the depression between the mastoid process and the mandible. Perpendicularly puncture to a depth of 0.8–1.2 *cun*; moxibustion is also applicable. Indications include wry eyes and mouth, red and white nebula and membrane, photophobia and tearing, headache and dizziness, blurred vision, double vision, and many other internal eye diseases.

8) **GB 12 (*wán gǔ*)**: In the depression just posterior and inferior to the mastoid process. Perpendicularly puncture to a depth of 0.5–1 *cun*; moxibustion is also applicable. Indications include tearing, clouded vision, and many other internal eye diseases. This acupoint could be applied alternatively with GB 20 (*fēng chí*).

9) **SJ 16 (*tiān yǒu*)**: Anterior and posterior to the mastoid process, on the posterior border of sternocleidomastoid muscle and the level of the mandibular angle. Perpendicularly puncture to a depth of 0.8–1.2 *cun*. Indications include clouded vision, double vision, glaucoma, and sudden blindness.

10) **GB 15 (*tóu lín qì*)**: Directly above GB 14 (*yáng bái*), 0.5 *cun* within the natural hair line. Horizontally puncture to a depth of 0.5–0.8 *cun*; moxibustion is also applicable. Indications include headache and eye pain, red eye with profuse discharge, and cold tearing.

11) **GB 16 (*mù chuāng*)**: 1 *cun* behind GB 15 (*tóu lín qì*). Horizontally puncture to a depth of 0.5–0.8 *cun*; moxibustion is also applicable. Indications include redness and pain of the external canthus, white nebula of eye, optic atrophy, and myopia.

12) **GB 20 (*fēng chí*)**: In the depression between the upper ends of the sternocleidomastoid and trapezius muscles, at the level of DU 16 (*fēng fǔ*). Obliquely puncture 1–2 *cun* towards the fellow eye. Moxibustion is applicable. Indications include headache, dizziness, tearing, pain of the internal canthus,

squinting, drooping of the upper eyelids, double vision, seeing objects in altered color and shape, sudden blindness, optic atrophy, night blindness, senile cataract, blurred vision, and glaucoma.

13) **DU 16** (*fēng fǔ*): 1 *cun* directly above the midpoint of the posterior hairline. Slowly puncture towards the lower mandible to 0.5–1 *cun*. Indications include headache and eye pain, red sore swollen eyes, corneal nebula, and double vision.

14) **DU 20** (*bǎi huì*): 7 *cun* directly above the midpoint of the posterior hairline. Horizontally puncture to a depth of 0.5–0.8 *cun*. Indications include headache, acute conjunctivitis, and all kinds of internal eye diseases.

15) **DU 23** (*shàng xīng*): 1 *cun* directly above the midpoint of the anterior hairline. Horizontally puncture to a depth of 0.5–0.8 *cun*. Moxibustion is applicable. Indications include tearing on exposure to wind, red sore swollen eyes, and blurred vision.

16) **Shén cōng** (神聪): 1 *cun* anterior, posterior and lateral to DU 20 (*bǎi huì*). Horizontally puncture to a depth of 0.5–0.8 *cun*. Indications include blindness due to cerebral palsy and blepharospasm.

17) **Yì míng** (翳明): 1 *cun* posterior to SJ 17 (*yì fēng*). Perpendicularly puncture to a depth of 0.5–0.8 *cun*. Indications include initial cataract, retinitis pigmentosa, optic atrophy, sudden blindness, myopia, hyperopia, and double vision.

18) **LI 2** (*èr jiān*): In the depression of the radial side of index finger, distal to the metacarpophalangeal joint. Perpendicularly puncture to a depth of 0.2–0.3 *cun*. Indications include blurred vision, wry eyes and mouth, marginal blepharitis, and photophobia.

19) **LI 4** (*hé gǔ*): In the depression between the first and second metacarpophalangeal joint. Perpendicularly puncture to a depth of 0.5–0.8 *cun*. Indications include headache, wry eyes and mouth, tearing on exposure to wind, acute conjunctivitis, eye screen, night blindness in children, and many other external and internal eye diseases.

20) **LI 11** (*qū chí*): With the elbow flexed, in the depression at the lateral end of the transverse cubital crease. Perpendicularly puncture to a depth of 0.8–1 *cun*. Indications include redness and pain of the eye and blurred vision.

21) **LI 14** (*bì nào*): On the line connecting LI 11 (*qū chí*) and LI 15 (*jiān yú*), 7 *cun* above LI 11. Perpendicularly puncture to a depth of 0.5–1 *cun*, or obliquely puncture to a depth of 0.8–1.2 *cun*. Moxibustion is applicable. Indications include optic atrophy, dry eyes, and corneal nebula.

22) **HT 7** (*shén mén*): At the posterior-root of the metacarpus, in the depression of the radial side of the tendon of the ulnal flexor muscle of the wrist. Perpendicularly puncture to a depth of 0.3–0.4 *cun*. Moxibustion is applicable. Indications include dizziness, blurred vision, and hallucination.

23) **SI 3** (*hòu xī*): At the ulnar end of the distal transverse crease proximal to the fifth

matacarpophalangeal joint, when the fist is slightly clenched. Perpendicularly puncture to a depth of 0.5–0.8 *cun*. Moxibustion is applicable. Indications include eye nebula, headache and eye pain, tearing, and blepharitis.

24) **BL 6** (*chéng guāng*): 1.5 *cun* posterior to BL 5 (*wǔ chù*). Horizontally puncture to a depth of 0.3–0.5 *cun*. Indications include optic atrophy, myopia, dizziness, pain of the eye, and eye nebula.

25) **Dà gǔ kōng** (大骨空): On the dorsal crease of the thumb, at the center of the finger joint. Moxibustion is primarily applied. Indications include blepharitis, red sore swollen eye, dry eyes, photophobia, corneal nebula, glaucoma, and blurred vision.

26) **Xiǎo gǔ kōng** (小骨空): On the dorsal crease of the little finger, at the center of the proximal interphalangeal joint. Moxibustion is primarily applied. Indications include blepharitis, red sore swollen eye, eye nebula, and tearing on exposure to wind.

27) **PC 6** (*nèi guān*): 2 *cun* above the transverse crease of the wrist, between the two tendons of the palmaris longus muscle and flexor carpi radialis muscle. Perpendicularly puncture to a depth of 0.5–1 *cun*. Moxibustion is applicable. Indications include dizziness, blurred vision, hallucination, vitreous opacity, migraine, squinting, and glaucoma.

28) **SJ 5** (*wài guān*): On the dorsal side of the forearm, 2 *cun* above the transverse crease of the wrist, opposite to PC 6 (*nèi guān*). Perpendicularly puncture to a depth of 0.5–1 *cun*. Moxibustion is applicable. Indications include tearing on exposure to wind, blepharitis, actute redness and pain of the eye, myopia, eye nebula, dry eyes, and double vision.

29) **BL 18** (*gān shù*): On the back, below the spinous process of the 9th thoracic vertebra, 1.5 *cun* lateral to the posterior midline. Perpendicularly puncture to a depth of 0.5–1 *cun*. Moxibustion is applicable. Indications include redness and nebula of the eye, canthus blepharitis, tearing and discharge, up-turned eyes, night blindness, clouded vision, and many other internal eye diseases.

30) **BL 22** (*sān jiāo shù*): On the lower back, below the spinous process of the 1st lumbar vertebra, 1.5 *cun* lateral to the posterior midline. Perpendicularly puncture to a depth of 0.5–1 *cun*. Moxibustion is applicable. Indications include liver and kidney deficiency, blurred vision, optic atrophy, and night blindness.

31) **Bl 23** (*shèn shù*): On the lower back, below the spinous process of the 2nd lumbar vertebra, 1.5 *cun* lateral to the posterior midline. Perpendicularly puncture to a depth of 0.8–1 *cun*. Moxibustion is applicable. Indications include dizziness, blurred vision, optic atrophy, myopia, hyperopia, color blindness, and many other internal eye diseases.

32) **ST 36** (*zú sān lǐ*): On the anterior-lateral side of the leg, 3 *cun* below ST 35 (*dú bí*), one finger-breadth (middle finger) from the anterior crest of the tibia.

Perpendicularly puncture to a depth of 1.5–2 *cun*. Moxibustion is applicable. Indications include blepharospasm, drooping of the upper eyelid, visual fatigue, double vision, furuncle of the eyelid, and optic atrophy.

33) **SP 6 (*sān yīn jiāo*)**: On the medial side of the leg, 3 *cun* above the tip of the medial malleolus, posterior to the medial border of the tibia. Perpendicularly puncture to a depth of 0.5–1 *cun*. Moxibustion is applicable. Indications include yin deficiency of the liver, spleen and kidney, drooping of the upper eyelid, blurred vision, and other internal eye diseases.

34) **BL 62 (*shēn mài*)**: In the depression directly below the midpoint of the inferior border of the external malleolus. Perpendicularly puncture to a depth of 0.3–0.5 *cun*. Moxibustion is applicable. Indications include wry eyes and mouth, itching and pain of the medial canthus, red sore swollen eye, and squinting.

35) **KI 3 (*tài xī*)**: In the depression at the midpoint of the line connecting the tip of the medial malleolus and the Achilles tendon. Perpendicularly puncture to a depth of 0.5–0.8 *cun*. Moxibustion is applicable. Indications include clouded vision and dry eyes.

36) **GB 37 (*guāng míng*)**: 5 *cun* above the tip of the external malleolus, on the anterior border of the fibula. Perpendicularly puncture to a depth of 0.5–1 *cun*. Moxibustion is applicable. Indications include itching and pain of the eye, eye nebula, optic atrophy, retinitis pigmentosa, and other internal eye diseases.

37) **GB 38 (*yáng fǔ*)**: 4 *cun* above the tip of the external malleolus, slightly anterior to the border of the fibula. Perpendicularly puncture to a depth of 0.5–1 *cun*. Moxibustion is applicable. Indications include redness and pain of the lateral canthus, migraine and eye pain, tearing, and photophobia.

38) **LV 1 (*dà dūn*)**: On the lateral side of the big toe, 0.1 *cun* from the corner of the nail. Obliquely puncture to a depth of 0.1–0.2 *cun*. Indications include sudden blindness, intraocular bleeding, and acute angle closure glaucoma.

39) **LR 2 (*xíng jiān*)**: On the dorsum of the foot between the 1st and 2nd toes, proximal to the margin of the web. Perpendicularly puncture to a depth of 0.5–0.8 *cun*. Moxibustion is applicable. Indications include photophobia, wry eyes and mouth, retinitis pigmentosa, and optic atrophy.

40) **LR 3 (*tài chōng*)**: On the dorsum of the foot between the 1st and 2nd toes, in the depression 1.5 *cun* to LR 2. Perpendicularly puncture to a depth of 0.5–0.8 *cun*. Moxibustion is applicable. Indications include wry eyes and mouth, red sore swollen eye, and eye nebula.

41) **LR 5 (*lí gōu*)**: On the midline of the medial surface of the tibia, 5 *cun* above the tip of the medial malleolus. Horizontally puncture to a depth of 0.5–0.8 *cun*. Moxibustion is applicable. Indications include red sore swollen eye, dry eyes, and retinitis pigmentosa.

42) **RN 4 (*guān yuán*)**: 3 *cun* below the center of the umbilicus. Perpendicularly

puncture to a depth of 0.5–1 *cun*. Moxibustion is applicable. Indications include all kinds of internal eye diseases caused by deficiency, blurred vision, dry eyes, and retinitis pigmentosa. Moxibustion of the acupoint has effects of optic health care.

43) **DU 4 (*mìng mén*)**: In the depression below the spinous process of the 2nd lumbar vertebra. Perpendicularly puncture to a depth of 0.5–1 *cun*. Moxibustion is applicable. Indications include blurred vision, retinitis pigmentosa, optic atrophy, and forward-staring eyes.

44) **DU 14 (*dà zhuī*)**: In the depression below the spinous process of the 7th lumbar vertebra. Obliquely puncture to a depth of 0.3–0.5 *cun*. Bloodletting, venesection, cupping glass as well as moxibustion is applicable. Indications include blepharospasm, red eye and tearing, blepharitis, optic atrophy, glaucoma, blurred vision, and clouded vision due to taxation damage and deficiency detriment.

2. Acupuncture

■ **Point Selection**

The principle of selecting acupoints in the practice of TCM ophthalmic acupuncture is based on diagnosis and pattern differentiation, usually using whole-body pattern differentiation combined with local acupoints to obtain the goal of supporting healthy qi, dispelling pathogen, relieving sickness by dredging the channels and collaterals, regulating *zang-fu* organs, and regulating qi and blood. All the essence of the five *zang* and six *fu* flows upward to the eyes. Therefore, all the patholological conditions of the *zang*, *fu*, qi, blood, channels and collaterals should be taken into consideration when making a pattern differentiation.

All the vessels are related to the eyes. The eyes are abundant with channels, collaterals, qi and blood, and thus they may become vulnerable to disease. Therefore, needling the local acupoints around the eyes can have a direct and rapid impact on vision. Moreover, for certain types of local eye diseases without changes in the tongue and pulse, it is advisable to select local acupoints around the eyes. In clinical practice, we commonly select local points in combination with body acupoints; however, local points can be used alone in some cases, depending on the patient's condition.

■ **Needling Methods**

It was recorded in *The Yellow Emperor's Inner Classic* that needling channels which connect with the eye may cause blindness. It is well known that the eye is a delicate tissue, sensitive to algesia, and that there are many blood vessels in the orbital cavity. Improper needling may result in intraocular bleeding and traumatic cataract if the wall of the eyeball is penetrated by a needle. Therefore, point location must be extremely accurate and manipulation should be minimal and precise when needling the acupoints around the eyes. It is not advisable to use twirling, lifting and thrusting methods, especially for patients with hyperthyreosis, severe myopia, and adolescent glaucoma or post intraocular surgeries; doing so will cause ocular proptosis and thinning of the eyeball wall. After withdrawl of the needle, press the acupoint to prevent bleeding. Once there is subcutaneous bleeding or intraorbital bleeding, pressure dress after cold compress. Ordinarily, the bleeding will not cause more damage or aggravate the primary condition, or influence the therapeutic effect.

The eye contains the spirit water and spirit jelly; it is also abundant in essence and blood. Because it is a yin organ but acts as yang organ, it is easily damaged by heat pathogen; therefore, moxibustion was contraindicated in ancient times. Moreover, damage to the eye can easily occur when applying moxibustion carelessly around the eye, and thus it is not advisable to apply moxibustion around the eye unless necessary.

3. Scalp Acupuncture

Scalp acupuncture is a modern acupuncture method combining traditional Chinese acupuncture and the modern medical theory of the functional localization of the cerebral cortex. The scalp acupuncture positions of the optic area originate 1 cm lateral to the midpoint of the occipital protuberance and runs for 4 cm parallel to the anterior-posterior line in an anterior direction. Indications include hysterical blindness, cortical blindness, retinitis pigmentosa, optic atrophy, and other diseases of the visual pathway.

Manipulation: Arrange patients in a sitting or lateral decubitus position, localize the acupuncture area, and horizontally puncture a needle about 2.5–3 *cun* in length into the scalp area. With the shaft of the needle at the subcutaneous area, apply twisting but do not let the tip of the needle reach the periosteum. Then, twist the needle rapidly without lifting and thrusting; after the arrival of the needling sensation (tingling, numbness, and distention), retain the needle for 15–30 minutes. Apply twisting stimulation two times during the period of needle retention. After withdrawl of the needle, press the needle hole for several minutes to prevent bleeding.

4. Ear Acupuncture

Ear acupuncture treats eye diseases by simulating certain (tender) points on the auricle with filiform-needle, circular needle acupuncture, or ear seed pressing. This treatment modality is easy to administer, has a wide scope of indications, and provides some reference value in diagnosis.

■ **Commonly Used Auricular Points**

The locations and indications of commonly used auricular acupoints are shown in table 5-1:

Table 5-1 Location and Indications of Commonly Used Auricular Acupoints

Acupoints	Location	Indications
Eye (yǎn, LO5, 眼)	Center of the fifth area of the meatus auditorius	Acute inflammation of the eyelids, canthi, conjunctiva, cornea and iris; glaucoma; retinal diseases; adolescent myopia, hyperopia; and amblyopia
Artery of the fundus (yǎn dǐ dòng mài, 眼底动脉)	Midpoint of the inferior part of the third area of the ear lobe	Obstruction and inflammation of the retinal vessels
Fundus (yǎn dǐ, 眼底)	Midpoint of the superior part of the second area of the ear lobe	Acute, chronic, or old retinal diseases
Eye 2 (mù 2, 目2)	Anterior-posterior to the intertragic notch	Inflammation of the outer eye, glaucoma, refraction error, and amblyopia
Eye 1 (mù 1, 目1)	Anterior-inferior to the intertragic notch	Inflammation of the outer eye, glaucoma, refraction error, and amblyopia
Endocrine (nèi fēn mì, 内分泌)	In the tragic notch	Phlyctenular conjunctivitis, allergic eyelid dermatitis, conjunctivitis, glaucoma, retinal diseases
Brain (nǎo, 脑)	Medial surface of the antihelix	Paralytic ectropion, drooping of the upper eyelid, visual pathway diseases
Lung (fèi, 肺)	Superior, inferior, and posterior to the heart acupoint, in the shape of a horseshoe	Acute or chronic conjunctivitis, scleritis, edema of the retina and macula
Subcortex (pí zhì xià, 皮质下)	Medial surface of the antihelix	Paralytic ectropion, drooping of the upper eyelid, visual pathway diseases
Adrenal gland (shèn shàng xiàn, 肾上腺)	Tip of the lower border of the tragus	Retinal diseases, refraction error, amblyopia
Heart (xīn, 心)	In the central depression of the cavum concha	Ischemic optic neuropathy, retinal vasculopathy, myopia, amblyopia
Stomach (wèi, 胃)	Area where helix crus terminates	Drooping of the upper eyelid, hordeolum, hypopyon
Spleen (pí, 脾)	Inferior to the liver acupoint, adjacent to the edge of the antihelix	Drooping of the upper eyelid, hordeolum, retinal disease, myopia

continued

Acupoints	Location	Indications
Eyelid (*yǎn jiǎn*, 眼睑)	On the antihelix, at the same level of the supratragic notch	Drooping of the upper eyelid, stye, hordeolum, blepharitis, blepharospasm, paralytic ectropion
Liver (*gān*, 肝)	Posterior to the acupoints of stomach and duodenum	Acute or chronic keratitis, iritis, optic neuritis, myopia, amblyopia
Kidney (*shèn*, 肾)	The inferior margin of the inferior antihelix crus	Senile cataract, retinal diseases, myopia
Sympathesis (*jiāo gǎn*, 交感)	Tip of the inferior antihelix	Uveitis, glaucoma, retinal diseases, myopia
Cornea (*jiǎo mó*, 角膜)	In the triangular fossa of the auricle, close to the midpoint of the superior antihelix crus	Corneal disases
Optic nerve (*shì shén jīng*, 视神经)	Tip of the superior antihelix crus	Optic neuropathy
Inner canthus (*mù nèi zì*, 目内眦)	Scapha part, superior to the helix tubercle	Acute or chronic dacryocystisis, stenosis of lacrimal passage, pterygium, esotropia
Lens (*jīng zhuàng tǐ*, 晶状体)	Between the superior and inferior crura of the antihelix	Cataract
Lacrimal sac (*lèi náng*, 泪囊)	In the helix, close to the tip of superior antihelix crus	Acute or chronic dacryocystisis, stenosis of lacrimal passage
Ear apex (*ěr jiān*, 耳尖)	At the tip of the helix	Acute conjunctivitis, chalazion

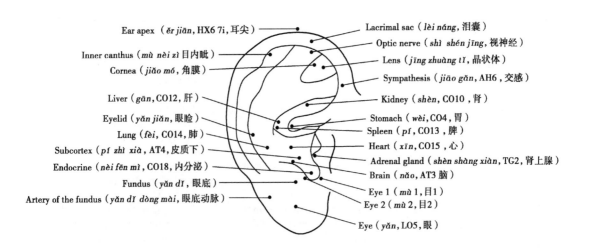

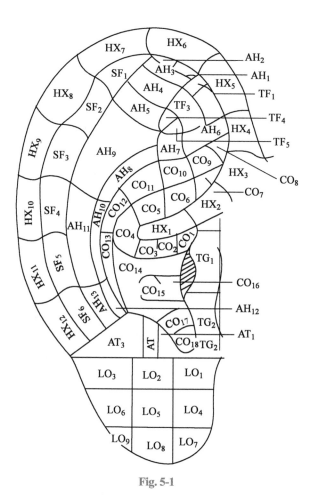

Fig. 5-1

■ **Manipulation**

Assess the patient in sitting position and locate the acupoints, looking for the tender points by pressing the auricle lightly with a filiform needle. Puncture the acupoints or tender points and twist the needle rapidly. The desired reaction is the intense but endurable pain felt by the patient. Retain the needle for 1–2 hours and twist it intermittently. Or, embed the specially made circular needle at the acupoint, but do not retain the needle for too long (usually 3–5 days is a treatment course, and there is a 5- to 7-day interval between courses). It is also applicable to compress the acupoints with tiny, hard seeds (such as vaccaria seed or mung bean), which are stuck on the adhesive plaster first before application. It is suggested to massage the acupoints several times a day; 3–7 days is a treatment course, with a 2- to 3-day interval of rest between courses.

Do not pierce the auricle when puncturing. It is forbidden to use this method on patients with chilblains on the ear or inflammation of the auricle and on pregnant women with habitual miscarriage. For elderly patients with hypertension, hypotension or heart disease, it is suggested to use a gentle manipulation and a shorter duration of needle retention; the patient should get some rest before or after acupuncture. Remove the ear seed promptly if the patient is allergic to the adhesive plaster.

5. Acupoint Injection

Acupoint injection is a method to treat eye diseases by injecting herbs into selected acupoints, and this method combines both herbal medicine and acupuncture in one treatment. It is primarily used to treat chronic internal diseases such as cataract, vitreous opacity, optic atrophy, old retinochoroiditis, retinitis pigmentosa, and ischemic oculopathy.

Commonly used drugs include Vitamin B_{12}, *Dāng Guī Zhù Shè Yè* (Angelica Injection, 当归注射液), *Fù Fāng Dān Shēn Zhù Shè Yè* (Compound Salviae Miltiorrhiza Injection, 复方丹参注射液), and *Fù Fāng Zhāng Liǔ Jiǎn Zhù Shè Yè* (Compound Anisodine Hydrobromide Injection, 复方樟柳碱注射液).

Manipulation: Choose 3–5 acupoints each time based on the patient's condition. It is advisable to combine methods of pattern-based point selection and local point selection when choosing acupoints. After routine disinfection, inject 0.3–2 ml of the chosen drug solution into each acupoint. Treatment is administered once a day or every other day, and generally 10 sessions equal a treatment course, with a 3- to 5-day period of rest in between courses.

6. Plum-Blossom Needle Therapy

A plum-blossom needle is a group of needles organized into the shape of a plum blossom. There are usually seven needles fixed on the top of an elastic needle handle. It gives shallow puncture through tapping the chosen skin area and acupoints. This method is applicable to many kinds of eye diseases, such as conjunctivitis, squinting, drooping of the upper eyelids, paralytic ectropion, myopia, cataract, glaucoma, optic atrophy, and retinitis pigmentosa. It treats eye diseases by moving qi and activating blood, dredging channels and collaterals, and supporting healthy qi and dispelling pathogen.

■ **Acupuncture Area**
➢ Head: Along the *du mai,* bladder channel, and gallbladder channel from the anterior hair line to the posterior hair line, and from the central to the lateral region of the head.
➢ Neck: Along the gallbladder channel, behind the ear, at the bilateral sides of the neck.
➢ Eye:
　• First line: From the inner side of the eyebrow to the tip of the eyebrow.
　• Second line: From the inner canthus to GB 1 (*tóng zǐ liáo*) over the closed upper eyelid.
　• Third line: From the inner canthus to GB 1 (*tóng zǐ liáo*) through the infraorbital margin.
➢ Back:

• First line: First line of the bladder channel along both sides of the spine.

• Second line: Second line of the bladder channel along both sides of the spine.

■ **Manipulation**

Tap the above parts with a plum-blossom needle. Manipulation and tapping is divided into mild, moderate, and heavy applications. In the mild tapping application, we tap lightly to hit the skin as lightly as possible; heavy tapping uses more strength and heavier impact on the skin for a longer period of time. A moderate tapping force is between the mild tapping and heavy tapping.

Tapping the skin with your wrist's movement and the elasticity of the needle handle, paying attention to keeping the needle perpendicular to the skin. Avoid oblique puncturing to prevent pain and bleeding. The tapping should be done with an even strength, rate of tapping, and area of coverage.

P A R T

II

Specific
Applications

Chapter 6
Eyelid Disorders

Section 1 Hordeolum (Stye)

Hordeolum, also commonly known as a stye, appears on the eyelid like a small boil in the shape of a wheat seed. Hordeolum is a common inflammatory condition of the eyelid glands. If the infection occurs in the sebaceous glands (Glands of Zeis) or sweat glands (Glands of Moll), it is called external hordeolum. If the infection occurs in the tarsal plate (Meibomian Glands), it is called internal hordeolum. Most hordeola are caused by Staphylococcus aureus infection. Hordeolum presents with pain, redness, swelling, and a nodule with pronounced tenderness of the infected area. It is more common in children and adolescents, but can also be seen in adults. The infection may be unilateral or bilateral with recurrent infections. In Western medicine, therapy for hordeola includes topical antibiotic eye drops or surgical care, depending on the extent of the condition.

In Chinese medicine, the disease is called *zhēn yǎn* (needle eye, 针眼), also known as *tǔ gān* (土疳), or *tǔ yáng* (土疡). The cause of the disease is associated with the invasion of pathogenic wind-heat at the site of the eyelid, excess heat in the spleen and stomach, and/or weakness of spleen qi. The main mechanism is the occurrence of pathogenic qi invading upward causing qi and blood stagnation on the eyelid. Because the disease is associated with pathogenic wind-heat invasion, poor dietary habits, and a constitutionally weak condition, it may be treated by regulating the whole body through pattern differentiation and treatment with flexible modification based on the principles of Chinese medicine, especially for severe and recurrent cases.

Clinical Manifestation

1. External Hordeolum

At the early stage, pain, redness, and swelling occur at the edge of the eyelid with marked tenderness. Later, the edema becomes localized and forms a hard nodule. If the condition is mild, all the symptoms may resolve spontaneously in a few days. If the condition is severe, a yellowish pustule may develop at the center of the affected area within 3 to 5 days. The lesion ruptures and discharge the pus spontaneously, thereby relieving pain and resolving the soreness and swelling. During the acute period, an external hordeolum may be accompanied by a tender pre-auricular lymph node. If the lesion is close to the outer canthus, it can cause reactive chemosis (inflammatory swelling of the conjunctiva) and severe pain.

2. Internal Hordeolum

Symptoms are the same as that of external hordeolum, except there might be a small abscess due to restriction of the tarsal plate. The affected palpebral conjunctiva shows localized hyperemia and swelling, and a yellowish pustule may develop within 2 to 3 days. Later, the pustule ruptures towards the conjunctival sac, relieving symptoms.

Treatment

1. Pattern Differentiation and Treatment

At the initial stage, the treatment principle is to clear heat, remove swelling, and dissipate redness, so as to resolve the severe inflammation, swelling, and soreness. If the pus is mature, the treatment should be to accelerate the pus to rupture on its own or expel it by means of drainage. For young patients with multiple recurrences due to weakness of the spleen-stomach, the treatment principle is to regulate the spleen and stomach, and to clear the remaining pathogenic heat.

(1) Wind-heat Invading the Eyelid

〖 Syndrome Characteristics 〗

Pain, redness, and swelling of the eyelid with a palpable nodule at the affected area, some accompanied by headache, red tongue with thin yellow coating, and a floating-rapid pulse.

〖 Treatment Principle 〗

Disperse wind and clear heat; resolve swelling and dissipate the mass

〖 Representative Formula 〗

Modified *Yín Qiào Sǎn* (Lonicera and Forsythia Powder, 银翘散)

〖 Prescription 〗

金银花	*jīn yín huā*	10 g	Flos Lonicerae Japonicae
连翘	*lián qiào*	10 g	Fructus Forsythiae
淡竹叶	*dàn zhú yè*	10 g	Herba Lophatheri
牛蒡子	*niú bàng zǐ*	10 g	Fructus Arctii
芦根	*lú gēn*	10 g	Rhizoma Phragmitis

荆芥	*jīng jiè*	10 g	Herba Schizonepetae
薄荷（后下）	*bò he (hòu xià)*	6 g	Herba Menthae (added later)
赤芍	*chì sháo*	10 g	Radix Paeoniae Rubra
夏枯草	*xià kū cǎo*	10 g	Spica Prunellae

【Modifications】
➢ For cases with severe swelling, add *huáng qín* (黄芩, Radix Scutellariae) 10 g to clear heat and disperse swelling.
➢ For cases with severe pain caused by stasis, add *zhì rǔ xiāng* (制乳香, Prepared Olibanum) 6 g and *mò yào* (没药, Myrrha) 6 g to break up stasis and relieve pain, dissipate blood stasis and disperse swelling.
➢ For cases with severe itching, add *fáng fēng* (防风, Radix Saposhnikoviae) 10 g, combined with *jīng jiè* (荆芥, Herba Schizonepetae) in the formula to disperse wind and stop itching.

(2) Heat Toxin Congestion and Exuberance
【Syndrome Characteristics】
Severe pain and redness, large palpable nodule with a burning sensation, tenderness and a visible yellow-white pus, often accompanied by fever, thirst, and constipation. Dark urine, red tongue with yellow coating, and a rapid pulse.
【Treatment Principle】
Clear heat and remove toxin, resolve swelling and stop pain
【Representative Formula】
Modified *Huáng Lián Jiě Dú Tāng* (Coptis Toxin-Resolving Decoction, 黄连解毒汤)
【Prescription】

黄芩	*huáng qín*	10 g	Radix Scutellariae
黄连	*huáng lián*	10 g	Rhizoma Coptidis
黄柏	*huáng bǎi*	10 g	Cortex Phellodendri Chinensis
栀子	*zhī zǐ*	10 g	Fructus Arctii
野菊花	*yě jú huā*	10 g	Flos Chrysanthemi Indici
牡丹皮	*mǔ dān pí*	10 g	Cortex Moutan
赤芍	*chì sháo*	10 g	Radix Paeoniae Rubra

【Modifications】
➢ For cases with constipation, add *dà huáng* (大黄, Radix et Rhizoma Rhei) 6 g to relieve constipation by purgation, invigorate blood and disperse swelling.
➢ For cases with thirsty feeling, add *tiān huā fěn* (天花粉, Radix Trichosanthis) 10 g, *lú gēn* (芦根, Rhizoma Phragmitis) 15 g to clear heat and promote fluid generation, resolve swelling, and evacuate pus.
➢ For cases with pus, add *chuān shān jiǎ* (穿山甲, Squama Manitis) 10 g and *zào jiǎo cì*

(皂角刺, Spina Gleditsiae) 10 g to express toxin and expel pus, invigorate blood, and disperse swelling.

(3) Spleen Deficiency Complicated by Excess

【 Syndrome Characteristics 】

Common in children, mild symptoms with multiple recurrence or multiple nodules at bilateral lids; accompanied by lusterless complexion, lack of strength and low food intake, poor appetite and digestion, loose stool, pale tongue, thready pulse.

【 Treatment Principle 】

Invigorate spleen and replenish qi, remove blood stasis and dissipate mass

【 Representative Formula 】

Modified *Sì Jūn Zǐ Tāng* (Four Gentlemen Decoction, 四君子汤)

【 Prescription 】

党参	*dǎng shēn*	10 g	Radix Codonopsis
白术	*bái zhú*	10 g	Rhizoma Atractylodis Macrocephalae
茯苓	*fú líng*	10 g	Poria
炙甘草	*zhì gān cǎo*	6 g	Radix et Rhizoma Glycyrrhizae Praeparata cum Melle
赤芍	*chì sháo*	10 g	Radix Paeoniae Rubra
刘寄奴	*liú jì nú*	10 g	Herba Artemisiae Anomalae
浙贝母	*zhè bèi mǔ*	10 g	Bulbus Fritillariae Thunbergii

【 Modifications 】

➢ For cases with prolonged swelling and stasis, add *zào jiǎo cì* (皂角刺, Spina Gleditsiae) 10 g, *hóng huā* (红花, Flos Carthami) 10 g to remove blood stasis and resolve swelling.

➢ For cases with poor digestion, add *shén qū* (神曲, Massa Medicata Fermentata) 10 g, *shān zhā* (山楂, Fructus Crataegi) 15 g, *jī nèi jīn* (鸡内金, Endothelium Corneum Gigeriae Galli) 10 g to invigorate the spleen and harmonize the stomach by dispersing and transforming food stagnation, which indirectly helps to disperse the stye.

2. Acupuncture

(1) Filiform Needling

Use a reduction method with moderate stimulation. Acupuncture points include:

tài yáng (太阳)	BL 2 (*cuán zhú*)	SJ 23 (*sī zhú kōng*)
GB 1 (*tóng zǐ liáo*)	*yú yāo* (鱼腰)	GB 14 (*yáng bái*)
ST 2 (*sì bái*)	ST 1 (*chéng qì*)	SJ 5 (*wài guān*)
LI 4 (*hé gǔ*)	LV 3 (*tài chōng*)	

Note: When selecting points around the eye, one should needle outside of the stye area.

(2) Pricking Method

Look for the pale red anthema along the two sides of T1–T7 thoracic vertebrae between the two scapulas. Prick the red anthema with a filiform needle, then squeeze and press to cause a little bleeding; wipe up the blood with a sterilized dry cotton ball, and repeat the bloodletting 3–5 times.

(3) Ear Acupuncture

Using the method of intermittent manipulation of the needle, Auricular points include eye (*yǎn*), liver (*gān*), spleen (*pí*), retaining the needle for 20 minutes, once a day. Or, induce bleeding with a three-edged needle at ear apex (*ěr jiān*) to break up stasis and resolve swelling.

3. Chinese Patent Medicines

(1) *Shuāng Huáng Lián Kǒu Fú Yè* (Honeysuckle Flower and Coptis Oral Solution, 双黄连口服液)

10 ml each time, three times a day; or take *Yín Qiào Jiě Dú* Tablet, four tablets each time, three times a day. Applicable to wind-heat invading the eyelid.

(2) *Huáng Lián Shàng Qīng Wán* (Coptis Upward-clearing Pill, 黄连上清丸)

6 g (6 tablets) each time, two times a day; applicable to heat toxin congestion and exuberance.

(3) *Shēn Líng Bái Zhú Sǎn* (Ginseng, Poria and Atractylodes Macrocephalae Powder, 参苓白术散)

6 g each time, two times a day; applicable to the pattern of spleen-stomach weakness.

4. Simple and Proven Recipes

(1) 9 g powder of raw *dǎn nán xīng* (胆南星, Arisaema cum Bile) and 15 g of *xiān dì huáng* (鲜地黄, Radix Rehmanniae Recens) are pounded into an ointment. Apply the ointment on *tài yáng* (太阳). Or, apply a powder made of green tea blended with rape oil on the infected area, 2–3 times per day. This therapy is applicable to hordeolum at the early stage.

(2) *Jīn yín huā* (金银花, Flos Lonicerae Japonicae) 15 g, *yě jú huā* (野菊花, Flos Chrysanthemi Indici) 15 g, *zǐ huā dì dīng* (紫花地丁, Herba Violae) 10 g, *pú gōng yīng* (蒲公英, Herba Taraxaci) 10 g, decocted with water for oral consumption; one batch per day divided into two doses. The method is applicable to patients with severe redness, swelling, and pain.

5. External Treatment

(1) Moist Heat Compress: Apply a moist, warm compress to the affected eye with hot water or the heated solution from dregs of the oral medicinal decoction.

(2) Crush fresh *pú gōng yīng* (Herba Taraxaci) and apply it to the affected area.

6. Treatment with Western Medicine

Please consult your physician or ophthalmologist for medical treatment.

Common therapies may include:

(1) Eye Drops: Antibiotic eye drops can be applied in severe cases, 3–4 times per day. Antibiotic ointment may also be used at night before bedtime, in order to prevent secondary conjunctival and/or corneal infection.

(2) Surgical Care: The veins of the eyelids (and face) have no vein valves, so do not squeeze or rub the stye before the abscess has formed, otherwise it can make the bacterial infection spread to the blood and can be potentially fatal. After the abscess forms, an incision and drainage should be done. For the external type, an incision is made through the skin parallel with the margin. For the internal type, an incision is made through the tarsal conjunctiva vertical to the margin.

7. Dietary Therapy and Preventive Care

(1) Generally, the digestive function of the spleen and stomach is weak in children and the elderly, so the emphasis should be on eating less food that may be difficult to digest. Examples include raw-cold foods, spicy foods, and fatty foods. These dietary adjuncts can help prevent the occurrence of styes.

(2) Never squeeze, rub, or prick the stye, as this may spread the infection.

(3) If the lesion ruptures and discharge pus, clean the pus right away to avoid direct exposure to the eye in order to reduce the potential for spreading the infection.

Case Studies

Zhang, a 4-year-old boy

【 Chief Complaint 】

The boy had recurrent hordeola on both eyelids for three months. He has had two unsuccessful surgeries after which the infections continue to return.

【 Examination 】

Two external hordeola about the size of mung beans were present on the upper lid of the right eye and the lower lid of the left eye, respectively, with mild tenderness.

【Medical History】

Other signs and symptoms included pale complexion, poor appetite with preference for sweet foods and cold drinks, loose stool, pale tongue with thin-white coating, thready pulse.

【Diagnosis】

TCM diagnosis: *Zhēn yǎn* (needle eye, 针眼)

Western medical diagnosis: Hordeolum

【Pattern Differentiation】

The spleen governs the muscles, which includes the eyelids. Poor diet damages the spleen and cause a deficiency of the spleen and stomach. Consequently, the eyelid is easily attacked by pathogens, resulting in hordeolum.

【Treatment Principles】

Fortify the spleen and promote digestion, transform phlegm, and dissipate mass.

【Prescription】

党参	*dǎng shēn*	6 g	Radix Codonopsis
茯苓	*fú líng*	6 g	Poria
炒白术	*chǎo bái zhú*	6 g	Rhizoma Atractylodis Macrocephalae (stir-fried)
陈皮	*chén pí*	3 g	Pericarpium Citri Reticulatae
川贝母	*chuān bèi mǔ*	6 g	Bulbus Fritillariae Cirrhosae
连翘	*lián qiào*	3 g	Fructus Forsythiae
白僵蚕	*bái jiāng cán*	3 g	Bombyx Batryticatus

The above medicinals were decocted. One batch was taken each day in two intervals for a total of 5 batches.

【Follow-up】

After three subsequent visits, the patient recovered. No recurrence was reported during a six-month follow-up.

Classic Quotes

《银海精微·睑生偷针》："人之患，目睑生小疖。俗曰偷针者何也。答曰：阳明胃经之热毒也。或因食壅热之物，或饮食太过，使胃经上充于眼目，故睑眦之间时发疮毒，俗名偷针。"

"What is the cause of small boils on the eyelid, commonly called needle eye? It is due to heat toxin in the *yangming* stomach channel, which is caused by excessive consumption of spicy and fatty food. The heat toxin attacks the eyelids through the stomach channel, producing sores, a condition commonly called 'needle eye'."

Essentials from the Silver Sea – Needle Eye (*Yín Hǎi Jīng Wēi – Jiǎn Shēng Tōu Zhēn*, 银海精微·睑生偷针)

Section 2 Blepharitis

Blepharitis is a kind of subacute or chronic inflammation of the surface of the palpebral margin, eyelash follicles, and its accessory glands. It is a common ocular surface disorder characterized by persistent and annoying irritation. Generally, the symptoms are more severe than the clinical signs. Blepharitis often attacks both eyes and is hard to cure. The disease may linger for a very long period and the intensity of the manifestations may range from intermittently mild to severe.

In TCM, blepharitis pertains to red ulceration of the palpebral margin (*jiǎn xián chì làn*, 睑弦赤烂) or wind palpebral margin and red eye (*fēng xián chì yǎn*, 风弦赤眼). The cause is associated with the accumulation of heat or damp-heat in the spleen and stomach with a co-existing attack of either external in the spleen and the stomach. Heart fire hyperactivity combined with wind pathogen may be another causative factor. The pathogenesis is due to wind-fire flaming upward and burning the canthi. Because the disease is hard to cure, it is better to combine Western medicine and TCM treatment modalities, which can both alleviate the symptoms and promote recovery.

Clinical Manifestation

Based on the underlying cause and clinical manifestation, blepharitis is divided into three types Table 6-1:

Table 6-1   Etiology and Diagnosis of Three Types of Blepharitis

Type	Squamous Blepharitis	Ulcerative Blepharitis	Angular Blepharitis
Cause	Meibomian glands secrete excessive amounts of oil, and bacteria decomposes the lesion into irritative free fatty acids	Inflammation of the ciliary follicles and accessory glands, mostly caused by staphylococcus aureus	Infected by Morax-Axenfield bacteria, or can be related to vitamin B_2 deficiency
Risk factors	Ametropia, asthenopia, malnutrition, bad cosmetics	Malnutrition, chronic systemic diseases, anemia, poor hygiene	Poor hygiene, malnutrition
Clinical manifestation	Unbearable itching, prickly pain, hyperemia and redness and swelling of the margin of the eyelid, gray-white flakes or scales around eyelash roots	Burning pain. ulcerations and crust at the root of eyelashes, trichiasis or alopecia palpebralis	Itching, hyperemia, swelling or erosion mainly on the lateral canthus

The condition may cause complications including:
➤ Abnormalities of the eyelashes such as trichiasis, eyelash whitening, or loss of eyelashes

➢ Styes or recurrent chalazion
➢ Brandy nose (red acne), eczema of lower eyelid
➢ Lower eyelid ectropion, epiphora due to dacryon swelling and blockage
➢ Peripheral corneal infiltration and ulcer
➢ Corneal scar and neovascularization especially on the bottom area
➢ Dry eyes due to dysfunction of tear film

Treatment

1. Pattern Differentiation and Treatment

(1) Wind-heat (Squamous)

【 Etiology & Pathomechanism 】
Accumulated heat in the spleen-stomach and recurring attack by pathogenic wind, resulting in dryness caused by consumption of body fluids

【 Syndrome Characteristics 】
Redness and swelling of the eyelid margin, stinging itching, prickly pain, white flakes or scales around eyelash root, red tongue with yellow coating, floating-rapid pulse.

【 Treatment Principle 】
Dispel wind and arrest itching, clear heat, and cool the blood

【 Representative Formula 】
Modified *Yín Qiào Sǎn* (Lonicera and Forsythia Powder, 银翘散)

【 Prescription 】

金银花	*jīn yín huā*	10 g	Flos Lonicerae Japonicae
连翘	*lián qiào*	10 g	Fructus Forsythiae
淡竹叶	*dàn zhú yè*	10 g	Herba Lophatheri
牛蒡子	*niú bàng zǐ*	10 g	Fructus Arctii
芦根	*lú gēn*	10 g	Rhizoma Phragmitis
荆芥	*jīng jiè*	10 g	Herba Schizonepetae
薄荷（后下）	*bò he (hòu xià)*	6 g	Herba Menthae (added later)
赤芍	*chì sháo*	10 g	Radix Paeoniae Rubra
生甘草	*shēng gān cǎo*	10 g	Radix et Rhizoma Glycyrrhizae
桔梗	*jié gěng*	10 g	Radix Platycodonis
淡豆豉	*dàn dòu chǐ*	10 g	Semen Sojae Praeparatum

【 Modifications 】
➢ For cases with severe redness and burning sensation, add *chì sháo* (赤芍, Radix Paeoniae Rubra) 10 g, *mǔ dān pí* (牡丹皮, Cortex Moutan) 10 g to clear heat, cool

blood and eliminate stasis.

➤ For cases with abnormal exuberance of wind and severe itching, add *chán tuì* (蝉蜕, Periostracum Cicadae) 6 g, *wū shāo shé* (乌梢蛇, Zaocys) 6 g to calm wind and relieve itching.

➤ For cases with eye aningeresting, add *tiān huā fěn* (天花粉, Radix Trichosanthis) 10 g to promote fluid production and moisten dryness.

(2) Damp-heat (Ulcerative)
【 Etiology & Pathomechanism 】
Damp-heat of the spleen and stomach, external contraction of external wind, wind-damp-heat attacking the peripheral margin
【 Syndrome Characteristics 】
Itching, burning pain of the limbus palpebrails, redness and erosion, trichiasis or alopecia palpebralis, red tongue with yellow and greasy coating, soft-rapid pulse.
【 Treatment Principle 】
Clear heat and remove dampness, dispel wind and arrest itching
【 Representative Formula 】
Modified *Chú Shī Tāng* (Dampness-Eliminating Decoction, 除湿汤)
【 Prescription 】

防风	*fáng fēng*	10 g	Radix Saposhnikoviae
荆芥	*jīng jiè*	10 g	Herba Schizonepetae
黄芩	*huáng qín*	10 g	Radix Scutellariae
黄连	*huáng lián*	6 g	Rhizoma Coptidis
连翘	*lián qiào*	10 g	Fructus Forsythiae
茯苓	*fú líng*	10 g	Poria
滑石（包煎）	*huá shí (bāo jiān)*	6 g	Talcum (wrap)
车前子（包煎）	*chē qián zǐ (bāo jiān)*	10 g	Semen Plantaginis (wrap)
枳壳	*zhǐ qiào*	10 g	Fructus Aurantii
陈皮	*chén pí*	10 g	Pericarpium Citri Reticulatae
炒白术	*chǎo bái zhú*	10 g	Rhizoma Atractylodis Macrocephalae (dry-fried)
甘草	*gān cǎo*	6 g	Radix et Rhizoma Glycyrrhizae

【 Modifications 】
➤ For cases with severe cauterization, add *jīn yín huā* (金银花, Flos Lonicerae Japonicae) 10 g, *pú gōng yīng* (蒲公英, Herba Taraxaci) 10 g, *zhī zǐ* (栀子, Fructus Gardeniae) 10 g to clear heat.
➤ For cases with diabrosis and erosion of the affected part, add *cāng zhú* (苍术, Rhizoma Atractylodis) 10 g, *huáng bǎi* (黄柏, Cortex Phellodendri Chinensis) 10 g to

reinforce the function of eliminating dampness.

(3) Up-flaming Heart Fire (Angular)

【 Etiology & Pathomechanism 】

Excess heart fire and external contraction of pathogen wind flaming upward and burning the canthus

【 Syndrome Characteristics 】

Redness, itching, and swelling of the canthus, may be accompanied by erosion, red tongue tip, thin coating, rapid pulse.

【 Treatment Principle 】

Clear heart heat and reduce fire

【 Representative Formula 】

Modified *Dǎo Chì Sǎn* (导赤散, Red Guiding Powder) combined *Huáng Lián Jiě Dú Tāng* (黄连解毒汤, Coptis Toxin-Resolving Decoction)

【 Prescription 】

生地	*shēng dì*	15 g	Radix Rehmanniae
金钱草	*jīn qián cǎo*	10 g	Herba Lysimachiae
黄芩	*huáng qín*	10 g	Radix Scutellariae
黄连	*huáng lián*	6 g	Rhizoma Coptidis
黄柏	*huáng bǎi*	10 g	Cortex Phellodendri Chinensis
生甘草	*shēng gān cǎo*	3 g	Radix et Rhizoma Glycyrrhizae
栀子	*zhī zǐ*	6 g	Fructus Gardeniae

【 Modification 】

➢ For cases with severe hyperemia of the affected part, add *chì sháo* (赤芍, Radix Paeoniae Rubra) 10 g, *mǔ dān pí* (牡丹皮, Cortex Moutan) 10 g to cool blood and relieve redness.

➢ For cases with unbearable itching, add *dì fū zǐ* (地肤子, Fructus Kochiae) 10 g, *bái xiān pí* (白鲜皮, Cortex Dictamni) 10 g, *fáng fēng* (防风, Radix Saposhnikoviae) 10 g, *chuān xiōng* (川芎, Rhizoma Chuanxiong) 6 g to calm wind and relieve itching.

2. Chinese Patent Medicines

Blepharitis is a disease with a long course, and high rate of recurrence. Chinese patent formulas are easy to take and readily accessible, and they retain their potency. It has, for the most part, the same effect as the traditional decoction form if prescribed with the correct pattern differentiation.

(1) *Yín Qiào Jiě Dú Wán* (Lonicera and Forsythia Toxin-Resolving Pill, 银翘解毒丸)

1 pill, two to three times a day, taken with warm water; applicable to wind-heat.

(2) *Chái Yín Kǒu Fú Yè* (Bupleurum, Lonicera and Forsythia Oral Drink, 柴银口服液)

20 ml (a vial), three times a day; applicable to wind-heat.

(3) *Lóng Dǎn Xiè Gān Wán* (Gentian Liver-Draining pill, 龙胆泻肝丸)

6 g, three times a day, applicable to damp-heat.

(4) *Zhī Zǐ Jīn Huā Wán* (Fructus Gardeniae and Flos Lonicerae Japonicae Pill, 栀子金花丸)

9 g, once a day; applicable to up-flaming heart fire.

(5) *Niú Huáng Jiě Dú Wán* (Bovine Bezoar Toxin-Expelling Tablets, 牛黄解毒丸)

1 pill (3 g), three times a day; applicable to up-flaming heart fire.

3. External Treatment

(1) Fumigation and Washing

Expose the lesion thoroughly so that the external medicinal application can reach the affected area. Common washing solutions include 0.9% sodium chloride injection and 3% boric acid. Warm boiled water or cooled boiled water can also be used to clean scales and pus scabs in the palpebral margin as well as interfollicular pus. Chinese medicinal therapy is another good option. The following are the ingredients of a representative formula: *Qiān lǐ guāng* (千里光, Herba Senecionis Scandentis) 30 g, *bái xiān pí* (白鲜皮, Cortex Dictamni) 15 g, *kǔ shēn* (苦参, Radix Sophorae Flavescentis) 30 g, *yě jú huā* (野菊花, Flos Chrysanthemi Indici) 15 g, *pú gōng yīng* (蒲公英, Herba Taraxaci) 30 g, and *shé chuáng zǐ* (蛇床子, Fructus Cnidii) 30 g. Fumigate and wash the affected eye with the decoction, 2 or 3 times a day.

(2) Eye Drop or Eye Ointment

Apply 0.5% zinc sulfate eye drops and antibiotic eye drops in the affected eye, 3–4 times a day. It is also applicable to smear yellow mercury oxide ophthalmic ointment on the cleaned palpebral margin with a cotton swab.

4. Dietary Therapy and Preventive Care

(1) Keep good ocular hygiene and avoid exposure to wind, sand, and flue dust.

(2) Correct ametropia and avoid excessive use of the eyes.

(3) Limit smoking, alcohol, and spicy food.

(4) Treat the underlying systemic diseases promptly.

(5) Adjust the diet, adding sufficient vegetables and fruits as well as foods rich in protein and vitamins.

(6) Do not use highly perfumed shampoo and soap; limit or stop the use of eye makeup.

Case Studies

Qiao, a 34-year-old-female

Initial visit: March 21, 1991

【 Chief Complaint 】

Eyelid itching, a prickly-burning sensation, and shedding of flakes

【 Medical History 】

She had been treated for an allergy of the eyelid skin and blepharitis in another hospital. The disease was intermittently light to severe, alternately. In the two weeks prior to this visit, she felt unbearable itching and heat sensations after working overtime (the patient was a chef at a restaurant). She had expressed that she felt a state of constant anxiety, along with dry eyes and a dry mouth.

【 Examination 】

Normal vision, redness of the upper and lower eyelids on both eyes, white flakes in the eyelash roots, red and irritated eyelid, conjunctival congestion, normal cornea and fundus. Floating and wiry pulse, red tongue with little fluid and thin white coating.

【 Diagnosis 】

Western diagnosis: Red ulceration of palpebral margin (squamous blepharitis)

【 Pattern Differentiation 】

Wind and heat contend with each other, transforming into dryness and damaging fluid, then causing blood and fluid deficiency.

【 Treatment Principles 】

Dispel wind and clear heat, nourish yin and moisten dryness.

【 Prescription 】

Modified *Chái Hú Sǎn* (Bupleurum Powder, 柴胡散)

柴胡	*chái hú*	10 g	Radix Bupleuri
防风	*fáng fēng*	10 g	Radix Saposhnikoviae
荆芥	*jīng jiè*	10 g	Herba Schizonepetae
羌活	*qiāng huó*	6 g	Radix et Rhizoma Notopterygii
赤芍	*chì sháo*	10 g	Radix Paeoniae Rubra
生地	*shēng dì*	10 g	Radix Rehmanniae
当归	*dāng guī*	10 g	Radix Angelicae Sinensis
玄参	*xuán shēn*	10 g	Radix Scrophulariae
天花粉	*tiān huā fěn*	10 g	Radix Trichosanthis
生甘草	*shēng gān cǎo*	6 g	Radix et Rhizoma Glycyrrhizae

All medicinals were decocted with water; 1 dose each day and seven doses in total. The patient was also asked to stop the use of Western medicine.

【 Follow-up 】

After seven days of treatment by TCM, the patient visited our clinic again on April 6, 1991. She felt the symptoms of itching were greatly improved, and she no longer had a dry mouth. The eyelid margin was slightly red, the flakes among eyelash roots were diminished. So, the formula was again administered with modifications. At her last visit, the redness of the eyelid had disappeared, and flakes were barely noticeable. The patient had no complaints of discomfort. She was asked to take the decoction twice a week, for an additional 2–3 weeks, for a full recovery.

Questions for Consideration

1. What are the complications of blepharitis?

2. A patient presents with itching, burning pain of limbus palpebrails, redness and erosion, trichiasis or alopecia palpebralis, a red tongue with yellow and greasy coating, and a soft and rapid pulse. Write out the TCM treatment principle and representative formula.

3. State the dietary treatment and Preventive Care for blepharitis.

Section 3 Blepharoptosis

The upper lid normally rests approximately midway between the superior limbus and the pupillary margin. Blephroptosis is a condition in which one or both upper lids assume an abnormally low position due to partial or complete functional loss of the levator muscles (innervated by oculomotor nerve) and Müller muscles (innervated by cervical sympathetic). The classification and treatment principles of blepharoptosis are in the table below.

In Chinese medicine, this disease is called drooping of the upper eyelid (上胞下垂), also known as *zhuī mù* (睢目), *qīn fēng* (侵风), and in severe cases, *jiǎn fèi* (睑废). The cause and pathogenesis of the disease can be associated with levator maldevelopment due to prenatal essence deficiency, which results in drooping of the upper eyelid. Another cause is associated with middle qi insufficiency due to spleen deficiency, which results in clear yang failing to ascend and failure of yang qi to ascend to the upper eyelid. Eyelid muscle retardation and apaxia are caused by wind-phlegm obstruction in the collaterals due to accumulation of dampness and phlegm. It is suggested that patients see a Western doctor first to identify the underlying cause of the disease. Neostigmine test is needed if myasthenia gravis is suspected.

Congenital ptosis is mainly treated by surgical treatment. For the cases caused by nervous system dysfunction, or ocular and other systemic disorders, besides the necessary etiotropic Western therapies, TCM treatment (including medicinals and acupuncture) is

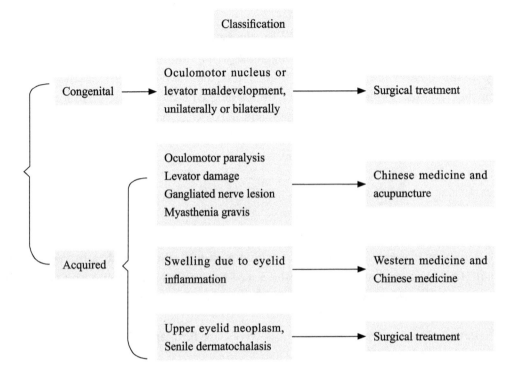

Classification

highly effective with few side effects.

Clinical Manifestation

1. Gradings of Blepharoptosis

Based on the position of lid margin at the orthophoria state, blepharoptosis is divided into three grades:

Mild: the upper limbus of the cornea is covered by the lid more than 3 mm

Moderate: 1/2 of the cornea is covered

Severe: more than 1/2 of the cornea is covered

2. Other Manifestations

(1) Blepharoptosis patients present with an obvious elevated eyebrow and wrinkles in the forehead on the affected side; this is due to the contraction of the frontalis muscle to compensate for the insufficient function of the levator. For those patients with bilateral ptosis, they may often need to tip their heads back into a chin-up position to see. Some congenital ptosis patients may also present with limited eyeball superducts when combined with functional defect or paralysis of the attolens oculi.

(2) The acquired blephroptosis patients may often have other underlying medical histories and symptoms. For example, the patients suffering from myasthenia gravis present with mild drooping of the eyelids in the morning and severe drooping in the afternoon. The cases caused by Horner syndrome due to cervical sympathetic nerve compression present with a light drooping of the eyelid (< 2mm) resulting from Müller muscle paralysis, accompanied by miosis at the same side and reduction of sweat secretion.

Treatment

1. Pattern Differentiation and Treatment

(1) Congenital Insufficiency
【Syndrome Characteristics】
Bilateral ptosis and persistent wrinkles in the forehead, possibly accompanied by fatigue and weakness, lusterless complexion, fear of cold and cold limbs, long voidings of clear urine, dusky tongue with thin coating, and deep-thready pulse.
【Treatment Principle】
Warm the kidney and strengthen the spleen
【Representative Formula】
Modified *Yòu Guī Yǐn* (Right-Restoring Drink, 右归饮)
【Prescription】

熟地	*shú dì*	12 g	Radix Rehmanniae Praeparata
淮山药	*huái shān yào*	6 g	Rhizoma Dioscoreae
山茱萸	*shān zhū yú*	3 g	Fructus Corni
枸杞子	*gǒu qǐ zǐ*	6 g	Fructus Lycii
杜仲	*dù zhòng*	6 g	Cortex Eucommiae
肉桂	*ròu guì*	3 g	Cortex Cinnamomi
制附子	*zhì fù zǐ*	3 g	Radix Aconiti Lateralis Praeparata
炙甘草	*zhì gān cǎo*	3 g	Radix et Rhizoma Glycyrrhizae Praeparata cum Melle
党参	*dǎng shēn*	6 g	Radix Codonopsis

【Modifications】
➢ For cases without cold limbs and fear of cold, remove *zhì fù zǐ* (制附子, Radix Aconiti Lateralis Praeparata).
➢ For cases with diarrhea, add *zhì huáng qí* (炙黄芪, Radix Astragali Praeparata cum Melle) 12 g, *chǎo bái zhú* (炒白术, dry-fried Rhizoma Atractylodis Macrocephalae) 6 g to replenish qi, invigorate the spleen, and stop diarrhea.

(2) Spleen Qi Deficiency

【 Syndrome Characteristics 】

Ptosis is mild in the early morning and aggravated in the afternoon or after exertion. The severe cases may have difficulties in moving the eyeballs and diplopia. The patients may often present with mental fatigue and poor appetite, pale tongue with whitish thin coating, and weak pulse.

【 Treatment Principle 】

Benefit qi and elevate yang

【 Representative Formula 】

Modified *Bǔ Zhōng Yì Qì Tāng* (Center-Supplementing and Qi-Boosting Decoction, 补中益气汤)

【 Prescription 】

炙黄芪	*zhì huáng qí*	15 g	Radix Astragali Praeparata cum Melle
人参(或党参)	*rén shēn* (or *dǎng shēn*)	10 g (15 g)	Radix et Rhizoma Ginseng (Radix Codonopsis)
炒白术	*chǎo bái zhú*	10 g	Rhizoma Atractylodis Macrocephalae (dry-fried)
陈皮	*chén pí*	6 g	Pericarpium Citri Reticulatae
当归	*dāng guī*	10 g	Radix Angelicae Sinensis
升麻	*shēng má*	3 g	Rhizoma Cimicifugae
柴胡	*chái hú*	3 g	Radix Bupleuri
炙甘草	*zhì gān cǎo*	5 g	Radix et Rhizoma Glycyrrhizae Praeparata cum Melle

【 Modifications 】

➢ For cases with oculogyria difficulties and diplopia, add *mù guā* (木瓜, Fructus Chaenomelis) 10 g, *bái jiāng cán* (白僵蚕, Bombyx Batryticatus) 10 g, *quán xiē* (全蝎, Scorpio) 3 g to subdue wind and dredge the collaterals.

➢ For cases with poor appetite, add *huái shān yào* (淮山药, Rhizoma Dioscoreae) 10g, *biǎn dòu* (扁豆, Semen Lablab Album) 10 g, *shā rén* (砂仁, Fructus Amomi) 3g to strengthen the spleen and stimulate the appetite.

(3) Wind-phlegm Obstructing Collaterals

【 Syndrome Characteristics 】

Sudden onset of ptosis, accompanied by oculogyria limitation, anorthopia, and diplopia. Other symptoms may include dizziness, nausea, upwelling and spitting of sputum, thick-greasy tongue coating, and thready, slippery pulse.

【 Treatment Principle 】

Expel wind and resolve phlegm, relax the channels and dredge the collaterals

【 Representative Formula 】
Modified *Zhèng Róng Tāng* (正容汤, Face-Restoring Decoction)
【 Prescription 】

羌活	*qiāng huó*	5 g	Radix et Rhizoma Notopterygii
防风	*fáng fēng*	5 g	Radix Saposhnikoviae
秦艽	*qín jiāo*	6 g	Radix Gentianae Macrophyllae
胆南星	*dǎn nán xīng*	3 g	Arisaema cum Bile
白附子	*bái fù zǐ*	5 g	Rhizoma Typhonii
姜半夏	*jiāng bàn xià*	9 g	Rhizoma Pinelliae Praeparatum
木瓜	*mù guā*	6 g	Fructus Chaenomelis
白僵蚕	*bái jiāng cán*	6 g	Bombyx Batryticatus
黄松节（抱木茯神）	*huáng sōng jié (bào mù fú shén)*	6 g	Lignum Pini Nodi
炙甘草	*zhì gān cǎo*	3 g	Radix et Rhizoma Glycyrrhizae Praeparata cum Melle
生姜	*shēng jiāng*	3 sheets	Rhizoma Zingiberis Recens

【 Modifications 】
> For cases with prolonged eye movement disorder, add *dāng guī* (当归, Radix Angelicae Sinensis) 10 g, *dān shēn* (丹参, Radix et Rhizoma Salviae Miltiorrhizae) 10 g to enhance the effects of nourishing the blood and dredging the collaterals.
> For cases with dizziness, upwelling and spitting of sputum, add *gōu téng* (钩藤, Radix Uncariae Macrophyllae) 10 g, *zhú lì* (竹沥, Succus Bambusae) 10 g to calm the liver, extinguish wind, and dissolve phlegm.

2. Acupuncture

(1) For cases with insufficiency of essence and decline of the fire from the gate of life, use a reinforcing method; acupuncture points include:

BL 2 (*cuán zhú*)	LV 2 (*xíng jiān*)	KI 1 (*yǒng quán*)
KI 3 (*tài xī*)		

(2) For cases with spleen qi deficiency with clear yang failing to ascend, choose acupuncture points below, still use a reinforcing method; it can be combined with moxibustion at acupuncture points including RN 8 (*shén què*), RN 6 (*qì hǎi*), and DU 20 (*bǎi huì*).

| ST 36 (*zú sān lǐ*) | SP 6 (*sān yīn jiāo*) | GB 14 (*yáng bái*) |

(3) For cases with obstruction of collaterals caused by wind-phlegm, use a neutral reinforcement and reduction method; acupuncture points include:

| GB 20 (*fēng chí*) | ST 40 (*fēng lóng*) | LV 3 (*tài chōng*) |
| BL 62 (*shēn mài*) | | |

The acupuncture may be used once daily or every other day; 10 sessions is a course of treatment.

The therapeutic effects can be strengthened by using the point-joining method, such as joining GB 14 (*yáng bái*) to *yú yāo* (鱼腰), joining GB 14 (*yáng bái*) to BL 2 (*cuán zhú*). Or, use transverse needling from BL 2 (*cuán zhú*) and SJ 23 (*sī zhú kōng*) to *yú yāo* (鱼腰).

Point-pricking with plum-blossom needle at the affected eyelid and around orbital skin can also be used every day or every other day as an additional treatment; 10 sessions is a course.

3. Chinese Patent Medicines

(1) *Bǔ Zhōng Yì Qì Wán* (Center-Supplementing and Qi-Boosting Pill, 补中益气丸)

6 g each time, twice a day; applicable to spleen qi deficiency.

(2) *Yòu Guī Wán* (Right-Restoring Pill, 右归丸)

1 pill each time, three times a day; applicable to patterns of congenital insufficiency, but avoid excessive intake in case of damage to yin. For children, the dose is 1/2 pill each time.

4. Dietary Therapy and Preventive Care

(1) For children and the elderly with severe bilateral ptosis, they should be cautious to avoid collision and any type of "falling injury" due to poor visual field. It is suggested to lift the upper eyelid with transparent rubber cement during the daytime to facilitate daily activities before the treatment takes effect or if the surgical method is unsuitable.

(2) Ptosis often leads to conjunctivitis because of abnormal blinking, so it may be applicable to use antibiotic eye drops for prevention.

(3) For the patients with spleen qi deficiency, the foods with the function of fortifying the spleen and increasing appetite, such as common yam rhizome, coix seed, water caltrop, lotus root, and common jujube, are should be added to their diet.

Case Studies

Liu, a 28-year-old female

Initial visit: May 29, 1992

【Chief Complaint】

Heavy drooping of the right upper lid. The symptom is mild in the early morning and more severe in the evening.

【Examination】

Her visual acuities were 20/17 on both eyes. The palpebral fissures were 6 mm wide on the right side and 10 mm wide on the left side at orthophoria state. Neostigmine test: The palpebral fissure of right eye was increased to 9.5 mm 20 minutes later after the injection.

Findings from the four examinations of TCM: Poor appetite; normal activities of sleep, urine, stool, and menstruation; pale tongue with thin-white coating; thready pulse

【Diagnosis】

Ocular myasthenia gravis

【Pattern Differentiation】

Insufficiency of center qi, failure of spleen yang to ascend

【Treatment Principles】

Supplement the middle and replenish qi, elevate yang and raise the drooping

【Prescription】

生黄芪	shēng huáng qí	15 g	Radix Astragali
炒白术	chǎo bái zhú	10 g	Rhizoma Atractylodis Macrocephalae (dry-fried)
党参	dǎng shēn	10 g	Radix Codonopsis
当归	dāng guī	10 g	Radix Angelicae Sinensis
陈皮	chén pí	10 g	Pericarpium Citri Reticulatae
升麻	shēng má	6 g	Rhizoma Cimicifugae
柴胡	chái hú	6 g	Radix Bupleuri
炙甘草	zhì gān cǎo	6 g	Radix et Rhizoma Glycyrrhizae Praeparata cum Melle
防风	fáng fēng	10 g	Radix Saposhnikoviae
羌活	qiāng huó	10 g	Radix et Rhizoma Notopterygii
丹参	dān shēn	10 g	Radix et Rhizoma Salviae Miltiorrhizae
钩藤	gōu téng	10 g	Ramulus Uncariae Cum Uncis

【Follow-up】

After taking the decoction for two weeks, the symptoms of the fatigue and heavy feeling on the right was reduced, and the palpebral fissure was increased to 7.5mm wide. Due to inconvenience for taking decoction, the prescription was processed into watered pill, and given every other day with alternation of the Chinese patent medicines *Shēng*

Mài Yǐn (Pulse-Engendering Decoction, 生脉饮) and *Huó Xuè Tōng Luò Piàn* (Blood-Invigorating and Collateral-Freeing Tablet, 活血通络片). The patient returned on July 10. The palpebral fissure of the right eye was increased to 9.5 mm wide (same as the left eye). The symptom recurred because the patient had stopped the medication on her own due to a busy work schedule, but improved after she continued the treatment again. The palpebral fissures were kept at 9.5 mm wide when she returned for her third follow-up visit on April 17, 1993.

Questions for consideration

1. What is the classification of blephroptosis? What are the main treatment principles for blephroptosis?

2. What are the patterns of blephroptosis? Please write out the main syndrome characteristics, acupuncture treatment (acupoints and manipulation) for two patterns.

Section 4   Blepharospasm

Blepharospasm, also called essential blepharospasm or benign blepharospam, is a local myodystonia disease. The cause is still not clear, but there are several studies suggesting that the abnormality or variation of the encephalic vessels, abnormality of basal ganglia and its electrical activity, deficiency or dysfunction of dopamine in corpora striatum, and genetic factors can be associated with blepharospasm. Head trauma, contact with toxic substances, and mental stress may also be risk factors.

Blepharospasm is characterized by repeated, uncontrolled, and progressively aggravated eyelid twitching. Although there are no obvious pathological changes in the eyes, some patients may be rendered functionally blind by the severity of the blepharospasm and its impact on watching TV, reading, and other daily activities. In TCM, blepharospasm is called *bāo lún zhèn tiào* (twitching eyelid, 胞轮振跳), *mù shùn* (目眴), or *pí lún zhèn tiào* (睥轮振跳). The underlying cause may originate from endogenous wind caused by prolonged liver-spleen blood deficiency, which results in the eyelid twitching. Another causative factor is the depletion of nutrients to the eyelid due to deficiency of the heart and spleen, or deficiency of qi and blood caused by excess fatigue. For those patients whom surgical therapies are unsuitable, and/or those patients who do not respond to Western treatments, TCM may help to resolve the symptoms and improve the overall condition, especially if combining Chinese medicinal therapy with acupuncture.

Clinical Manifestation

Based on the severity of blepharospasm, the disease is divided to 5 grades:

0: no eyelid twitch

Ⅰ: Increased frequency of involuntary blinking under stimulus

Ⅱ (mild): Slight eyelid twitching without dysfunction

Ⅲ (moderate): Obvious eyelid twitching accompanied by mild dysfunction

Ⅳ: Besides obvious eyelid twitching, patients always have difficulty reading and driving

The symptoms above may be exacerbated by fatigue, reading for long periods of time, insufficient sleep, or emotional fluctuation, some accompanied by twitching of facial muscles and angle of mouth.

Treatment

In Western medicine, the direct causes and pathogenesis of blepharospasm are still unclear. All conventional treatments including drugs, botulinum toxin injection, and surgery do not focus directly on the underlying causes, therefore they cannot cure the disease and/or prevent the recurrence. In many cases, due to the major side-effects and limitations of conventional medical treatments, it may be necessary to treat blepharospasm with TCM.

1. Pattern Differentiation and Treatment

(1) Blood Insufficiency Generating Wind

【Syndrome Characteristics】

Involuntary eyelid twitching, may be accompanied by contraction of facial muscles and angle of mouth. Other manifestations include lightheadedness, lusterless facial complexion, light red tongue with thin coating, and a wiry and thready pulse.

【Treatment Principle】

Nourish blood to extinguish wind

【Representative Formula】

Dāng Guī Huó Xuè Yǐn (Chinese Angelica Blood-Invigorating Decoction, 当归活血饮)

【Prescription】

当归	*dāng guī*	10 g	Radix Angelicae Sinensis
白芍	*bái sháo*	10 g	Radix Paeoniae Alba
熟地黄	*shú dì huáng*	10 g	Radix Rehmanniae Praeparata
川芎	*chuān xiōng*	10 g	Rhizoma Chuanxiong
炙黄芪	*zhì huáng qí*	15 g	Radix Astragali (stir-fried with liquid adjuvant)
苍术	*cāng zhú*	10 g	Rhizoma Atractylodis

防风	fáng fēng	10 g	Radix Saposhnikoviae
羌活	qiāng huó	10 g	Rhizoma et Radix Notopterygii
甘草	gān cǎo	6 g	Radix et Rhizoma Glycyrrhizae
薄荷（后下）	bò he (hòu xià)	6 g	Herba Menthae (added later)

【Modifications】
➢ For cases with sustained eye twitching, add *tiān má* (天麻, Rhizoma Gastrodiae) 10 g, *jiāng cán* (僵蚕, Bombyx Batryticatus) 10 g, and *gōu téng* (钩藤, Ramulus Uncariae Cum Uncis) 10 g to pacify the liver, extinguish wind, and stop convulsions.
➢ For cases with forceful closure of eyelids, add *dǎng shēn* (党参, Radix Codonopsis) 10 g, *shēng má* (升麻, Rhizoma Cimicifugae) 10 g to replenish qi and elevate yang to raise the eyelids.

(2) Heart and Spleen Deficiency
【Syndrome Characteristics】
Mild or severe eyelid twitching, aggravated by fatigue and insomnia; some cases may be accompanied by vexation and sleeplessness, fearful throbbing and forgetfulness, decreased food intake and fatigue, pale tongue, and weak, thready pulse.
【Treatment Principle】
Supplement the heart and spleen
【Representative Formula】
Modified *Guī Pí Tāng* (Spleen-Restoring Decoction, 归脾汤)
【Prescription】

黄芪	huáng qí	9 g	Radix Astragali
白术	bái zhú	9 g	Rhizoma Atractylodis Macrocephalae
茯神	fú shén	9 g	Sclerotium Poriae Pararadicis
人参	rén shēn	9 g	Radix et Rhizoma Ginseng
龙眼肉	lóng yǎn ròu	9 g	Arillus Longan
炒枣仁	chǎo zǎo rén	9 g	Semen Ziziphi Spinosae (dry-fried)
当归	dāng guī	9 g	Radix Angelicae Sinensis
木香	mù xiāng	9 g	Radix Aucklandiae
远志	yuǎn zhì	9 g	Radix Polygalae
炙甘草	zhì gān cǎo	5 g	Radix et Rhizoma Glycyrrhizae Praeparata cum Melle
木瓜	mù guā	9 g	Fructus Chaenomelis
钩藤	gōu téng	9 g	Ramulus Uncariae Cum Uncis

【Modifications】
➢ For cases with vexation and insomnia, add *sāng shèn* (桑椹, Fructus Mori) 9 g and *dēng xīn cǎo* (灯心草, Medulla Junci) 3 g to nourish yin and tonify blood, clear heart heat

and eliminate heat vexation.

➢ For cases with poor appetite and anorexia, add *shén qū* (神曲, Massa Medicata Fermentata) 9 g, *gǔ yá* (谷芽, Fructus Setariae Germinatus) 10 g and *mài yá* (麦芽, Fructus Hordei Germinatus) 9 g to promote digestion, harmonize the middle, invigorate the spleen, and increase the appetite.

2. Acupuncture

(1) Filiform Needling
A reinforcing method is indicated in most cases; retain the needles for 30 minutes after the arrival of qi, one time per day or every other day. 15 sessions is a treatment course.

BL 2 (*cuán zhú*)	SJ 23 (*sī zhú kōng*)	ST 8 (*tóu wéi*)
ST 2 (*sì bái*)	GB 14 (*yáng bái*)	GB 20 (*fēng chí*)
LI 4 (*hé gǔ*)	ST 36 (*zú sān lǐ*)	BL 20 (*pí shù*)

(2) Row Needling
Insert 6–8 needles along the row 3–5 mm up or below the superior eyelid or inferior eyelid; the depth of needling is at the orbicular muscles. Once a day, retain 30 minutes each time; 15 sessions is a course.

(3) Plum-blossom Needling
Point-pricking with a plum-blossom needle at the affected eyelid and around orbital skin can also be used every day or every other day; 10 sessions is a course.

(4) Ear Acupuncture
Eye (*yǎn*), liver (*gān*), spleen (*pí*), spirit gate (*shén mén*), heart (*xīn*), and gallbladder (*dǎn*) are effective ear acupucture points.

(5) Roll Needling
Choose the head points of the *du mai*, bladder channel, liver channel, and gall bladder channel; roll over the rolling needle from the proximal points to the distal points, back and forth, for 100–200 turns every time, according to patients' sensation. Once a day; 15 days is a treatment course.

3. Chinese Patent Medicines

(1) *Dāng Guī Bǔ Xuè Wán* (Chinese Angelica Blood-Supplementing Pill, 当归补血丸) or *Dāng Guī Bǔ Xuè Kǒu Fú Yè* (Chinese Angelica Blood-Supplementing Oral Drink, 当归补血口服液)
1 pill (9 g) or 10 ml, two times per day; useful for patients with qi and blood deficiency.

(2) *Guī Pí Wán* (Spleen-Restoring Pill, 归脾丸) or *Guī Pí Hé Jì* (Spleen-Restoring Mixture, 归脾合剂)

8–10 pills or 10–20 ml, three times per day; useful for patients with heart and spleen deficiency. Or, the patient can also take this formula alternately every other day with *Guī Pí Tāng* (Spleen-Restoring Decoction, 归脾汤).

(3) *Quán Tiān Má Jiāo Náng* (Whole Rhizoma Gastrodiae Capsule, 全天麻胶囊)

4–6 capsules, three times per day; useful for severe cases.

4. Dietary Therapy and Preventive Care

(1) Avoid excitant food like spicy food, shallot, and onion. Quit smoking and limit alcohol consumption.

(2) Reconcile work with rest. Avoid stress and extreme emotional fluctuations.

Classic Quotes

《证治准绳·七窍门》: "谓目睥不待人之开合而自谦搜振跳也。乃气分之病，属肝脾二经络牵振之患，人皆呼为风，殊不知血虚而气不顺，非纯风也。"

Eyelid twitching is involuntary blinking, and belongs to a qi-level pattern. It is a disorder of the liver and spleen collateral pulling and shaking the eyelids. Pathogenic wind causes the symptoms of this disease; however, the underlying causative factor is due to deficiency of blood and the abnormal flow of qi, which is not external wind.

Standards for Diagnosis and Treatment – Seven Orifices (*Zhèng Zhì Zhǔn Shéng – Qī Qiào Mén*, 证治准绳·七窍门). Wang Ken-tang 王肯堂 (Styles: Wang Yu-tai 王宇泰, Wang Sun-an 王损俺), 1602 (Ming).

Questions for Consideration

1. What is blepharospasm called in the TCM classics?

2. If the patient has involuntary eyelid twitching, contraction of facial muscle and angle of mouth, lightheadedness, lusterless facial complexion, light red tongue with thin coating, wiry and thready pulse, what is the TCM pattern?

3. Write out 3 kinds of acupuncture methods for the disease.

Section 5   Herpes Zoster of the Eyelid

Herpes zoster of the eyelid is also called herpes zoster ophthalmicus, which is a common unilateral, viral blister disorder of the eyelid. Herpes zoster ophthalmicus is caused by a varicella-zoster virus infection in the semilunar ganglion or the first branch of the trigeminal nerve. This disease is commonly seen in the elderly, or those who are in an immune-deficient state or whose immunity is suppressed. The condition is always severe in patients with immunity disorders.

In TCM, this disease pertains to the classification of *fēng chì chuāng yí* (wind red sore, 风赤疮痍). The causes and pathogenesis are mainly associated with wind-heat pathogen attacking upward at the eyelid with an underlying weak constitution and insecurity of the *wei qi* (卫气; a.k.a. defensive qi), or wind-damp-heat pathogen attacking upward to the eyelid as a result of attack by external wind combined with damp-heat in the spleen and stomach. The damp-heat arises from excessive consumption of spicy food, or excess heat in the spleen channel. If the diagnosis is made, it is typically treated with oral or topical antiviral drugs. However, treatment of symptoms is usually recommended in order to relieve pain, accelerate healing, and prevent the virus from spreading and causing a second outbreak. Chinese medicine has good results with treating viral diseases. Combined treatment of both Chinese medicine and Western medicine can have a better effect of relieving pain, reducing complications, and shortening the course.

Clinical Manifestation

This disease occurs along the skin area where the first branch of the trigeminal nerve is located, with the lesion settling on one side of the head, forehead, and upper and lower eyelids. In some cases it may involve the same side on the nose, but it does pass the facial midline. The characteristics of the lesion are described as the following:

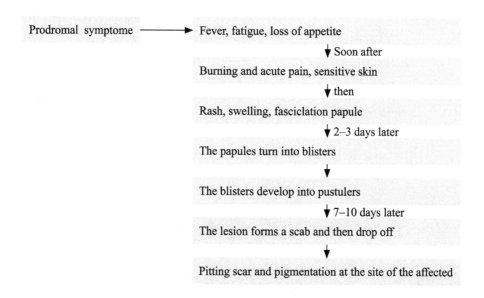

It should be noted that this viral disease may cause complications such as keratitis, iridocyclitis, or even glaucoma, posterior scleritis, and ophthalmoplegia, if it is not controlled in time.

Treatment

1. Pattern Differentiation and Treatment

(1) Wind-heat Attacking the Exterior
【Syndrome Characteristics】
Eyelid redness, itching, burning pain, papule and blisters; may be accompanied by fever, aversion to cold, headache, red tongue with thin yellow coating, and a floating and rapid pulse.
【Treatment Principle】
Disperse wind and dissipate pathogens, discharge and clear spleen heat
【Representative Formula】
Chú Fēng Qīng Pí Yǐn (Wind-Eliminating Spleen Heat-Clearing Decoction, 除风清脾饮)
【Prescription】

陈皮	*chén pí*	10 g	Pericarpium Citri Reticulatae
连翘	*lián qiào*	10 g	Fructus Forsythiae
防风	*fáng fēng*	10 g	Radix Saposhnikoviae
知母	*zhī mǔ*	10 g	Rhizoma Anemarrhenae
玄明粉	*xuán míng fěn*	12 g	Natrii Sulfas Exsiccatus
黄芩	*huáng qín*	10 g	Radix Scutellariae
玄参	*xuán shēn*	10 g	Radix Scrophulariae
黄连	*huáng lián*	5 g	Rhizoma Coptidis
荆芥	*jīng jiè*	10 g	Spica Schizonepetae
大黄	*dà huáng*	10 g	Radix et Rhizoma Rhei
桔梗	*jié gěng*	10 g	Radix Platycodonis

【Modifications】
➤ For cases accompanied by dampness, add *cāng zhú* (苍术, Rhizoma Atractylodis) 10 g and *kǔ shēn* (苦参, Radix Sophorae Flavescentis) 10 g to clear heat and dry dampness. For cases with severe burning pain of the skin, add *mǔ dān pí* (牡丹皮, Cortex Moutan) 10 g and *chì sháo* (赤芍, Radix Paeoniae Rubra) 10g to cool blood, disperse stasis, and relieve pain.
➤ If the patient has no sign of constipation, remove *xuán míng fěn* (玄明粉, Natrii Sulfas) and reduce *dà huáng* (大黄, Radix et Rhizoma Rhei) to 5g.

(2) Wind-Damp-Heat Toxin

【 Syndrome Characteristics 】

Eyelid redness, pain, blister and pustules, tearing, extreme itching; may be accompanied by sticky and greasy sensation in the mouth, intake of fluid failing to resolve thirst, oppression in the chest, poor appetite and digestion, red tongue with greasy coating, and a slippery and rapid pulse.

【 Treatment Principle 】

Dispel wind and remove dampness, discharge fire and resolve toxin

【 Representative Formula 】

Modified *Chú Shī Tāng* (Dampness-Dispelling Decoction, 除湿汤)

【 Prescription 】

防风	*fáng fēng*	10 g	Radix Saposhnikoviae
荆芥	*jīng jiè*	6 g	Herba Schizonepetae
茯苓	*fú líng*	10 g	Poria
滑石	*huá shí*	10 g	Talcum
车前子	*chē qián zǐ*	10 g	Semen Plantaginis
黄芩	*huáng qín*	10 g	Radix Scutellariae
黄连	*huáng lián*	6 g	Rhizoma Coptidis
连翘	*lián qiào*	10 g	Fructus Forsythiae
枳壳	*zhǐ qiào*	10 g	Fructus Aurantii
陈皮	*chén pí*	6 g	Pericarpium Citri Reticulatae
炒白术	*chǎo bái zhú*	10 g	Rhizoma Atractylodis Macrocephalae (dry-fried)
苍术	*cāng zhú*	10 g	Rhizoma Atractylodis
甘草	*gān cǎo*	6 g	Radix et Rhizoma Glycyrrhizae

【 Modifications 】

➢ For cases with severe damp-heat, add *tǔ fú líng* (土茯苓, Rhizoma Smilacis Glabrae) 10 g, *yì yǐ rén* (薏苡仁, Semen Coicis) 15 g and *jīn yín huā* (金银花, Flos Lonicerae Japonicae) 10 g to enhance the function of removing dampness and clearing heat.

➢ For cases with large pustules and extreme itching, add *dì fū zǐ* (地肤子, Fructus Kochiae) 10 g, *bái xiān pí* (白鲜皮, Cortex Dictamni) 10 g and *kǔ shēn* (苦参, Radix Sophorae Flavescentis) 10 g to clear damp-heat and stop itching.

(3) Excess Heat Toxin

【 Syndrome Characteristics 】

Marked eyelid redness, acute pain, blisters, pustules and skin eruptions, and fever. Other signs include red tongue with dry yellow coating, and a forceful, rapid pulse.

【 Treatment Principle 】
Clear heat and resolve toxin, disperse wind and dissipate pathogen
【 Representative Formula 】
Pǔ Jì Xiāo Dú Yǐn (Universal Relief Toxin-Removing Decoction, 普济消毒饮)
【 Prescription 】

黄连	*huáng lián*	10 g	Rhizoma Coptidis
黄芩	*huáng qín*	10 g	Radix Scutellariae
牛蒡子	*niú bàng zǐ*	10 g	Fructus Arctii
玄参	*xuán shēn*	10 g	Radix Scrophulariae
甘草	*gān cǎo*	5 g	Radix et Rhizoma Glycyrrhizae
桔梗	*jié gěng*	10 g	Radix Platycodonis
板蓝根	*bǎn lán gēn*	10 g	Radix Isatidis
柴胡	*chái hú*	10 g	Radix Bupleuri
升麻	*shēng má*	10 g	Rhizoma Cimicifugae
马勃	*mǎ bó*	3 g	Lasiosphaera seu Calvatia
陈皮	*chén pí*	5 g	Pericarpium Citri Reticulatae
薄荷	*bò he*	3 g	Herba Menthae
僵蚕	*jiāng cán*	3 g	Bombyx Batryticatus
连翘	*lián qiào*	10 g	Fructus Forsythiae

【 Modifications 】

➢ For cases with constipation, add *dà huáng* (大黄, Radix et Rhizoma Rhei) 6 g to resolve constipation by purgation, heat-clearing, and resolution of toxin.

➢ For cases with unbearable aching, add *rǔ xiāng* (乳香, Olibanum) 6 g and *mò yào* (没药, Myrrha) 6 g to activate blood to stop pain, disperse swelling, and engender flesh.

2. Acupuncture

(1) Filiform Needling

Use reduction method; the commonly used acupoints include:

LI 4 (*hé gǔ*)	ST 2 (*sì bái*)	PC 6 (*nèi guān*)
LI 11 (*qū chí*)	SP 10 (*xuè hǎi*)	GB 34 (*yáng líng quán*)
ST 36 (*zú sān lǐ*)	LR 3 (*tài chōng*)	

(2) Ear Acupuncture

It is optional to select the corresponding sensitive points like spleen (*pí*), stomach (*wèi*), liver (*gān*), eye (*yǎn*), and gallbladder (*dǎn*). Choose 2–4 points each time; twirl the needle to give strong stimulation, and then retain the needles for 20–30 minutes.

3. Chinese Patent Medicines

(1) *Yín Qiào Jiě Dú Piàn* (Lonicera and Forsythia Toxin-Expelling Tablets, 银翘解毒片)

4 tablets, three times a day. Applicable to wind-heat attacking the exterior.

(2) *Lóng Dǎn Xiè Gān Wán* (Gentian Liver-Draining Pill, 龙胆泻肝丸)

3–6 g each time for water pills, twice a day. 4–6 tablets for tablets, 2–3 times a day. It is applicable for patients with wind-damp-heat toxin.

(3) *Qīng Rè Jiě Dú Kē Lì* (Heat-Clearing Toxin-Expelling Granules, 清热解毒颗粒)

1 pouch each time (18 g), two times a day. It can be an assistant method to treat excess heat toxin.

4. Simple and Proven Recipes

Qīng dài (青黛, Indigo Naturalis, natural indigo) 30 g, *huáng bǎi* (黄柏, Cortex Phellodendri Chinensis) 30 g and *bīng piàn* (冰片, Borneolum Syntheticum) 0.5 g are ground together into a powder, then blended with a *jú huā* (Flos Chrysanthemi) decoction to make a paste. Apply the paste to the affected skin, three times a day.

5. External Treatment

(1) Apply Aldrich's mixture and Calamine lotion to the affected area, twice a day. If the conjunctiva and cornea are involved, it is suggested to apply antiviral eye drops (such as acyclovir drops or ganciclovir drops) frequently, and to consult an ophthalmologist for further treatment.

(2) For patients with skin ulceration, treat with 0.1% Ethacridine wet compress and antibacterial ointment.

6. Treatment for Complications

If the condition becomes complicated with keratitis and iridocyclitis, insist the patient see an ophthalmologist as soon as possible.

7. Dietary Therapy and Preventive Care

(1) Take bed rest during the acute period of onset, and drink more water.

(2) Avoid eating lamb, seafood, spicy food and food in rich flavor; take more bland foods that are easy to digest. Consume more fresh fruit and juice as needed.

(3) Keep the lesion area clean and dry. Do not scratch the affected area, and keep the lesion exudates from flowing into the eye to prevent complications and spreading the infection.

(4) Avoid excess fatigue and catching cold. Open the window and get fresh air frequently. Keep the room dry and clean.

Case Studies

Yang, a 56-year-old female

Initial visit: May 12, 2005.

【 Chief Complaint 】

Upper eyelid redness, blistering and unbearable pain, accompanied by a fever for the last 4 days

【 Examination 】

Redness and swelling of the left upper eyelid and forehead, clustering transparent blisters, red tongue with yellow coating, and a soggy and rapid pulse.

【 Diagnosis 】

Herpes zoster of the eyelids

【 Pattern Differentiation 】

Damp-heat in the spleen and stomach

【 Treatment Principles 】

Clear spleen heat and remove dampness

【 Prescription 】

Modified *Qīng Pí Chú Shī Yǐn* (Spleen Heat-Clearing and Dampness-Removing Decoction, 清脾除湿饮)

茵陈	*yīn chén*	10 g	Herba Artemisiae Scopariae
泽泻	*zé xiè*	10 g	Rhizoma Alismatis
生地	*shēng dì*	10 g	Radix Rehmanniae
栀子	*zhī zǐ*	10 g	Fructus Gardeniae
黄芩	*huáng qín*	10 g	Radix Scutellariae
连翘	*lián qiào*	10 g	Fructus Forsythiae
苍术	*cāng zhú*	10 g	Rhizoma Atractylodis
白术	*bái zhú*	10 g	Rhizoma Atractylodis Macrocephalae
枳壳	*zhǐ qiào*	10 g	Fructus Aurantii
茯苓	*fú líng*	10 g	Poria
麦冬	*mài dōng*	10 g	Radix Ophiopogonis

甘草	*gān cǎo*	5 g	Radix et Rhizoma Glycyrrhizae
玄明粉	*xuán míng fěn*	10 g	Natrii Sulfas Exsiccatus
黄连	*huáng lián*	15 g	Rhizoma Coptidis

【Follow-up】

At her second visit, we added *jīng jiè* (荆芥, Herba Schizonepetae) 10 g, *fáng fēng* (防风, Radix Saposhnikoviae) 10 g and *bǎn lán gēn* (板蓝根, Radix Isatidis) 10 g to the primary formula, and prescribed oral acyclovir, 500 mg, four times a day. *Qīng Dài Ruǎn Gāo* (Natural Indigo Ointment, 青黛软膏) was prescribed for external use. The lesion dried up and formed a scab ten days later.

Classic Quotes

《秘传眼科龙木论》："风赤生于脾脏家，疱生面睑似朱砂，乌珠洁净未为事。"

"Wind redness originates from the spleen, presenting with papules like cinnabar at the face and eyelids. It is not a severe condition if the cornea looks clean with luster."

The Secret Transmission of Long-mu's Ophthalmology (Mì Chuán Yǎn Kē Lóng Mù Lùn, 秘传眼科龙木论); Author unknown, 13th Century.

Questions for Consideration

1. What is the cause of *fēng chì chuāng yí* (herpes zoster ophthalmicus)?

2. Which pattern requires the application of the formula *Pǔ Jì Xiāo Dú Yǐn* (Universal Relief Toxin-Removing Decoction, 普济消毒饮)?

3. Write out the main syndrome characteristics of the pattern.

Chapter 7
Conjunctival Diseases

Section 1   Acute Catarrhal Conjunctivitis

Acute catarrhal conjunctivitis, commonly called "pink eye", is typically seen in the autumn and summer months. Because the disease is highly contagious, it is more likely to occur at densely-populated places like schools and factories. The disease presents as an acute onset with a latency period of 1 to 3 days; it can either attack bilaterally or one eye at a time, with a one- or two-day interval before both eyes are affected. Symptoms are most severe during the third or fourth days after the initial onset. The condition gradually improves and recovery typically occurs within 1–2 weeks. The most common pathogenic microbes are viruses and bacteria, including diplococcus pneumoniae, staphylococcus aureus, and haemophilus influenzae strains.

In Chinese medicine, pink eye is called "*Bào Fēng Kè Rè*" (fulminant wind and invading fever, 暴风客热). The cause of the disease is primarily attributed to externally contracted wind-heat and/or constrained heat in the interior. Pathogenic wind and heat contend with each other, stagnate in the lung, and then attack upward to affect the conjunctiva.

Clinical Manifestation

Tearing, itching, pain, profuse sticky discharge, edema, fever, nasal obstruction, headache, dark urine, and dry stool.

Treatment

1. Pattern Differentiation and Treatment

(1) Wind Outweighing Heat
[Syndrome Characteristics]
Itching, prick pain, photophobia, tearing, conjunctival congestion and edema, headache, nasal obstruction, aversion to wind, red tongue with white thin coating, a

floating pulse or a floating and rapid pulse.

【Treatment Principle】

Dissipate wind and clear heat, reduce swelling and relieve pain

【Representative Formula】

Modified *Yín Qiào Sǎn* (Lonicera and Forsythia Powder, 银翘散)

【Prescription】

连翘	*lián qiào*	10 g	Fructus Forsythiae
金银花	*jīn yín huā*	10 g	Flos Lonicerae Japonicae
桔梗	*jié gěng*	10 g	Rhizoma Phragmitis
薄荷（后下）	*bò he (hòu xià)*	10 g	Herba Menthae (added later)
淡竹叶	*dàn zhú yè*	10 g	Herba Lophatheri
甘草	*gān cǎo*	3 g	Radix et Rhizoma Glycyrrhizae
荆芥穗	*jīng jiè suì*	10 g	Spica Schizonepetae
淡豆豉	*dàn dòu chǐ*	10 g	Semen Sojae Praeparatum
牛蒡子	*niú bàng zǐ*	10 g	Fructus Arctii

【Modifications】

➢ For cases with marked conjunctival congestion, add *jú huā* (菊花, Flos Chrysanthemi) 10 g, *pú gōng yīng* (蒲公英, Herba Taraxaci), *zǐ cǎo* (紫草, Radix Arnebiae) 10 g, *mǔ dān pí* (牡丹皮, Cortex Moutan) 10 g to clear heat, cool blood, and eliminate stasis.

(2) Heat Overweighing Wind

【Syndrome Characteristics】

Eye pain, aversion to heat, photophobia, profuse yellow sticky discharge, hot tearing, conjunctival congestion and edema, thirst, dark urine and dry stool, red tongue with yellow coating, rapid pulse.

【Treatment Principle】

Clear heat and remove toxins, dissipate wind and relieve pain

【Representative Formula】

Modified *Xiè Fèi Yǐn* (Lung-Draining Decoction, 泻肺饮)

【Prescription】

石膏	*shí gāo*	10 g	Gypsum Fibrosum
赤芍	*chì sháo*	10 g	Radix Paeoniae Rubra
黄芩	*huáng qín*	3 g	Radix Scutellariae
桑白皮	*sāng bái pí*	10 g	Cortex Mori

枳壳	zhǐ qiào	10 g	Fructus Aurantii
木通	mù tōng	10 g	Caulis Akebiae
连翘	lián qiào	10 g	Fructus Forsythiae
荆芥	jīng jiè	10 g	Herba Schizonepetae
防风	fáng fēng	10 g	Radix Saposhnikoviae
栀子	zhī zǐ	10 g	Fructus Arctii
白芷	bái zhǐ	10 g	Radix Angelicae Dahuricae
羌活	qiāng huó	10 g	Radix et Rhizoma Notopterygii
甘草	gān cǎo	3 g	Radix et Rhizoma Glycyrrhizae

【Modifications】

➢ For cases with marked conjunctival congestion and edema, add *jié gěng* (桔梗, Radix Platycodonis) 10 g, *tíng lì zǐ* (葶苈子, Semen Lepidii) 10 g, *shēng dì* (生地, Radix Rehmanniae) 10 g and *mǔ dān pí* (牡丹皮, Cortex Moutan) 10 g.

➢ For cases with constipation, add *dà huáng* (大黄, Radix et Rhizoma Rhei) 10 g.

(3) Equal Wind and Heat

【Syndrome Characteristics】

Eye pain, itching, photophobia, conjunctival congestion and edema, thirst for fluids, dark urine and dry stool, red tongue with white coating, a thready and rapid pulse or a wiry and thready pulse.

【Treatment Principle】

Clear heat and remove toxins, dissipate wind and expel the pathogen

【Representative Formula】

Modified *Shuāng Jiě Tāng* (Double Resolution Decoction, 双解汤)

【Prescription】

金银花	jīn yín huā	15 g	Flos Lonicerae Japonicae
蒲公英	pú gōng yīng	15 g	Herba Taraxaci
天花粉	tiān huā fěn	10 g	Radix Trichosanthis
黄芩	huáng qín	10 g	Radix Scutellariae
枳壳	zhǐ qiào	5 g	Fructus Aurantii
龙胆草	lóng dǎn cǎo	10 g	Radix et Rhizoma Gentianae
荆芥	jīng jiè	10 g	Herba Schizonepetae
防风	fáng fēng	10 g	Radix Saposhnikoviae
桑白皮	sāng bái pí	6 g	Cortex Mori
甘草	gān cǎo	3 g	Radix et Rhizoma Glycyrrhizae

【 Modifications 】

➢ For cases with constipation, add *dà huáng* (大黄, Radix et Rhizoma Rhei) 10 g.

➢ For cases with loose stool, remove *lóng dǎn cǎo* (龙胆草, Radix et Rhizoma Gentianae), add *cāng zhú* (苍术, Rhizoma Atractylodis) 10 g and *bái zhú* (白术, Rhizoma Atractylodis Macrocephalae) 10 g.

➢ For cases with severe wind-heat, manifesting as marked eye itching, add *qiāng huó* (羌活, Rhizoma et Radix Notopterygii) 10 g.

2. Acupuncture

(1) Filiform Needling:

ST 1 (*chéng qì*)	*tài yáng* (太阳)	GB 20 (*fēng chí*)
BL 1 (*jīng míng*)	LI 11 (*qū chí*)	LI 4 (*hé gǔ*)

Choose 3–4 points every treatment, use a 1-*cun* needle, and retain the needle for 30–40 minutes after arrival of qi. Treat daily.

(2) Bloodletting

Prick the points of superciliary arch, tip of eyebrow, *tài yáng* (太阳) and ear apex, and squeeze out several drops of blood.

(3) Ear Acupuncture

Choose eye (*yǎn*), liver (*gān*), and lung (*fèi*); retain the needle for 30 minutes during each treatment. Treat daily.

3. Chinese Patent Medicines

(1) *Qīng Rè Jiě Dú Ruǎn Jiāo Náng* (Heat-Clearing and Toxin-Expelling Soft Capsule, 清热解毒软胶囊)

3 capsules, three times a day.

(2) *Niú Huáng Jiě Dú Piàn* (Bovine Bezoar Toxin-Expelling Tablet, 牛黄解毒片)

3 tablets a time, three times a day.

(3) *Sān Huáng Piàn* (Three Yellow Tablets, 三黄片)

3 tablets, three times a day.

(4) *Shuāng Huáng Lián Kǒu Fú Yè* (Honeysuckle and Coptis Oral Solution, 双黄连口服液)

10–20 ml, three times a day.

4. Simple and Proven Recipes

Jīn yín huā (Flos Lonicerae Japonicae) 30 g, *jú huā* (Flos Chrysanthemi) 30 g, *jué míng zǐ* (Semen Cassiae), *pàng dà hǎi* (Semen Sterculiae Lychnophorae) 30 g: wrap the medicinals individually using 1 g of each medicinal for each dose, put into a teapot and steep to make a tea with boiled water. Take 6–9 times every day until the symptoms are gone.

5. Treatment by Western Medicine

(1) Sulfacetamide Sodium Eye Drops 15%: 1 gtt (drop), 6 times a day. 1 gtt every 30 minutes for severe cases.

(2) Rifampicin 0.1%: 1 gtt (drop), 6 times a day. 1 gtt every 30 minutes for severe cases.

(3) Chloramphenicol Eye Drops 0.5%: 1 gtt (drop), 6 times a day. 1 gtt every 30 minutes for severe cases.

(4) Tobramycin Eye Drops: 1 gtt (drop), 6 times a day. 1 gtt every 30 minutes for severe cases.

6. Dietary Therapy and Preventive Care

Pay attention to personal hygiene. Do not rub the eyes with dirty hands and/or dirty towels. Sterilize handkerchiefs, towels, sinks, etc. Serious consideration should be given to the unaffected eye when only one eye has been infected. One should avoid contaminating the healthy eye with the discharge from the infected eye. The doctor should wash and disinfect his/her hands after examination of patients with conjunctivitis in order to prevent cross-infection.

Case Studies

Zhang, a seven-year-old girl

【 Chief Complaint 】

Redness, pain and profuse sticky secretion of both eyes for 1 day

【 Examination 】

Moderate redness and swelling of both eyes, marked congestion of the bulbar conjunctiva, red tongue with light yellow coating.

【 Treatment Principles 】

The following formula was prescribed:

大黄	*dà huáng*	10 g	Radix et Rhizoma Rhei
炒栀子	*chǎo zhī zǐ*	6 g	Fructus Gardeniae (dry-fried)
菊花	*jú huā*	6 g	Flos Chrysanthemi
密蒙花	*mì méng huā*	10 g	Flos Buddlejae

| 连翘 | *lián qiào* | 10 g | Fructus Forsythiae |
| 草决明 | *cǎo jué míng* | 10 g | Semen Cassiae |

The medicinals were decocted with water and taken orally, 1 dose every day, for a total of three doses. In addition, one bottle of *Xī Huáng Sǎn* (Bovine Bezoar Powder, 犀黄散) was administered topically, applied as a tiny grain-sized powder into the conjunctiva sac three times a day; the eyes were closed for 5 minutes after each application.

【Follow-up】

After three days of treatment, the bulbar conjunctival hyperemia disappeared and the subjective symptoms subsided.

Classic Quotes

《秘传眼科龙木论·第五十九·暴风客热外障》:"此眼初患之时,忽然白睛胀起,都覆乌睛和瞳人,红肿,或痒或痛,泪出难开。"

"At the initial stage of the disease, the white of the eye gets red and swollen suddenly, and may cover the black of the eye; may be accompanied by itching, soreness, or tearing."

The Secret Transmission of Long-mu's Ophthalmology – Fifty Ninth – Fulminant Wind and Invading Fever (Mì Chuán Yǎn Kē Lóng Mù Lùn – 59th – Bào Fēng Kè Rè Wài Zhàng, 秘传眼科龙木论·第五十九·暴风客热外障); author unknown, 13th century.

Questions for Consideration

1. The patient has eye pain, itching, photophobia, conjunctival congestion and edema, thirst for fluids, dark urine and dry stool, red tongue with white coating, a thready and rapid pulse or a wiry and thready pulse. What is the presenting pattern?

2. What is the treatment principle and representative formula?

3. State briefly the dietary treatment and Preventive Care for acute catarrhal conjunctivitis.

Section 2　Vernal Keratoconjunctivitis

Vernal keratoconjunctivitis (VKH), also called conjunctivitis catarrhalis aestiva or seasonal conjunctivitis, is a kind of allergic disorder. Generally, VKH presents at preadolescence and often attacks both eyes. It typically occurs during spring months, and the symptoms decrease during autumn and winter. The main clinical characteristic of VKH is intense itching of the eyes. The disease is more common in the Middle East and Africa; it is rare in cold climates. The allergens may include pollen, antigenic components of various microorganisms, dirt, dander of animals, feathers, sunlight, and temperature change.

In ophthalmology of TCM, VKH pertains to *shí fù mù yǎng* (seasonal eye itching, 时复目痒) or *yǎng ruò chóng xíng zhèng* (itching like worm crawling, 痒若虫行症). The disease can be caused by invasion of pathogenic wind, which then flees hither and thither in the striae and interstitial space of the eyelid and the canthus. It may also be caused by wind, dampness, and heat contending with one other and then leading to stagnation of pathogens at the eyelids. Stirring wind due to deficiency of liver blood can be another causative factor.

Clinical Manifestation

Extreme itching in both eyes may be accompanied by photophobia, tearing, burning and a sensation of a foreign body in the eye with a little stringy discharge. It is a seasonal recurrent disease, always occuring in spring and summer. The symptoms become remittent and disappears in autumn and winter. Clinically, it has three subtypes:

1. Palpebral Type

The most common characteristic is a lot of "giant" and flat papillae in the upper palpebral conjunctiva, of different sizes and pinkish in color, arranged like cobblestones, accompanied by conjunctival congestion and white mucous discharge.

2. Corneal Limbus Type

There are some small papillae in the upper and lower palpebral conjunctiva, and yellow-brown or dirty red colloid tubercles surrounding the cornea with marked hyperemia of the conjunctiva near the upper corneal limbus.

3. Mixed Types

The symptoms and signs of the above two types are coexistent.

Treatment

1. Pattern Differentiation and Treatment

(1) Wind-Heat
[Syndrome Characteristics]
Unbearable itching, burning sensation and mild pain, white mucous discharge, lots

of papillae in the palpebral conjunctiva arranged like cobblestones, hyperemia of the conjunctiva, light red tongue with thin white coating, floating and rapid pulse.

【 Treatment Principle 】
Dispel wind and stop itching

【 Representative Formula 】
Modified Xiāo Fēng Sǎn (Wind-Dispersing Powder, 消风散)

【 Prescription 】

荆芥穗	*jīng jiè suì*	10 g	Spica Schizonepetae
羌活	*qiāng huó*	10 g	Radix et Rhizoma Notopterygii
防风	*fáng fēng*	10 g	Radix Saposhnikoviae
川芎	*chuān xiōng*	10 g	Rhizoma Chuanxiong
白僵蚕	*bái jiāng cán*	10 g	Bombyx Batryticatus
蝉蜕	*chán tuì*	10 g	Periostracum Cicadae
茯苓	*fú líng*	10 g	Poria
陈皮	*chén pí*	10 g	Pericarpium Citri Reticulatae
厚朴	*hòu pò*	10 g	Cortex Magnoliae Officinalis
炙甘草	*zhì gān cǎo*	3 g	Radix et Rhizoma Glycyrrhizae Praeparata cum Melle
藿香叶	*huò xiāng yè*	10 g	Herba Agastachis

【 Modifications 】
➢ For cases with marked itching, add *sāng yè* (桑叶, Folium Mori) 10 g, *jú huā* (菊花, Flos Chrysanthemi) 10 g and *cì jí lí* (刺蒺藜, Fructus Tribuli) 10 g to enhance the effect of dispelling wind and arresting itching.

➢ For cases with prominent conjunctival hyperemia and burning sensation, add *mǔ dān pí* (牡丹皮, Cortex Moutan) 10 g, *chì sháo* (赤芍, Radix Paeoniae Rubra) 10 g and *yù jīn* (郁金, Radix Curcumae) 10 g to cool blood, disperse stagnation, and abate redness.

(2) Damp-Heat with Wind

【 Syndrome Characteristics 】
Unbearable itching, symptoms may be aggravated by wind exposure, sunshine, and rubbing the eyes; tearing, mucous discharge, lots of papillae in the palpebral conjunctiva arranged like cobblestones, dirty yellow bulbar conjunctiva, colloid tubercles at corneal limbus, red tongue, yellow and greasy coating, rapid pulse.

【 Treatment Principle 】
Clear heat and resolve dampness, dispel wind and arrest itching

【 Representative Formula 】
Modified *Chú Shī Tāng* (Dampness-Eliminating Decoction, 除湿汤)

【Prescription】

连翘	lián qiào	10 g	Fructus Forsythiae
滑石	huá shí	10 g	Talcum
车前子	chē qián zǐ	10 g	Semen Plantaginis
枳壳	zhǐ qiào	10 g	Fructus Aurantii
黄连	huáng lián	10 g	Rhizoma Coptidis
黄芩	huáng qín	10 g	Radix Scutellariae
木通	mù tōng	10 g	Caulis Akebiae
甘草	gān cǎo	10 g	Radix et Rhizoma Glycyrrhizae
陈皮	chén pí	10 g	Pericarpium Citri Reticulatae
荆芥	jīng jiè	10 g	Herba Schizonepetae
茯苓	fú líng	10 g	Poria
防风	fáng fēng	10 g	Radix Saposhnikoviae

【Modifications】

➤ For cases with marked itching, add *bái xiān pí* (白鲜皮,Cortex Dictamni) 10 g, *dì fū zǐ* (地肤子, Fructus Kochiae) 10 g and *yīn chén* (茵陈, Herba Artemisiae Scopariae) 15 g to enhance the effect of dispelling wind and arresting itching.

➤ For cases with lots colloid tubercles at the corneal limbus, add *qīng pí* (青皮, Pericarpium Citri Reticulatae Viride) 10 g and *chuān xiōng* (川芎, Rhizoma Chuanxiong) 10 g to break stagnant qi and eliminate stasis.

(3) Blood Deficiency Engendering Wind

【Syndrome Characteristics】

Mild intermittent itching of eye, slight redness of the conjunctiva, lusterless complexion or shallow yellow complexion, pale tongue, and thready pulse.

【Treatment Principle】

Nourish blood and extinguish wind

【Representative Formula】

Modified *Sì Wù Tāng* (Four Substances Decoction, 四物汤)

【Prescription】

当归	dāng guī	10 g	Radix Angelicae Sinensis
川芎	chuān xiōng	10 g	Rhizoma Chuanxiong
白芍	bái sháo	10 g	Radix Paeoniae Alba
熟地黄	shú dì huáng	10 g	Radix Rehmanniae Praeparata
白僵蚕	bái jiāng cán	10 g	Bombyx Batryticatus

白蒺藜	*bái jí lí*	10 g	Fructus Tribuli
荆芥	*jīng jiè*	6 g	Herba Schizonepetae
防风	*fáng fēng*	6 g	Radix Saposhnikoviae

【 Modifications 】

➤ For cases with mental fatigue and lack of strength, add *chǎo bái zhú* (炒白术, Rhizoma Atractylodis Macrocephalae) 10 g, *fú líng* (茯苓, Poria) 10 g and *dǎng shēn* (党参, Radix Codonopsis) 10 g to replenish qi and fortify the spleen, thereby strengthening the source of qi and blood production.

2. Acupuncture

| ST 1 (*chéng qì*) | *tài yáng* (太阳) | BL 2 (*cuán zhú*) |
| SJ 5 (*wài guān*) | LI 4 (*hé gǔ*) | |

Retain the needle for 30 minutes after arrival of qi, once a day; 10 sessions is a course of treatment.

3. Chinese Patent Medicines

(1) *Chuān Xīn Lián Piàn* (穿心莲片 , Herba Andrographis Tablets)
1–2 tablets, three times a day; applicable to externally contracted wind-heat.
(2) *Shuāng Huáng Lián Kǒu Fú Yè* (双黄连口服液 , Flos Lonicerae Japonicae and Rhizoma Coptidis Oral Drink)
30 ml, three times a day.

4. Simple Proven Recipes

Jīn yín huā (金银花, Flos Lonicerae Japonicae) 30 g, *jú huā* (菊花, Flos Chrysanthemi) 30 g, *jué míng zǐ* (决明子, Semen Cassiae) 30 g, *pàng dà hǎi* (胖大海, Semen Sterculiae Lychnophorae) 30 g, wrap the medicinals individually, take 1 g of each, put in a teapot and add some boiled water to make medicinal tea, take 6–9 times each day.

5. External Treatment

For patients with red swelling and papule of eyelid, apply moist compress with 2%–3% boric acid.

6. Treatment with Western Medicine

Try to identify and avoid the allergens that cause symptoms. Topical corticosteroids (0.1% Dexamethasone Eye Drop) and angiotonics (0.1% Epinephrine or 1% Efedrina) are helpful to alleviate itching and redness. According to the condition, application of Ketorolac Tromethamine 0.5%, Emedastine Difumarate 0.05%, or Nedocromil sodium 2% can reduce the symptoms markedly. For severe cases, medication including Chlorphenamine, Astemizole, antihistaminics or glucocorticoid may be indicated.

7. Dietary Therapy and Preventive Care

During the period of onset, wear UV-protection sunglasses when outdoors. Do not rub harshly when there is extreme itching. Consume less or completely avoid spicy and fatty food to prevent aggravating the condition. During remission, eat foods which have the function of replenishing qi and fortifying the spleen, including *dà zǎo* (大枣, Fructus Jujubae), *shān yào* (山药, Rhizoma Dioscoreae), etc. This may be helpful in preventing recurrence and/or relieving the symptoms.

Case Studies

Ding, an 18-year-old man

【Chief Complaint】

Intense itching of the eyelids that feels like worms crawling, which has occurred every spring during the past four years.

【Examination】

Lots of papillae in the shapes of pepper and millet were presented in the upper palpebra conjunctiva. Other signs included a red tongue and an excess pulse.

【Pattern Differentiation】

Wind-fire invading upward; qi and blood stagnating at the eyelids

【Treatment Principles】

Dispel wind and clear heat, activate blood and move stagnation

【Prescription】

Modified *Guǎng Dà Chóng Míng Tāng* (Great Sight-Restoring Decoction, 广大重明汤)

防风	*fáng fēng*	8 g	Radix Saposhnikoviae
龙胆草	*lóng dǎn cǎo*	8 g	Radix et Rhizoma Gentianae
甘草	*gān cǎo*	6 g	Radix et Rhizoma Glycyrrhizae
细辛	*xì xīn*	3 g	Radix et Rhizoma Asari

黄芩	*huáng qín*	8 g	Radix Scutellariae
赤芍	*chì sháo*	8 g	Radix Paeoniae Rubra
牡丹皮	*mǔ dān pí*	8 g	Cortex Moutan
浮萍	*fú píng*	8 g	Herba Spirodelae
地肤子	*dì fū zǐ*	8 g	Fructus Kochiae

5 batches were prescribed (with another 2–5 batches at the second and third follow-up visits).

By the fourth follow-up visit, the intense itching had disappeared and the papillae in the palpebra conjunctiva had decreased; he had a red tongue, and a thready-rapid pulse. Because the condition was prolonged for years, the healthy qi had been damaged though the pathogen was been removed; therefore, the treatment principle should be changed to securing healthy qi and removing pathogen. Formula: Modified *Dāng Guī Yǎng Róng Tāng* (Chinese angelica Supporting and Nourishing Decoction, 当归养荣汤). Prescription: *dāng guī* (当归, Radix Angelicae Sinensis), *bái sháo* (白芍, Radix Paeoniae Alba), *shēng dì* (生地, Radix Rehmanniae), *chuān xiōng* (川芎, Rhizoma Chuanxiong), *bái zhǐ* (白芷, Radix Angelicae Dahuricae), *qiāng huó* (羌活, Rhizoma et Radix Notopterygii), *fáng fēng* (防风, Radix Saposhnikoviae), *huáng qín* (黄芩, Radix Scutellariae), *huáng bǎi* (黄柏, Cortex Phellodendri Chinensis), *dì fū zǐ* (地肤子, Fructus Kochiae) and *chì sháo* (赤芍, Radix Paeoniae Rubra); 7 doses in total.

Classic Quotes

《眼科菁华录·时复之病》："类似赤热,不治自愈,及期而发,过期又愈,如花如潮,久而不治,遂成其害。"

"It presents with redness and heat and resolves on its own without treatment, but reoccurs at the same of next year and the patient recovers after the season, like flowers and tides. If left untreated for a long time, it will damage the body."

Ophthalmology Essence Records – Seasonal Disease (*Yǎn Kē Jīng Huá Lù – Shí Fú Zhī Bìng*, 眼科菁华录·时复之病)

Questions for Consideration

1. What are the clinical manifestations of vernal keratoconjunctivitis?

2. State briefly the main syndrome characteristics of the damp-heat with wind pattern, along with its treatment principle and formula.

Section 3 Phlyctenular Keratoconjunctivitis

Phlyctenular keratoconjunctivitis is a hypersensitivity reaction caused by a microprotein. The common pathogenetic microorganisms include: tubercle bacillus, staphylococcus aureus, white candida, coccidioides, and type L1, L2, L3 serotype chlamydia trachomatis. This condition occurs commonly in spring and summer, and is most often seen in children and teenagers. Females are more prone to it than males. Phlyctenular keratoconjunctivitis is a spontaneous disease that comes and goes rather quickly, but does recur easily. In Chinese medical ophthalmology, this condition is named *jīn gān* (金疳, golden gan). If the lesion is at the cornea with radial neovascular vessels invading, it is called *fēng lún chì dòu* (风轮赤豆, wind wheel red bean). The cause and pathogenesis of this disease is due to dry heat in the lung channel, which results in delinquency of descending and dispersion of qi. Abundant lung fire is attacking the eyes, causing qi and fire toxin to stagnate. Another causative factor may be associated with deficiency of lung yin causing deficiency fire to rise upward to the whites of the eyes. Dysfunction of the spleen and stomach could be another possible causative factor. The pathogenesis is due to an inability of earth to generate metal, which results in loss of nourishment to the lung channel and dysfunction of lung qi.

Clinical Manifestation

Genarally, the patient may only feel a mild sensation of a foreign object in the eye. When the cornea is affected, photophobia, tearing, and aching may be present. During the initial stages, a hard, elevated, translucent nodule (1–3 mm in size) may appear on the conjunctiva or cornea, surrounded by redness and swelling. Latterly, the ulcer erupts and heals usually within 10–12 days without scarring. If the lesion is at the limbus, one or several nodules may present, accompanied by local congestion. There may be residual minor nebulas left over when the lesion is healed, which can make the limbus irregular. This condition may recur with aggravating factors such as reactive conjunctivitis and acute bacterial conjunctivitis. After recurrences, the lesion may migrate towards the center of the cornea, accompanied by neovascularization, which is called fasicular keratitis. There will typically be a residual girdle-shaped nebula.

Treatment

1. Pattern Differentiation and Treatment

(1) Dry Heat in the Lung Channel

【 Syndrome Characteristics 】

Eye pain, hot tearing, hyperemia and tortuosity of conjunctival vessels, thirst, dry nose, constipation, dark urine, red tongue with thin yellow coating, rapid pulse.

【 Treatment Principle 】

Clear lung heat, dissipate masses, and reduce swelling

【 Representative Formula 】

Modified *Xiè Fèi Tāng* (Lung-Draining Decoction, 泻肺汤)

【 Prescription 】

桑白皮	*sāng bái pí*	15 g	Cortex Mori
黄芩	*huáng qín*	10 g	Radix Scutellariae
地骨皮	*dì gǔ pí*	12 g	Cortex Lycii
知母	*zhī mǔ*	10 g	Rhizoma Anemarrhenae
麦冬	*mài dōng*	10 g	Radix Ophiopogonis
桔梗	*jié gěng*	10 g	Radix Platycodonis

【 Modifications 】

➢ For cases with severe conjunctival congestion, add *chì sháo* (赤芍, Radix Paeoniae Rubra) 10 g, *mǔ dān pí* (牡丹皮, Cortex Moutan) 10 g, *lián qiào* (连翘, Fructus Forsythiae) 10 g and *xià kū cǎo* (夏枯草, Spica Prunellae) 10 g to clear heat, cool blood, and remove redness.

➢ For cases with constipation, add *dà huáng* (大黄, Radix et Rhizoma Rhei) 6 g to purge the *fu* and clear heat.

(2) Lung Yin Deficiency

【 Syndrome Characteristics 】

Mild eye pain of the affected eye, dry and thick secretions, conjunctival congestion, dry cough, dry throat, a red tongue with a thin coating, and a thready and rapid pulse.

【 Treatment Principle 】

Nourish yin and clear lung heat; clear heat and rectify stagnation

【 Representative Formula 】

Modified *Yǎng Yīn Qīng Fèi Tāng* (Yin-Nourishing and Lung-Clearing Decoction, 养阴清肺汤)

【Prescription】

甘草	gān cǎo	10 g	Radix et Rhizoma Glycyrrhizae
白芍	bái sháo	10 g	Radix Paeoniae Alba
生地	shēng dì	10 g	Radix Rehmanniae
薄荷	bò he	10 g	Herba Menthae
玄参	xuán shēn	10 g	Radix Scrophulariae
麦冬	mài dōng	10 g	Radix Ophiopogonis
贝母	bèi mǔ	10 g	Bulbus Fritillaria
牡丹皮	mǔ dān pí	10 g	Cortex Moutan
夏枯草	xià kū cǎo	10 g	Spica Prunellae
连翘	lián qiào	10 g	Fructus Forsythiae

【Modifications】
➢ For cases with marked thirst and dry throat, add *běi shā shēn* (北沙参, Radix Glehniae) 10 g and *lú gēn* (芦根, Rhizoma Phragmitis) 10 g to nourish yin and promote fluid production.

(3) Lung and Spleen Deficiency

【Syndrome Characteristics】
Mild congestion around the conjunctiva, chronic course and/or recurrence, lack of energy, poor appetite, abdominal distention and discomfort, pale tongue with thin white coating, thready and weak pulse.

【Treatment Principle】
Benefit qi and strengthen the spleen.

【Representative Formula】
Modified *Shēn Líng Bái Zhú Sǎn* (Ginseng, Poria and Atractylodes Macrocephalae Powder, 参苓白术散)

【Prescription】

党参	dǎng shēn	10 g	Radix Codonopsis
炒白术	chǎo bái zhú	15 g	Rhizoma Atractylodis Macrocephalae (dry-fried)
茯苓	fú líng	10 g	Poria
甘草	gān cǎo	6 g	Radix et Rhizoma Glycyrrhizae
山药	shān yào	10 g	Rhizoma Dioscoreae
桔梗	jié gěng	10 g	Radix Platycodonis
白扁豆	bái biǎn dòu	10 g	Semen Lablab Album
莲子肉	lián zǐ ròu	10 g	Semen Nelumbinis
薏苡仁	yì yǐ rén	10 g	Semen Coicis
陈皮	chén pí	10 g	Pericarpium Citri Reticulatae

Modification: For cases with severe conjunctival congestion and pain, add *chì sháo* (赤芍, Radix Paeoniae Rubra) 10 g and *sāng bái pí* (桑白皮, Cortex Mori) 10 g to clear heat and stop pain.

【 Modifications 】

For cases with severe conjunctival congestion and pain, add *chì sháo* (赤芍, Radix Paeoniae Rubra) 10 g and *sāng bái pí* (桑白皮, Cortex Mori) 10 g to clear heat and stop pain.

2. Acupuncture

ST 1 (*chéng qì*)	BL 2 (*cuán zhú*)	*tài yáng* (太阳)
yú yāo (鱼腰)	GB 20 (*fēng chí*)	LI 4 (*hé gǔ*)

Choose 3–4 points each treatment, use 1 *cùn* size filiform needle, retain the needles for 30–50 minutes; 12 sessions is a treatment course.

3. Chinese Patent Medicines

(1) **Qīng Rè Jiě Dú Ruǎn Jiāo Náng (Heat-clearing and Toxin-Expelling Soft Capsules, 清热解毒软胶囊)**

3 capsules, three times a day.

(2) **Shuāng Huáng Lián Kǒu Fú Yè (Honeysuckle flower, Coptis Oral Liquid, 双黄连口服液)**

10–20ml, three times a day.

(3) **Yín Qiào Jiě Dú Piàn (Lonicera and Forsythia Toxin-Expelling Tablets, 银翘解毒片)**

3 tablets, three times a day.

4. Simple and proven recipes:

Jīn yín huā (金银花, Flos Lonicerae Japonicae) 30 g, *jú huā* (菊花, Flos Chrysanthemi) 30 g, *jué míng zǐ* (决明子, Semen Cassiae) 30 g, *pàng dà hǎi* (胖大海, Semen Sterculiae Lychnophorae) 30 g, wrap the medicinals individually, take 1 g of each every time, put in a teapot and add some boiled water to make medicinal tea, take 6–9 times each day.

5. External Treatment

(1) *Zhēn Zhū Míng Mù Yè* (珍珠明目液, Pearl Eye-Brightening Drop): 1–2 drops, 6 times a day.

(2) *Zhēn Shì Míng Yǎn Yào Shuǐ* (珍视明眼药水, Precious Eye-Brightening Drop): 1–2

drops, 6 times a day.

(3) *Xióng Dǎn Yǎn Yào Shuǐ* (熊胆眼药水, Bear Gallbladder Eye Drop): 1–2 drops each time, 6 times a day.

6. Treatment with Western Medicine

Treat the underlying conditions of phlyctenular keratoconjunctivitis. Topical steroidal eye drops are effective. If caused by tubercle bacillus protein, eyes may be very sensitive to steroid treatment; symptoms will generally improve within 24 hours and disappear in another day or so. Steroid/antibiotics eye drops are recommended if there is a bacterial infection in the conjunctiva or cornea. Taking multiple vitamins, enhancing nutrition, and strengthening the immune system will be helpful as well. If corneal scarring causes severe vision loss, keratoplasty may be an option.

7. Dietary Therapy and Preventive Care

Intake of spicy and deep-fried food should be restrained because it may produce pathogenic heat and damage yin. Increase outdoor exercise to strengthen the constitution.

Case Studies

Ning, a 15-year-old girl
【Chief Complaint】
Photophobia, tearing, and pain at the left eye, accompanied by constipation.
【Examination】
Gray-white nodules at the lateral limbus about the size of a grain of rice surrounded by conjunctival congestion, thin white tongue coating, and a thready and rapid pulse.
【Diagnosis】
Phlyctenular keratoconjunctivitis
【Prescription】
Modified *Shuāng Jiě Tāng* (Double Resolution Decoction, 双解汤)

金银花	*jīn yín huā*	15 g	Flos Lonicerae Japonicae
蒲公英	*pú gōng yīng*	15 g	Herba Taraxaci
天花粉	*tiān huā fěn*	10 g	Radix Trichosanthis
黄芩	*huáng qín*	10 g	Radix Scutellariae
枳壳	*zhǐ qiào*	5 g	Fructus Aurantii
龙胆草	*lóng dǎn cǎo*	10 g	Radix et Rhizoma Gentianae
荆芥	*jīng jiè*	10 g	Herba Schizonepetae

防风	*fáng fēng*	10 g	Radix Saposhnikoviae
桑白皮	*sāng bái pí*	6 g	Cortex Mori
甘草	*gān cǎo*	3 g	Radix et Rhizoma Glycyrrhizae

【Follow-up】

After three batches of the formula, the redness was decreased significantly and the nodules had mostly resolved. After 5 more batches of the same formula, all symptoms disappeared. In order to strengthen the effect, she was administered a formula to help nourish the yin, clear heat, and regulate the spleen and stomach:

生地	*shēng dì*	15 g	Radix Rehmanniae
天花粉	*tiān huā fěn*	15 g	Radix Trichosanthis
麦冬	*mài dōng*	10 g	Radix Ophiopogonis
知母	*zhī mǔ*	6 g	Rhizoma Anemarrhenae
金银花	*jīn yín huā*	10 g	Flos Lonicerae Japonicae
枳壳	*zhǐ qiào*	5 g	Fructus Aurantii
槟榔	*bīng láng*	3 g	Semen Arecae
莱菔子	*lái fú zǐ*	5 g	Semen Raphani
甘草	*gān cǎo*	10 g	Radix et Rhizoma Glycyrrhizae

All the medicinals of the above were decocted with water; one batch a day, for a total of 7 batches. We continued our observation for 2 years and no recurrence was reported.

Classic Quotes

《证治准绳·杂病·七窍门》“金疳,初起与玉粒相似,至大方便出祸患······生于气轮者,则有珠痛泪流之苦。”

"Golden gan is similar to jade grain at the beginning; it hurts when it gets bigger....If it occurs at the qi wheel, the patient will suffer from pain and tearing."

Standards for Diagnosis and Treatment – Miscellaneous Diseases– Seven Orifices Sect (Zhèng Zhì Zhǔn Shéng – Zá Bìng – Qī Qiào Mén, 证治准绳·杂病·七窍门)

Question for Consideration

What is the cause and pathogenesis of phlyctenular keratoconjunctivitis?

Chapter 8

Ocular Surface Diseases

Dry Eyes

Keratoconjunctivitis sicca (dry eyes), is a lacrimal film abnormality caused by decreased lacrimal secretions, or hyperactive lacrimal evaporation. The condition is present with symptoms of discomfort in the eye which may accompany ocular surface diseases. If patients have isolated symptoms of dry eyes, they may recover with rest or short-term use of artificial tears. If there is no presence of ocular surface damage and/or any other local or systemic causes, it is called simple dry eyes. If patients have both symptoms and clinical signs of dry eyes, it is called xerophthalmia. If accompanied by systemic immunologic diseases, it is called dry eye syndrome. With the popularization of the computer and lifestyle habit changes, the incidence of dry eyes has gradually increased while the average age of onset is much lower than before. An investigation of 2,520 individuals (≥65 years old) in Salisbury, Maryland, USA, showed that 14.6% had the symptoms of dry eyes.

In Chinese medicine, the disease pertains to *bái sè zhèng* (white dry eye, 白涩症), or *shén shuǐ jiāng kū* (impending desiccation of spirit water, 神水将枯), belongs to *zào zhèng* (dryness pattern, 燥证). The causes and pathogenesis are insufficiency of lung yin or liver-kidney yin deficiency, which lead to nutritional deficiency of the eyes.

Clinical Manifestation

Common ocular symptoms include asthenopia, sensation of foreign bodies in the eyes, dryness, burning, swelling, ophthalmalgia, photophobia, redness, and so on. If there are symptoms, patients should be asked in detail their history, in order to find the underlying cause. For severe dry eyes, the patients should be asked if their condition is accompanied by dry mouth or joint pain, in order to rule out a simple diagnosis of dry eye syndrome. Signs of dry eye include vasodilatation, tarnished, thickening, edema and folds of bulbar conjunctiva, narrowing or interruption of lacrimal river, and occasional yellowish sticky silky secretions seen in the lower fornix, punctuate damages of corneal epithelium in the palpebral fissure area. When dry eye is suspected, relevant tests may be considered, including Schirmer test, break-up time of tear film (BUT), and so on. Dry eye may affect the visual acuity in early stages, and may further develop into filamentary keratitis, at later stages, lead to a corneal ulcer, corneal thinning, perforation, and in some cases a secondary bacterial infection.

Treatment

1. Pattern Differentiation and Treatment

(1) Insufficiency of Lung Yin
【 Syndrome Characteristics 】
Dry eyes, unable to see for an extended time, mild hyperemia of the conjunctiva, point lesions of the corneal superficial layer, relapse and poor recovery, dry cough with little phlegm, dry pharynx and constipation, red tongue with little moisture, thready rapid pulse.

【 Treatment Principle 】
Enrich yin and moisten the lung

【 Representative Formula 】
Yăng Yīn Qīng Fèi Tāng (Yin-Nourishing Lung-Clearing Decoction, 养阴清肺汤)

【 Prescription 】

牡丹皮	*mŭ dān pí*	10 g	Cortex Moutan
白芍	*bái sháo*	10 g	Radix Paeoniae Alba
生甘草	*shēng gān căo*	10 g	Radix et Rhizoma Glycyrrhizae
生地	*shēng dì*	15 g	Radix Rehmanniae
薄荷	*bò he*	6 g	Herba Menthae
玄参	*xuán shēn*	10 g	Radix Scrophulariae
麦冬	*mài dōng*	15 g	Radix Ophiopogonis
贝母	*bèi mŭ*	10 g	Bulbus Fritillaria
太子参	*tài zĭ shēn*	15 g	Radix Pseudostellariae
五味子	*wŭ wèi zĭ*	10 g	Fructus Schisandrae Chinensis

【 Modifications 】
➢ For cases with pronounced dry throat and mouth, add *bĕi shā shēn* (北沙参, Radix Glehniae) 15 g, *shí hú* (石斛, Caulis Dendrobii) 10 g to boost qi and nourish yin.

➢ For cases with constipation, add *jué míng zĭ* (决明子, Semen Cassiae) 15 g to moisten the intestines and free the stool.

➢ For cases with point lesions of the cornea, add *chán tuì* (蝉蜕, Periostracum Cicadae) 6 g, *jú huā* (菊花, Flos Chrysanthemi) 12 g, *mì méng huā* (密蒙花, Flos

Buddlejae) 10 g to clear heat, abate visual screens, and brighten the eyes.

(2) Liver-Kidney Yin Deficiency

〖 Syndrome Characteristics 〗

Dry eyes with discomfort, photophobia, symptoms increased after prolonged use, dry mouth with scant saliva, lumbago, weak and/or painful knees, dizziness and tinnitus, insomnia with profuse dreams, red tongue with little coating, thready pulse.

〖 Treatment Principle 〗

Nourish the liver and kidney

〖 Representative Formula 〗

Modified *Qǐ Jú Dì Huáng Wán* (Lycium Berry, Chrysanthemum and Rehmannia Pill, 杞菊地黄丸)

〖 Prescription 〗

枸杞子	*gǒu qǐ zǐ*	15 g	Fructus Lycii
菊花	*jú huā*	10 g	Flos Chrysanthemi
熟地	*shú dì*	10 g	Radix Rehmanniae Praeparata
山茱萸	*shān zhū yú*	10 g	Fructus Corni
山药	*shān yào*	15 g	Rhizoma Dioscoreae
泽泻	*zé xiè*	10 g	Rhizoma Alismatis
茯苓	*fú líng*	10 g	Poria
牡丹皮	*mǔ dān pí*	10 g	Cortex Moutan

〖 Modifications 〗

➤ For cases with dry mouth with scanty saliva, add *mài dōng* (麦冬, Radix Ophiopogonis) 10g, *xuán shēn* (玄参, Radix Scrophulariae) 10 g to nourish yin and engender liquid.

➤ For cases with obvious hyperemia of the conjunctiva, add *sāng bái pí* (桑白皮, Cortex Mori) 9 g, *dì gǔ pí* (地骨皮, Cortex Lycii) 10 g to clear heat and reduce congestion.

2. Acupuncture

ST 1 (*chéng qì*)	太阳 (*tài yáng*)	GB 20 (*fēng chí*)
BL 2 (*cuán zhú*)	鱼腰 (*yú yāo*)	SJ 23 (*sī zhú kōng*)
ST 2 (*sì bái*)	LV 3 (*tài chōng*)	GB 37 (*guāng míng*)
SP 6 (*sān yīn jiāo*)	LI 4 (*hé gǔ*)	DU 23 (*shàng xīng*)
DU 20 (*bǎi huì*)		

4–6 acupoints are selected each session; retain the needles for 20–30 minutes, treating once every day. 10 treatments constitute one course of treatment.

3. Chinese Patent Medicines

(1) *Qǐ Jú Dì Huáng Wán* (Lycium Berry, Chrysanthemum and Rehmannia Pill, 杞菊地黄丸)

6 pills, two times everyday; applicable to liver-kidney yin deficiency.

(2) *Zhī Bǎi Dì Huáng Wán* (Lycium Berry, Chrysanthemum and Rehmannia Pill, 知柏地黄丸)

6 pills, two times everyday; applicable to liver-kidney yin deficiency or effulgent yin-deficiency fire.

(3) *Yǎng Yīn Qīng Fèi Kǒu Fú Yè* (Yin-Nourishing Lung-Clearing oral liquid, 养阴清肺口服液)

10 ml, two times everyday; applicable to insufficiency of lung yin.

4. Simple and Proven Recipes

Jú huā (菊花, Flos Chrysanthemi), *mài dōng* (麦冬, Radix Ophiopogonis), *gǒu qǐ zǐ* (枸杞子, Fructus Lycii), *mù hú dié* (木蝴蝶, Semen Oroxyli), singly wrapped; drink a small amount each time, brew in a teapot with boiling water. Drink 6–9 times every day.

5. Treatment with Western Medicine

(1) 1% sodium hyaluronate eye drops; use 4–6 times a day.

(2) Carboxymethylcellulose Sodium Lubricant Eye Drops; 4–6 times every day.

(3) For cases with severe symptoms, seek advice or treatment from a conventional eye doctor; increase some methods like application of a local immunodepressant or plugging the opening to the lacrimal ducts.

6. Dietary Therapy and Preventive Care

(1) Do not use the eyes excessively. TV and computers should be placed in a position below eye level.

(2) Avoid air conditioning and flue dust, and be sure to maintain a certain degree of humidity in the room.

(3) Live regularly, pay attention to dietary regulations and healthy eating; eat fresh vegetables and fruits, while increasing intake of vitamin A, B_1, C, and E. Do not overeat spicy, greasy-fried, or irritating foods.

(4) Regulate the emotions and work on cultivating an optimistic mood; maintain proper balance between work and leisure.

Case Studies

Chen, a 45 year old male

Initial visit: November 11, 2008

【Chief Complaint】

Dryness of both eyes for 6 months

【Medical History】

Sometimes his symptoms were accompanied by dry stool. There was no history of arthritis. He also complained of dry mouth and dry nose, nosebleeding when tired or in an irregular life routine; stomachache and diarrhea would occur after ingesting cold food. Pale red tongue with thin white coating, thready moderate pulse.

【Examination】

Visual acuity: 20/25 on both eyes, fluorescein stain of cornea was positive, breakup time of tear film: 5 seconds (ou, oculus uterque), Schirmer test: 1mm in the left eye, 2mm in the right eye.

【Diagnosis】

Binocular dry eye

【Pattern Differentiation】

Deficiency of both qi and yin

【Treatment Principles】

Boost qi and nourish yin, supply the spleen and boost the kidney

【Prescription】

太子参	tài zǐ shēn	15 g	Radix Pseudostellariae
麦冬	mài dōng	15 g	Radix Ophiopogonis
五味子	wǔ wèi zǐ	6 g	Fructus Schisandrae Chinensis
生地	shēng dì	15 g	Radix Rehmanniae
熟地	shú dì	15 g	Radix Rehmanniae Praeparata
山茱萸	shān zhū yú	10 g	Fructus Corni
山药	shān yào	10 g	Rhizoma Dioscoreae
茯苓	fú líng	10 g	Poria
泽泻	zé xiè	10 g	Rhizoma Alismatis
牡丹皮	mǔ dān pí	10 g	Cortex Moutan
白蒺藜	bái jí lí	20 g	Fructus Tribuli
升麻	shēng má	10 g	Rhizoma Cimicifugae
葛根	gé gēn	10 g	Radix Puerariae Lobatae

【Follow-up】

The prescribed formula was modified over time and with changing symptoms. After 4 months of treatment, results of the Schirmer test were the following: 11 mm in the right eye, and 8 mm in the left eye. Dryness and astringent sensation of both eyes were much improved.

Classic Quotes

《审视瑶函·神水将枯症》："此症视珠外神水枯涩，而不润莹，最不易识。虽形于言而不审其状。乃火郁蒸于膏泽，故精不清，而珠不盈润，汁将内竭。"

"The disease was caused by desiccation of spirit water at the outer surface of the eyeball, and it is not easy to be recognized. Although the patients complain, clinical signs cannot be found. Pathogenesis of the disease was congestion of fire causing spirit jelly, thus essence cannot remain clear and becomes opaque, and the eyeball cannot be moistened, and liquid gets exhausted."

A Close Examination of the Precious Classic on Ophthalmology – Impending Desiccation of Spirit Water (*Shěn Shì Yāo Hán – Shén Shuǐ Jiāng Kū Zhèng*, 审视瑶函·神水将枯症)

Questions for Consideration

What are main points of pattern differentiation of dry eyes? Simply explain the pathogenesis.

Chapter 9
Scleritis

Scleritis is an inflammatory disease that affects the surface tissue of the sclera. If the infection occurs within the surface sclera tissue, it is called episcleritis. If the infection occurs in the stroma of the sclera, it is called scleritis. The cause of the disease is very complex, and is associated with autoimmune factors. Main clinical manifestations include eye pain, dark red hyperemia in the localized area of the sclera, and immobile nodule. Occurrence is more common in persons aged 20 to 60 years old. Female patients are more susceptible than males. More than half of the patients have bilateral attacks successively, and the condition easily becomes recurrent. Western medical therapy for this condition includes topical eye drops and/or medication that is taken internally. Glucocorticoids and non-steroidal anti-inflammatory drugs are commonly used.

In Chinese medicine, the disease is called *huǒ gān* (火疳, scleritis) because of the invasion and accumulation of pathogenic heat at the site of the sclera and conjunctiva. The main organ pathologies associated with this condition are those of the lung, heart, and liver. The disease is caused by pathogenic heat flourishing, fire constraint being unable to diffuse, thus ascending upward, causing qi and blood stagnation in the sclera and conjunctiva. General methods of treatment are aimed at clearing heat and promoting the flow of qi. The treatment principle is to regulate *zang-fu* organs, clear pathogenic heat, and diffuse congestion and constraint, so as to relieve the clinical symptoms. It is possible to cure this disease and control recurrences.

Clinical Manifestation

1. Episcleritis

The clinical features of episcleritis include rapid onset, with a disease course lasting about 10 to 20 days. During the period of the initial onset, there are symptoms of discomfort in the affected eye including photophobia, tearing and pain. The affected region shows redness and localized edema in the superficial layer of sclera. There can also be localized nodular bulging which presents itself as dark red, slightly movable, and appears in multiple quadrants, due to the recurrent attacks in different parts of the sclera. The disease has a partial self-limiting tendency, but recurrent attacks can last over a period of many years.

2. Scleritis

The clinical features of scleritis include rapid onset or gradual progression, severe pain in the affected eye, radiating pain to the affected side of the head, and edema in the conjunctiva. Hyperemia shows dark red or prunosus in the superficial as well as the deep layer. Single or multiple nodules may present in the sclera that are hard and immobile with tenderness. Some severe conditions may develop rapidly, or become complicated forms of uveitis. If vasculitis occurs in the outer vesicles of affected sclera area, some features may appear in the lesion or the surrounding area including non-perfusion capillary, infarction and necrosis, thinning and light blue coloring of the involved sclera. Severe scleritis may bring about staphyloma or perforations of the sclera.

Treatment

1. Pattern Differentiation and Treatment

The disease occurs in the inner layer of *bái jīng* (sclera and conjunctiva). The common causes of this disease are accumulation of pathogenic heat in the lung channel. Because the sclera and conjunctiva are relatively exterior and more closely related with (cornea), the main treatment principle is geared to clear and drain heat of the lung and liver channels. Excessive heat can damage blood and yin, so yin and blood should be protected and emphasis placed on invigorating blood as a means of dissipating the pathogenic accumulation.

(1) Heat Stagnation in the Lung Channel
【 Syndrome Characteristics 】
At the initial stage, the major local symptoms include mild eye pain, local red or dark purple color in the sclera and conjunctiva, with local bulging. Systemic symptoms include pharyngalgia, cough, yellow, thick phlegm, yellow urine, red tongue with thin yellow coating, rapid pulse.
【 Treatment Principle 】
Clear lung heat
【 Representative Formula 】
Modified *Xiè Fèi Tāng* (Lung-Draining Decoction, 泻肺汤)
【 Prescription 】

桑白皮	*sāng bái pí*	2 g	Cortex Mori
地骨皮	*dì gǔ pí*	12 g	Cortex Lycii
黄芩	*huáng qín*	10 g	Radix Scutellariae

知母	zhī mǔ	10 g	Rhizoma Anemarrhenae
麦冬	mài dōng	10 g	Radix Ophiopogonis
桔梗	jié gěng	8 g	Radix Platycodonis
葶苈子	tíng lì zǐ	8 g	Semen Lepidii; Semen Descurainiae
杏仁	xìng rén	8 g	Semen Armeniacae Amarum

【Modifications】

➢ For cases with redness in the sclera caused by excessive heat stasis, add *mǔ dān pí* (牡丹皮, Cortex Moutan) 10 g, *chì sháo* (赤芍, Radix Paeoniae Rubra) 12 g, *hóng huā* (红花, Flos Carthami) 10 g to relieve redness by cooling blood and resolving stasis.

➢ For cases with severe pain caused by stasis, add *shēng pú huáng* (生蒲黄, Pollen Typhae) 12 g, *wǔ líng zhī* (五灵脂, Faeces Trogopterori) 8 g to break up stasis, relieve pain, and dissipate nodules.

(2) Fire Toxin Exuberance

【Syndrome Characteristics】

Eye pain, orbital pain, photophobia, excessive tearing, nodule bulge in the sclera, hyperemia, dark purple coloring, bitter taste and dry mouth, yellow urine, red tongue with yellow coating, rapid pulse.

【Treatment Principle】

Purge fire and remove toxin, cool blood and dissipate masses

【Representative Formula】

Modified *Huán Yīn Jiù Kǔ Tāng* (Yin-Returning Bitterness-Relieving Decoction, 还阴救苦汤)

【Prescription】

黄芩	huáng qín	10 g	Radix Scutellariae
黄连	huáng lián	5 g	Rhizoma Coptidis
黄柏	huáng bǎi	10 g	Cortex Phellodendri Chinensis
龙胆草	lóng dǎn cǎo	5 g	Radix et Rhizoma Gentianae
连翘	lián qiào	10 g	Fructus Forsythiae
羌活	qiāng huó	8 g	Radix et Rhizoma Notopterygii
藁本	gāo běn	10 g	Rhizoma Ligustici
蔓荆子	màn jīng zǐ	12 g	Fructus Viticis
柴胡	chái hú	8 g	Radix Bupleuri
桔梗	jié gěng	5 g	Radix Platycodonis
知母	zhī mǔ	12 g	Rhizoma Anemarrhenae
生地	shēng dì	15 g	Radix Rehmanniae
川芎	chuān xiōng	12 g	Rhizoma Chuanxiong

当归尾	*dāng guī wěi*	10 g	Radix Angelicae Sinensis (extremities)
赤芍	*chì sháo*	12 g	Radix Paeoniae Rubra
升麻	*shēng má*	10 g	Rhizoma Cimicifugae
甘草梢	*gān cǎo shāo*	5 g	Radix Tenuis Glycyrrhizae

【Modifications】

➢ For cases with constipation, add *dà huáng* (大黄, Radix et Rhizoma Rhei) 5 g to relieve constipation by purgation, improve the clearing of heat and removal of toxin, invigorate blood, and disperse nodules.

➢ For cases with obvious redness of the sclera, add *sāng bái pí* (桑白皮, Cortex Mori) 15 g, *dì gǔ pí* (地骨皮, Cortex Lycii) 12g to purge the lung and promote qi flow.

➢ For cases with marked eye pain accompanied by orbital pain that is especially severe in the night, add *xià kū cǎo* (夏枯草, Spica Prunellae) 10 g, *zhì xiāng fù* (制香附, Rhizoma Cyperi) 12 g to soothe the liver, regulate qi, and alleviate pain.

(3) Wind-Damp-Heat Brewing and Binding

【Syndrome Characteristics】

Blurred vision, distending pain in the eyeball which refuses pressure, photophobia, tearing, red or dark purple color of the sclera, difficult recovery, recurrent attacks, multiple nodules on the sclera, arthralgia, limb swelling, difficulty bending and stretching (muscle tightness), dyspnea, gastric stuffiness, anorexia and loose stool, red tongue with yellow greasy coating, slippery and rapid pulse.

【Treatment Principle】

Dispel wind and clear heat, remove dampness and dissipate masses

【Representative Formula】

Modified *Qiāng Huó Tāng* (Notopterygium Decoction, 羌活汤)

【Prescription】

菊花	*jú huā*	10 g	Flos Chrysanthemi
决明子	*jué míng zǐ*	15 g	Semen Cassiae
木贼	*mù zéi*	8 g	Herba Equiseti Hiemalis
苍术	*cāng zhú*	10 g	Rhizoma Atractylodis
防风	*fáng fēng*	10 g	Radix Saposhnikoviae
羌活	*qiāng huó*	10 g	Radix et Rhizoma Notopterygii
川芎	*chuān xiōng*	10 g	Rhizoma Chuanxiong
滑石	*huá shí*	20 g	Talcum
柴胡	*chái hú*	5 g	Radix Bupleuri
青皮	*qīng pí*	8 g	Pericarpium Citri Reticulatae Viride
黄芩	*huáng qín*	10 g	Radix Scutellariae

栀子	*zhī zǐ*	10 g	Fructus Gardeniae
桔梗	*jié gěng*	5 g	Radix Platycodonis
枳壳	*zhǐ qiào*	8 g	Fructus Aurantii
陈皮	*chén pí*	10 g	Pericarpium Citri Reticulatae
甘草	*gān cǎo*	3 g	Radix et Rhizoma Glycyrrhizae

【Modifications】

➢ For cases with severe hyperemia of the sclera, which indicates heat is more pronounced than dampness, remove *fáng fēng* (防风, Radix Saposhnikoviae) and *qiāng huó* (羌活, Radix et Rhizoma Notopterygii), and add *chì sháo* (赤芍, Radix Paeoniae Rubra) 12 g, *mǔ dān pí* (牡丹皮, Cortex Moutan) 10 g, and *lóng dǎn cǎo* (龙胆草, Radix et Rhizoma Gentianae) 5 g to clear heat and dry dampness, and cool and activate blood.

➢ For cases with dyspnea, and tongue with thick greasy coating, manifesting of excess pathogenic dampness, add *tōng cǎo* (通草, Medulla Tetrapanacis) 10 g, *chē qián zǐ* (车前子, Semen Plantaginis) 10 g, and *yì yǐ rén* (薏苡仁, Semen Coicis) 15 g to eliminate dampness with bland medicinals.

(4) Deficiency Fire Flaming Upward

【Syndrome Characteristics】

Recurrent attacks in later stages of the disease, sore and uncomfortable eyes, dry and dim-vision, no obvious bulge of the nodule, purple and dark color, mild tenderness, oro-pharyngoxerosis, vexing heat in five centers, red cheeks and night sweats, red tongue with little coating, thready and rapid pulse.

【Treatment Principle】

Nourish yin and reduce fire

【Representative Formula】

Modified *Yǎng Yīn Qīng Fèi Tāng* (Yin-Nourishing and Lung-Clearing Decoction, 养阴清肺汤)

【Prescription】

生地	*shēng dì*	15 g	Radix Rehmanniae
玄参	*xuán shēn*	12 g	Radix Scrophulariae
麦冬	*mài dōng*	10 g	Radix Ophiopogonis
贝母	*bèi mǔ*	8 g	Bulbus Fritillaria
白芍	*bái sháo*	10 g	Radix Paeoniae Alba
牡丹皮	*mǔ dān pí*	12 g	Cortex Moutan
薄荷	*bò he*	5 g	Herba Menthae
甘草	*gān cǎo*	3 g	Radix et Rhizoma Glycyrrhizae

【 Modifications 】

➤ For the cases with marked hyperemia of the sclera, heat vexation, and night sweating, add *zhī mǔ* (知母, Rhizoma Anemarrhenae) 8 g, *huáng bǎi* (黄柏, Cortex Phellodendri Chinensis) 8 g, *dì gǔ pí* (地骨皮, Cortex Lycii) 10 g, and *shí hú* (石斛, Caulis Dendrobii) 10 g to nourish yin and reduce fire.

➤ For lingering nodules, add *yù jīn* (郁金, Radix Curcumae) 10 g, *dān shēn* (丹参, Radix et Rhizoma Salviae Miltiorrhizae) 12 g, *shēng mǔ lì* (生牡蛎, Ostreae Concha Cruda) 20 g, and *wǎ léng zǐ* (瓦楞子, Concha Arcae) 15 g to invigorate blood and dissipate pathogenic accumulation.

2. Acupuncture

LU 7 (*liè quē*)	LU 5 (*chǐ zé*)	LI 4 (*hé gǔ*)
LI 11 (*qū chí*)	ST 1 (*chéng qì*)	ST 2 (*sì bái*)
BL 1 (*jīng míng*)	BL 2 (*cuán zhú*)	*tài yáng* (太阳)
BL 13 (*fèi shù*)	BL 18 (*gān shù*)	

Use moderate reduction, and withdraw the needles after arrival of qi. Do not lift, thrust, and rotate the needle when puncturing the intraorbital acupoints.

3. Treatment with Western Medicine

The characteristics of the disease include many complex causes and systemic diseases. Scleral perforation may occur in severe cases, leading to further damage. The patients may seek advice or treatment from eye doctors.

Common therapies include:

(1) Eye Drops

Glucocorticoids such as dexamethasone, and cortisone. Combined with nonsteroid anti-inflammatory drops such as pranoprofen and diclofenac sodium. For severe conditions or occurrence with iridocyclitis, add mydriatics such as atropine eye ointment.

(2) Systemic Administration

According to the pathogenetic condition, patients may be administered glucocorticoids or nonsteroid anti-inflammatory drugs when necessary. If those do not work, cytotoxicity immunosuppressive agents, such as cyclophosphamide, and azathioprine, may be added to the treatment.

(3) Surgery

For severe cases such as scleral perforation, which develops from necrotizing scleritis, scleral transplant surgery should be considered.

(4) Etiological Treatment

Treat systemic collagenosis and metabolic diseases to decrease the incidence and recurrence rate of the disease.

4. Prevention and Health Care

Major importance is placed on improving nutrition, physical exercise, strengthening the body constitution, improving the overall body condition, and eating less spicy and fried food to avoid causing inflammation and damage to yin. The patient's residence should be carefully selected in order to avoid a damp environment.

Case Studies

Wu, 24-year-old male

Main signs included purple-colored sclera, bulging nodule, severe redness and swelling, eye pain and headache, ophthalmic discharge, and photophobia. Systemic signs showed dry mouth, scanty urination and dyschezia, floating and rapid pulse, red tongue with slightly yellow coating.

【Pattern Differentiation】

Flaring up of wind heat, due to depressed lung qi. Stasis due to pathogen being stronger than blood (defense), and blood coagulates leading to thickening and "sludging".

【Treatment Principles】

Dispel wind and dissipate heat, invigorate blood and purge fire

【Prescription】

Qū Féng Sàn Rè Yǐn (Wind-Dispelling and Heat-Dissipating Decoction, 驱风散热饮)

羌活	*qiāng huó*	8 g	Radix et Rhizoma Notopterygii
薄荷（后下）	*bò he (hòu xià)*	6 g	Herba Menthae (added later)
防风	*fáng fēng*	8 g	Radix Saposhnikoviae
牛蒡子	*niú bàng zǐ*	10 g	Fructus Arctii
金银花	*jīn yín huā*	12 g	Flos Lonicerae Japonicae
连翘	*lián qiào*	12 g	Fructus Forsythiae
栀子	*zhī zǐ*	10 g	Fructus Arctii
莲子心	*lián zǐ xīn*	8 g	Plumula Nelumbinis
当归	*dāng guī*	10 g	Radix Angelicae Sinensis
赤芍	*chì sháo*	10 g	Radix Paeoniae Rubra
川芎	*chuān xiōng*	10 g	Rhizoma Chuanxiong
甘草	*gān cǎo*	8 g	Radix et Rhizoma Glycyrrhizae

【Follow-up】

Second Visit: The pain eased and the conjunctival congestion and stasis symptoms were alleviated. Lingering signs included scanty urine, floating and rapid pulse, and red tongue. The condition indicated there was lingering internal heat, which needed to be cleared further.

Prescription: Modified *Dǎo Chì Sǎn* (Red Guiding Powder, 导赤散)

生地	*shēng dì*	15 g	Radix Rehmanniae
木通	*mù tōng*	10 g	Caulis Akebiae
甘草梢	*gān cǎo shāo*	10 g	Radix Tenuis Glycyrrhizae
黄连	*huáng lián*	5 g	Rhizoma Coptidis
黄芩	*huáng qín*	10 g	Radix Scutellariae
桃仁	*táo rén*	10 g	Semen Persicae
当归	*dāng guī*	10 g	Radix Angelicae Sinensis
金银花	*jīn yín huā*	12 g	Flos Lonicerae Japonicae
连翘	*lián qiào*	12 g	Fructus Forsythiae

Third Visit: Conjunctival swelling and nodules disappeared. Residual signs included minor congestion, red tongue, and rapid pulse. The indicated heat had not disappeared completely, and needed to be cleared further.

Prescription:

生地	*shēng dì*	15 g	Radix Rehmanniae
木通	*mù tōng*	10 g	Caulis Akebiae
甘草梢	*gān cǎo shāo*	10 g	Radix Tenuis Glycyrrhizae
黄连	*huáng lián*	5 g	Rhizoma Coptidis
黄芩	*huáng qín*	10 g	Radix Scutellariae

Excerpted from *Experience of the Patterns and Treatment of Ophthalmology* (*Yǎn Kē Zhèng Zhì Jīng Yàn*, 眼科证治经验)

Classic Quotes

《证治准绳·火疳证》:"生于睛眦气轮,在气轮为害尤急,盖火之实邪在于金部,火克金,鬼贼之邪,故害最急。初起如椒疮榴子一颗小而圆,或带横长而圆如小赤豆,次后渐大,痛者多,不痛者少。不可误以为轮上一颗如赤豆之证,因瘀积在外易消者。此则从内而生也。"

"This disease occurs at the canthi or qi wheen (the white of the eye, sclera and conjunctiva). If it occurs at the sclera, it would hurt with an acute onset, which is caused by excess fire pathogen attacking metal (the lung). At the initial stage, it is small and round or oval like pepper or pomegranate seed, and then gets bigger gradually, often accompanied by pain. Do not consider is as wind-orbiculus red bean (fascicular keratitis), which is caused by external stagnation and may vanish easily. This disease usually originates from the interior of the body."

Standards for Diagnosis and Treatment – Fire Gan Syndrome (*Zhèng Zhì Zhǔn Shéng– Huǒ Gān Zhèng,* 证治准绳·火疳证)

Question for Consideration

Please briefly describe the point selection and manipulation for the treatment of scleritis.

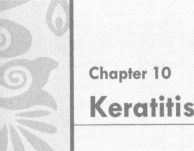

Chapter 10
Keratitis

Section 1   Herpes Simplex Keratitis

HSK (herpes simplex keratitis) is a common corneal infection caused by herpes simple virus. HSK often attacks one eye, although in some cases it may affect both eyes and can occur at any age. HSK occurs more often in the winter and autumn months with a relatively high recurrence rate. Because of recurrent attacks, the corneal opacity becomes more severe and can finally lead to blindness. Conventional Western medicine treats HSK with antiviral drugs; glucocorticoids can be used for disc interstitial keratitis caused by an immune reaction.

HSK is one of the commonest corneal disorders and the leading cause of cornea-related blindness in the world. Herpes simplex virus is highly infectious to humans. The serum HSV antibody test is positive in 90% of adults older than 20 of age; however, only 1%-10% of them have clinical symptoms. In China, corneal disease is the second most common cause leading to blindness, while HSK is the most common cause of blindness among corneal disorders at 42.8%.

In TCM, HSK is similar to *jù xīng zhàng* (clustered star nebula, 聚星障), *hǔn jīng zhàng* (murky eye nebula, 混睛障), and *huā yì bái xiàn* (petaloid nebula with a sunken center, 花翳白陷). The description of the clustered star nebula was first seen in *Standards for Diagnosis and Treatment – Seven Orifices* (*Zhèng Zhì Zhǔn Shéng – Qī Qiào Mén*, 证治准绳·七窍门). The etiology, pathomechanism, clinical features, and prescriptions are discussed thoroughly in *Treatise on Ophthalmology* (*Yuán Jī Qǐ Wēi*, 原机启微), which is very instructive to pattern differentiation and treatment. In contemporary Chinese ophthalmology, HSK pertains to *jù xīng zhàng* (clustered star nebula, 聚星障).

Chinese medicine considers the disease as being caused by wind-heat invading the exterior and the black of the eye (the cornea), or deep-lying heat in the liver channel combined with exterior wind pathogen attacking the eye. Another causative factor is damp-heat of the spleen and stomach due to disorders of the spleen and stomach resulting from dietary irregularities. Yin-fluid deficiency due to the consumption of yin caused by febrile disease or a constitutional yin deficiency, combined with a wind pathogen, is another causative factor.

At present, there is no effective drug to control recurrence. Chinese medicine emphasizes concepts of holistic health. TCM has the advantages of improving the symptoms, shortening the course of the disease, and reducing the rate of recurrence by regulating *zang-fu* function and balancing the dynamic interplay of yin and yang. Typically, therapy includes both systemic and local treatment. Through strengthening the qi, Chinese medicine may improve immune function and enhance the body's ability to fight off viral activity, thus reducing the incidence and even preventing recurrence.

Clinical Manifestation

1. Symptoms

When the body is in a state of lowered resistance, such as is the case when experiencing a cold, fever, trauma, fatigue, stress, menstruation, allergic reactions, and taking systemic glucocorticoids, the virus (which is hiding out and lying dormant in the basal ganglion after primary infection) will be reactivated. The reactivated virus migrates down the nerve axon to the sensory nerve endings and out to the ocular surface or the corneal epithelial cell. Symptoms vary from a sensational to mild irritation, photophobia, tearing in light cases to acute pain, burning sensation, blepharospasm and marked vision loss in severe cases.

2. Signs

Conjunctival congestion, corneal opacity, infiltration, and edema. The cornea lesions may appear altered due to the various pathological changes.

3. Complication

Corneal neogenesis pannus, iridocyclitis, corneal scar, corneal perforation, and secondary bacterial infection.

4. Clinical Typing

The disease is divided into primary infection and recurrent infection.

(1) **Primary infection:** Primary infection of HSV usually occurs in young children. It is generally self-limited with symptoms such as fever, enlarged preauricular lymph nodes, lips or skin lesion. When the eye is involved, it may present acute follicular conjunctivitis, pseudomembranous conjunctivitis, herpes simplex infection of the eyelid, and punctiform or dendritic keratitis in some cases. The incidence of interstitial keratitis and uveitis is lower than 10% of all patients.

(2) Recurrent infection: There are many patterns of manifestation. Common types include the following:

- Epithelial keratitis: Initial manifestation of corneal vesicles appears first. Several hours later, the vesicles enlarge and coalesce, then a central epithelium defect develops and forms dendritic ulcer. The epithelial borders contain activated live viruses. If the dendritic ulcer furtherly enlarges, it will form into geographic ulcer. The condition may also present with marginal ulcer. The typical manifestation is dendritic ulcer with shallow stromal infiltration and congestion of the neighboring corneal limbus.
- Neurotrophic keratopathy: The pathological change is neither immune, nor infectious. It is because of the nerve injury of the cornea and tear reduction. Extensive local application over time, especially antiviral drugs, can aggravate keratopathy. The cornea has a rough surface and loses the normal luster, followed by punctate epithelial erosions. It can develop into long-standing epithelial defects and stromal ulcers called neurotrophic ulcers.
- Stromal keratitis: It has two forms, necrotizing stromal keratitis and immune stromal keratitis. The necrotizing stromal keratitis is rarely seen in the clinic, and manifests as corneal ulcers, necrosis, dense stromal infiltration, and thinning or perforation of the cornea. Immune stromal keratitis usually has a history of epithelial keratitis, and the clinical findings include stromal infiltration and disc-shaped edema, often accompanied by an inflammatory reaction in the anterior chamber. An "immune ring" and stromal neovascularization may also be seen.
- Endotheliitis: It is characterized by stromal edema and keratic precipitates only at the site of the infected cornea, usually accompanied by iritis. The stromal edema may present like disc-shaped, diffuse, and fan-shaped or hemicycle-shaped (line-like distribution KP offering), corresponding to the three clinical types: disciform endotheliitis, diffuse endotheliitis, and linear endotheliitis.

Treatment

1. Pattern Differentiation and Treatment

(1) Wind-Heat

【Syndrome Characteristics】

Sudden appearance of tiny pupil nebula, ciliary hyperemia, photophobia, lacrimation, aversion to wind, fever, headache, nasal congestion, dry mouth and pharyngodynia, thin yellow tongue coating, floating-rapid pulse.

【Treatment Principle】

Disperse wind and clear heat

【Representative Formula】

Modified *Yín Qiào Sǎn* (Lonicera and Forsythia Powder, 银翘散)

【Prescription】

金银花	jīn yín huā	10 g	Flos Lonicerae Japonicae
连翘	lián qiào	10 g	Fructus Forsythiae
淡竹叶	dàn zhú yè	10 g	Herba Lophatheri
牛蒡子	niú bàng zǐ	10 g	Fructus Arctii
芦根	lú gēn	10 g	Rhizoma Phragmitis
荆芥	jīng jiè	10 g	Herba Schizonepetae
薄荷 (后下)	bò he (hòu xià)	6 g	Herba Menthae (added later)
赤芍	chì sháo	10 g	Radix Paeoniae Rubra
柴胡	chái hú	10 g	Radix Bupleuri
黄芩	huáng qín	10 g	Radix Scutellariae

【Modifications】
➢ For cases with pronounced ciliary hyperemia, add *dà qīng yè* (大青叶, Folium Isatidi) 10 g, *bǎn lán gē*n (板蓝根, Radix Isatidis) 10 g, and *zǐ cǎo* (紫草, Radix Arnebiae) 10 g to reinforce the effect of clearing heat and removing toxins.

➢ For cases with marked tearing and photophobia, ophthalmalgia, headache, and difficulty in opening the eyes, add *qiāng huó* (羌活, Radix et Rhizoma Notopterygii) 10 g and *fáng fēng* (防风, Radix Saposhnikoviae) 10 g to disperse wind and eliminate pathogen.

(2) Blazing Liver-Gallbladder Fire
【Syndrome Characteristics】
The vesicles of the cornea enlarge and coalesce, deepen, and form into dendritic or geographic ulcer in white or yellowish color. Other symptoms include turbid hyperemia of the conjunctiva, frequent tearing, photophobia and difficulty in opening the eye, ophthalmalgia, and astringent pain, and may be accompanied by reddish urine, flank pain, bitter taste in the mouth and dry throat, red tongue with yellow coating, and wiry-rapid pulse.
【Treatment Principle】
Clear the liver and drain fire
【Representative Formula】
Modified *Lóng Dǎn Xiè Gān Tāng* (Gentian Liver-Draining Decoction, 龙胆泻肝汤)
【Prescription】

龙胆草	lóng dǎn cǎo	10 g	Radix et Rhizoma Gentianae
柴胡	chái hú	10 g	Radix Bupleuri
黄芩	huáng qín	10 g	Radix Scutellariae
栀子	zhī zǐ	10 g	Fructus Arctii

生地	*shēng dì*	10 g	Radix Rehmanniae
赤芍	*chì sháo*	10 g	Radix Paeoniae Rubra
当归	*dāng guī*	10 g	Radix Angelicae Sinensis
泽泻	*zé xiè*	10 g	Rhizoma Alismatis
车前子 (包煎)	*chē qián zǐ (bāo jiān)*	20 g	Semen Plantaginis (decocting in wrapped condition)
野菊花	*yě jú huā*	10 g	Flos Chrysanthemi Indici
木贼	*mù zéi*	10 g	Herba Equiseti Hiemalis
甘草	*gān cǎo*	3 g	Radix et Rhizoma Glycyrrhizae

【Modifications】
➢ For cases with constipation, add *dà huáng* (大黄, Radix et Rhizoma Rhei) and *shí gāo* (石膏, Gypsum Fibrosum) to purge fire and relax the bowels.

(3) Damp-Heat Steaming
【Syndrome Characteristics】
Geographic corneal nebula and diabrosis, or disk-shaped swelling of the cornea with ciliary congestion, recurrent outbreaks, and slow healing. The systemic symptoms may include heavy head and oppression in the chest, reduced appetite, loose stool, red tongue with yellow-greasy coating, and slippery-rapid pulse.

【Treatment Principle】
Resolve dampness and clear heat

【Representative Formula】
Modified *Sān Rén Tāng* (Three Kernels Decoction, 三仁汤)

【Prescription】

薏苡仁	*yì yǐ rén*	10 g	Semen Coicis
杏仁	*xìng rén*	10 g	Semen Armeniacae Amarum
厚朴	*hòu pò*	10 g	Cortex Magnoliae Officinalis
茵陈	*yīn chén*	10 g	Herba Artemisiae Scopariae
栀子	*zhī zǐ*	10 g	Fructus Arctii
柴胡	*chái hú*	10 g	Radix Bupleuri
黄芩	*huáng qín*	10 g	Radix Scutellariae
黄连	*huáng lián*	10 g	Rhizoma Coptidis
法半夏	*fǎ bàn xià*	10 g	Rhizoma Pinelliae Praeparatum
陈皮	*chén pí*	10 g	Pericarpium Citri Reticulatae
秦皮	*qín pí*	10 g	Cortex Fraxini
藿香	*huò xiāng*	10 g	Herba Agastachis
甘草	*gān cǎo*	3 g	Radix et Rhizoma Glycyrrhizae

【Modifications】

➢ For cases with loose stool and poor appetite, decrease the bitter cold medicinals, such as *zhī zǐ* (栀子, Fructus Arctii) and *huáng lián* (黄连, Rhizoma Coptidis), and add *chǎo bái zhú* (炒白术, dry-fried Rhizoma Atractylodis Macrocephalae) 15 g and *dǎng shēn* (党参, Radix Codonopsis) 10 g to fortify the spleen and dry dampness.

(4) Yin Deficiency with Wind

【Syndrome Characteristics】

Slow healing or intermittent nebula on the cornea, mild ciliary congestion, dryness of the eye and mouth, red tongue with little moisture, thready pulse or thready-rapid pulse.

【Treatment Principle】

Nourish yin and dispel wind

【Representative Formula】

Modified *Dì Huáng Wán* (Modified Rehmannia Pill, 地黄丸)

【Prescription】

生地	*shēng dì*	15 g	Radix Rehmanniae
熟地黄	*shú dì huáng*	15 g	Radix Rehmanniae Praeparata
当归	*dāng guī*	10 g	Radix Angelicae Sinensis
羌活	*qiāng huó*	10 g	Radix et Rhizoma Notopterygii
防风	*fáng fēng*	10 g	Radix Saposhnikoviae
枳壳	*zhǐ qiào*	10 g	Fructus Aurantii
杏仁	*xìng rén*	6 g	Semen Armeniacae Amarum
知母	*zhī mǔ*	10 g	Rhizoma Anemarrhenae
黄柏	*huáng bǎi*	10 g	Cortex Phellodendri Chinensis
木贼	*mù zéi*	10 g	Herba Equiseti Hiemalis
蝉蜕	*chán tuì*	6 g	Periostracum Cicadae

【Modifications】

➢ Following a high fever, if the patient presents with shortness of breath and lack of strength, add *tài zǐ shēn* (太子参, Radix Pseudostellariae) 10 g and *mài dōng* (麦冬, Radix Ophiopogonis) 10 g to replenish qi and generate fluids.

2. Acupuncture

For the acupuncture treatment of all the patterns listed below, treat once a day; 10 days equals one course of treatment.

(1) Wind-Heat: Disperse wind and clear heat with the following acupoints:

| LI 4 (*hé gǔ*) | GB 20 (*fēng chí*) | *tài yáng* (太阳) |
| LU 11 (*shào shāng*) | BL 1 (*jīng míng*) | |

Bleed *tài yáng* and LU 11. For BL 1, needle slowly and carefully until mild arrival of qi. Retain the needle for 30 minutes.

(2) Blazing Liver and Gallbladder Fire: Clear the liver and drain fire with:

LV 2 (*xíng jiān*)	GB 43 (*xiá xī*)	*tài yáng* (太阳)
LI 4 (*hé gǔ*)	BL 1 (*jīng míng*)	LI 11 (*qū chí*)

Bleed the ear apex. Needle the above points and retain the needles for 30 minutes.

(3) Damp-Heat Steaming: Resolve dampness and clear heat with the following:

ST 36 (*zú sān lǐ*)	SP 9 (*yīn líng quán*)	LI 4 (*hé gǔ*)
ST 44 (*nèi tíng*)	*tài yáng* (太阳)	BL 1 (*jīng míng*)

Use reduction methods and retain the needles for 30 minutes.

(4) Yin Deficiency with Wind: Nourish yin and dispel pathogenic pathogenics with:

BL 1 (*jīng míng*)	*qiú hòu* (球后)	BL 18 (*gān shù*)
BL 23 (*shèn shù*)	KI 6 *(zhào hǎi)*	KI 3 (*tài xī*)

Use reinforcing method. Moxibustion is also applicable. Retain the needles for 30 minutes.

(5) Embedding seeds on ear points:

Eye (*yǎn*, 眼)	Eye 1 (*mù* 1, 目1)	Eye 2 (*mù* 2, 目2)
Liver (*gān*, 肝)	Kidney (*shèn*, 肾)	

Press and stick vaccaria seeds on the ear acupuncture points. Tell patients to massage the points 3–4 times per day. Press the points for 20 times at a time, and change the seeds every three days; alternate placing the seeds on either the left and right ear. Ten sessions is a course of treatment.

3. Chinese Patent Medicines

(1) *Qīng Kāi Líng Zhù Shè Yè* (Heat-Removing Injection, 清开灵注射液)
20–40 ml, added into 100ml 0.9% saline, intravenously guttae; once a day. Applicable to exogenous wind-heat, blazing liver and gallbladder fire, and damp-heat steaming.

(2) *Bǎn Lán Gēn Chōng Jì* (Radix Isatidis Granules, 板蓝根冲剂)

6–12 g, take after mixing with water, three times a day, applicable to exogenous wind-heat and blazing liver and gallbladder fire.

(3) *Qǐ Jú Dì Huáng Wán* or *Míng Mù Dì Huáng Wán* (Lycii and Chrysanthemi and Rehmanniae Pills or Eyesight-improving Rehmanniae Pills, 杞菊地黄丸 / 明目 地黄丸)

6 g, two times a day, applicable to yin deficiency with wind.

4. Simple and Proven Recipes

(1) *Gōng Yīng Sān Wèi Yǐn* (Mongolian Dandelion Three Medicinals Decoction, 公 英三味饮): *pú gōng yīng* (蒲公英, Herba Taraxaci) 50–80 g, *bǎn lán gēn* (板蓝根, Radix Isatidis) 20 g and *bò he* (薄荷, Herba Menthae) 10 g. Applicable to epithelial keratitis. For dendritic keratitis, add *bǎn lán gēn* (板蓝根, Radix Isatidis) to 30 g and *bò he* (薄荷, Herba Menthae) to 20 g; decoct each batch of medicinals with water and take in two equal doses per day, for a total of four batches.

(2) *Yù Píng Fēng Sǎn* (Jade Wind-Barrier Powder, 玉屏风散): *huáng qí* (黄芪, Radix Astragali) 20 g, *fáng fēng* (防风, Radix Saposhnikoviae) 15 g, *chǎo bái zhú* (炒白术, dry-fried Rhizoma Atractylodis Macrocephalae) 15 g. Applicable to herpes simplex keratitis with high recurrence rate. This formula can reduce the rate of recurrence.

5. External Treatment

(1) *Yú Xīng Cǎo Yǎn Yào Shuǐ* (Heartleaf Houttuynia Medicinal Eye Drops, 鱼腥草眼 药水): Topical application once every 2 hours.

(2) Fumigation and washing: Decoct *jīn yín huā* (金银花, Herba Lonicerae Delavayi) 15 g, *lián qiào* (连翘, Fructus Forsythiae) 10 g, *pú gōng yīng* (蒲公英, Herba Taraxaci) 30 g, *dà qīng yè* (大青叶, Folium Isatidis) 15 g, *bò he* (薄荷, Herba Menthae) 5 g, *zǐ cǎo* (紫草, Radix Arnebiae) 6 g, and *huáng qín* (黄芩, Radix Scutellariae) 10 g with water; fumigate first, then wash the infected eye twenty minutes each time, one to two times a day. Filter the dregs before using. This formula is also applicable for wet-warm compress therapy.

6. Western Medicine Treatment

Antiviral eye drops including ganciclovir and acyclovir are applicable based on the patient's condition. When necessary, corticosteroids can be added (for severe corneal stromal edema without obvious epithelium defect) as well as immunosuppressive medication. Consult an ophthalmologist for a detailed Western medicine strategy.

7. Dietary Therapy and Preventive Care

(1) Cassia Seed Porridge (决明子粥):

Actions: Clears away fire in the liver and gallbladder

Preparation: Get a decoction made of *chǎo jué míng zǐ* (炒决明子, dry-fried Semen Cassiae) 12 g and *bái jú huā* (白菊花, Flos Chrysanthemi) 9 g, then boiled it with *jīng mǐ* (粳米, Oryza Sativa L.) 50 g to make porridge. When it is done, add some crystal sugar and mix it evenly. Take it on an empty stomach.

(2) Lycium Berry, Chrysanthemum and Obtuseleaf Senna Seed Tea (杞菊决明子茶):

Ingredients: *Gǒu qǐ zǐ* (枸杞子, Fructus Lycii) 10 g, *jú huā* (菊花, Flos Chrysanthemi) 10 g, *chǎo jué míng zǐ* (炒决明子, Semen Cassiae) 10 g.

Actions: Eliminates pathogen and removes nebula; supports healthy qi and brightens the eyes.

Preparation: Steep all the ingredients with boiled water and take as a tea.

(3) Exercise regularly to strengthen the constitution, avoid catching a cold, getting sick, fatigue, and overtiredness. These are important ways to prevent HSK. See a doctor promptly if you feel discomfort in the eye upon catching a cold. You may have to use corticosteroids reasonably and properly to avoid permanent damage and/or to control the inflammation. Eat a healthy diet and avoid excitant foods like spicy food.

Case Studies

Bao, an eleven-year-old girl

Initial visit: January 26, 1966

【Chief Complaint】

Redness, pain, photophobia, and tearing of the right eye for about 30 days.

【Medical History】

The patient was diagnosed with "dendritic ulcer of the right eye" in another hospital and given symptomatic and mydriasis treatment. Five years ago, her right eye suffered from the same kind of disease and left corneal scarring after iodine tincture cauterization.

【Examination】

The vision acuity was 20/200 on the right eye. There was a gray, deep dendritic infiltration close to the cornea spot corresponding to the 7–8 o'clock position of the pupil with the diameter about 2 mm, with fluorescein staining (+). There was also an old nebula above it. Other signs included red tongue with thin-white coating and thready pulse.

【Diagnosis】

Petaloid nebula with a sunken center of the right cornea

【Pattern Differentiation】

Exuberant fire in the liver and the lung combined with external pathogens and toxins invading the eye

【 Treatment Principles 】

Dispel wind and clear heat, activate blood and nourish yin, remove nebula to improve vision

【 Prescription 】

生地	*shēng dì*	12 g	Radix Rehmanniae
赤芍	*chì sháo*	10 g	Radix Paeoniae Rubra
密蒙花	*mì méng huā*	6 g	Flos Buddlejae
白芷	*bái zhǐ*	10 g	Radix Angelicae Dahuricae
石决明 (先煎)	*shí jué míng (xiān jiān)*	15 g	Concha Haliotidis (to be decocted first)
赤石脂 (包煎)	*chì shí zhī (bāo jiān)*	10 g	Halloysitum Rubrum (wrap)
炒川芎	*chǎo chuān xiōng*	3 g	Rhizoma Chuanxiong (dry-fried)
夏枯草	*xià kū cǎo*	6 g	Spica Prunellae
炙甘草	*zhì gān cǎo*	5 g	Radix et Rhizoma Glycyrrhizae Praeparata cum Melle

Decoct for oral intake. External application: *Xī Huáng Sǎn* (犀黄散, Rhinoceros Bezoar Powder), one bottle, applied to the infected eye, three times a day.

Her second visit was on January 31. All the symptoms were markedly reduced, the ulcer became flat, but there was still congestion in the conjunctiva. She presented with a thready-rapid pulse and a thin-white coating.

The original prescription was modified into the following:

炒川芎	*chǎo chuān xiōng*	3 g	Rhizoma Chuanxiong (dry-fried)
生地	*shēng dì*	12 g	Radix Rehmanniae
赤芍	*chì sháo*	10 g	Radix Paeoniae Rubra
密蒙花	*mì méng huā*	6 g	Flos Buddlejae
白芷	*bái zhǐ*	10 g	Radix Angelicae Dahuricae
桑白皮	*sāng bái pí*	15 g	Cortex Mori
木通 (先煎)	*mù tōng (xiān jiān)*	15 g	Caulis Akebiae (to be decocted first)
赤石脂 (包煎)	*chì shí zhī (bāo jiān)*	10 g	Halloysitum Rubrum (wrap)
炙甘草	*zhì gān cǎo*	5 g	Radix et Rhizoma Glycyrrhizae Praeparata cum Melle
地骨皮	*dì gǔ pí*	10 g	Cortex Lycii

The patient took a total of 5 batches (1 batch a day).

Her last visit was on February 5, 1966. The eye pain disappeared completely. She presented with slight photophobia and some tearing, a thready-rapid pulse, and a red tongue with thin-white coating. The treatment principle was changed to dispelling wind and clearing liver heat, while removing nebula to improve vision. The prescription contained:

龙胆草	*lóng dǎn cǎo*	6 g	Radix et Rhizoma Gentianae
连翘	*lián qiào*	10 g	Fructus Forsythiae
夏枯草	*xià kū cǎo*	6 g	Spica Prunellae
草决明	*cǎo jué míng*	10 g	Semen Cassiae
密蒙花	*mì méng huā*	6 g	Flos Buddlejae
荆芥	*jīng jiè*	15 g	Herba Schizonepetae
白菊花	*bái jú huā*	10 g	Flos Chrysanthemi

The patient took a total of 12 batches (1 batch a day). She was told to continue the use of *Xī Huáng Sǎn* (Rhinoceros Bezoar Powder, 犀黄散). All symptoms eventually disappeared and the corneal ulcer healed.

(Selection from *Wei Wen-gui's Case Records*)

Classic Quotes

《证治准绳·杂病·七窍门》：“聚星障证，乌珠上有细颗，或白色，或微黄，微黄者急而变重。或联缀，或团聚，或散漫，或一同生起，或先后逐渐一而二，二而三，三而四，四而六七八十数余。如此生起者，初起者易治，生定者退迟，能大者有变，团聚生大而作一块者，有凝脂之变。联缀四散，傍风轮白际而起，变大而接连者，花翳白陷也。”

“Clustered stars nebula presents with tiny vesicles on the black of the eye (cornea), or (can be) white, or slightly yellow; the yellow one is more acute and severe. The vesicles are connected like a line, or gather together, or occur at the same time, or in sequence as two by one, three by two, then four, six, seven to more than ten. The initial lesion is easy to cure, while the chronic nebula is hard to resolve. If the vesicles enlarge and coalesce into a big piece, it is referred to as a congealed-fat nebula. If the vesicles at the peripheral cornea connect and enlarge, and are accompanied by a white infiltration in the center, it may develop into a petaloid nebula with a sunken center.”

Standards for Diagnosis and Treatment – Miscellaneous Diseases – Seven Orifices (*Zhèng Zhì Zhǔn Shéng – Zá Bìng – Qī Qiào Mén*, 证治准绳·杂病·七窍门)

Section 2   Bacterial Keratitis

Bacterial keratitis is caused by bacterial infection and is commonly seen after corneal trauma. The main symptoms include eye pain, photophobia, tearing, foreign body sensation, and decreased vision. Aeruginosus bacillus corneal ulcer is a severe keratitis with characteristics of acute onset, intense eye pain, vision loss accompanied by redness and swelling, photophobia, and tearing. Bacterial keratitis may occur in any season, but occurs most often in summer and autumn. Elderly and people with a weak constitution are more susceptible to this condition. Topical application of antibiotics is the most effective treatment method for bacterial keratitis.

In TCM, bacterial keratitis pertains to *níng zhī yì* (nongealed-fat nebula, 凝脂翳), which is described as an acute and severe eye disease. At the initial stage, it presents with star-like nebula on the cornea; soon afterward it extends to its surrounding and deep layers rapidly and form a coagulated, fat-like lesion on the corneal surface. In some cases, it may be accompanied by hypopyon. The pathogenesis is usually due to either injury of the corneal surface and external wind-heat toxin exploiting deficiency. At the initial stages, the treatment is mainly aimed at clearing heat and resolving toxins. If the condition lasts for a long time and the ulcer does not heal, it is suggested that it should be treated with the principle of reinforcing healthy qi and eliminating pathogens. The pathogenesis is associated with lingering of pathogens due to deficiency of healthy qi.

Clinical Manifestation

1. Symptoms

Acute onset, severe subjective symptoms, red eye, pain, photophobia, tearing, blurred vision, foreign body sensation, blepharospasm, and increased discharge.

2. Signs

Ciliary congestion, swelling of the eyelid, congestion and edema of the conjunctiva, corneal infiltration, corneal ulcer and edema, descemetocele, keratic precipitates, hypopyon, and corneal perforation.

3. The manifestation is not always the same if it is caused by a different bacterial microbe

(1) **Gram positive coccus infection:** Round or oval-shaped abscess lesion on the cornea, accompanied by gray-white stromal infiltration. If the keratitis is caused by pneumococcus, it presents with an oval-shaped ulcer, deep at the center area with creeping margin, usually accompanied by hypopyon.

(2) **Gram negative bacteria infection:** This is a group of keratitis characterized by rapid expansion of corneal liquefaction necrosis. If it is caused by Pseudomonas aeruginosa, the signs are characterized by mucosity necrosis, rapid expansion of the ulcer, large hypopyon, and yellow-green infiltrate and discharge. The other typical features include severe eye pain, marked ciliary congestion or mixed congestion accompanied by chemosis. If the inflammation is not controlled, the ulcer will cause corneal necrosis, finally bring about perforation and prolapse of eyeball contents or panophthalmitis. Cases

of Pseudomonas aeruginosa corneal ulcer may follow minor corneal abrasion or use of contact lenses. Some cases have reported following the use of contaminated fluorescein solution or eye drops.

(3) Gonococcal infection: It commonly occurs in infants following natural birth. The symptoms are photophobia, tearing, pain, blurred vision, and blepharospasm. The signs include ponderosus purulent secretion, ciliary congestion or mixed congestion, defect of corneal epithelium, stromal infiltrate, and ulcer. Hypopyon is common, and corneal perforation may present in some cases.

Treatment

Because the disease is acute and severe and the condition can change rapidly, in order to control the condition quickly and prevent or reduce complications, treat it with combined internal and external therapy or integrated medicine.

1. Pattern Differentiation and Treatment

(1) Wind-Heat
【 Syndrome Characteristics 】
At the initial stage, there is gray-white nebula on the cornea with muddy appearance and unclear border, ciliary congestion, mild swelling of the eyelid, pain, foreign body sensation, photophobia, tearing, and blurred vision. Other signs include thin yellow coating and a floating and rapid pulse.
【 Treatment Principle 】
Dispel wind and clear heat
【 Representative Formula 】
Xīn Zhì Chái Lián Tāng (New Bupleurum and Coptis Decoction, 新制柴连汤)
【 Prescription 】

柴胡	*chái hú*	10 g	Radix Bupleuri
黄连	*huáng lián*	6 g	Rhizoma Coptidis
黄芩	*huáng qín*	10 g	Radix Scutellariae
赤芍	*chì sháo*	10 g	Radix Paeoniae Rubra
蒲公英	*pú gōng yīng*	10 g	Herba Taraxaci
炒栀子	*chǎo zhī zǐ*	10 g	Fructus Gardeniae (dry-fried)
龙胆草	*lóng dǎn cǎo*	10 g	Radix et Rhizoma Gentianae
木通	*mù tōng*	10 g	Caulis Akebiae
荆芥	*jīng jiè*	10 g	Herba Schizonepetae
防风	*fáng fēng*	10 g	Radix Saposhnikoviae

大青叶	*dà qīng yè*	10 g	Folium Isatidis
野菊花	*yě jú huā*	10 g	Flos Chrysanthemi Indici
甘草	*gān cǎo*	3 g	Radix et Rhizoma Glycyrrhizae

【Modifications】

➢ For cases with severe mixed conjunctival congestion and ciliary congestion, add *sāng bái pí* (桑白皮, Cortex Mori) 10 g and *jié gěng* (桔梗, Radix Platycodonis) 10 g to purge lung heat.

(2) Blazing Fire of the Liver and Gallbladder

【Syndrome Characteristics】

Sheet of congealed-fat infiltration on the cornea, mixed congestion, difficulty in opening the eye due to severe eyelid swelling, intense eye pain, marked photophobia, hot water-like tearing; in severe cases there is turbid spirit water (aqueous humor), contracted pupil, and hypopyon. Other symptoms and signs include headache, excessive thirst, reddish urine and constipation, red tongue with thick yellow coating, rapid and forceful pulse.

【Treatment Principle】

Clear and purge liver heat

【Representative Formula】

Lóng Dǎn Xiè Gān Tāng (Gentian Liver-Draining Decoction, 龙胆泻肝汤)

【Prescription】

龙胆草	*lóng dǎn cǎo*	10 g	Radix et Rhizoma Gentianae
柴胡	*chái hú*	10 g	Radix Bupleuri
黄连	*huáng lián*	6 g	Rhizoma Coptidis
黄芩	*huáng qín*	10 g	Radix Scutellariae
炒栀子	*chǎo zhī zǐ*	10 g	Fructus Gardeniae (dry-fried)
泽泻	*zé xiè*	10 g	Rhizoma Alismatis
车前子 (包煎)	*chē qián zǐ (bāo jiān)*	20 g	Semen Plantaginis (wrapped)
赤芍	*chì sháo*	10 g	Radix Paeoniae Rubra
石膏 (先煎)	*shí gāo (xiān jiān)*	15 g	Gypsum Fibrosum (decocted first)
金银花	*jīn yín huā*	10 g	Flos Lonicerae Japonicae
蒲公英	*pú gōng yīng*	10 g	Herba Taraxaci
甘草	*gān cǎo*	3 g	Radix et Rhizoma Glycyrrhizae

【Modifications】

➢ For cases with hypopyon, add *yě jú huā* (野菊花, Flos Chrysanthemi Indici) 10 g, *zǐ huā dì dīng* (紫花地丁, Herba Violae) 10 g, and *bài jiàng cǎo* (败酱草, Herba Patriniae) 10 g to enhance the function of clearing heat and removing toxin.

(3) Intense Heat Toxin
【Syndrome Characteristics】

Deep and large congealed-fat lesion on the cornea (yellow-green color) and severe hypopyon covering the pupil. The topical symptoms are more intense than that of the liver and gallbladder blazing fire pattern; lesions usually develop towards the deep layer and may eventually lead to serious complications such as corneal perforation or iris emersion. Other symptoms and signs include headache, excessive thirst, reddish urine and constipation, and a rapid, forceful pulse.

【Treatment Principle】

Purge fire and remove toxins

【Representative Formula】

Sì Shùn Qīng Liáng Yǐn Zi (Four Favorable Cooling Decoction, 四顺清凉饮子)

【Prescription】

龙胆草	*lóng dǎn cǎo*	10 g	Radix et Rhizoma Gentianae
黄连	*huáng lián*	8 g	Rhizoma Coptidis
黄芩	*huáng qín*	10 g	Radix Scutellariae
桑白皮	*sāng bái pí*	12 g	Cortex Mori
熟大黄	*shú dà huáng*	10 g	Radix et Rhizoma Rhei
枳壳	*zhǐ qiào*	10 g	Fructus Aurantii
车前子	*chē qián zǐ*	12 g	Semen Plantaginis
羌活	*qiāng huó*	10 g	Radix et Rhizoma Notopterygii
防风	*fáng fēng*	10 g	Radix Saposhnikoviae
柴胡	*chái hú*	10 g	Radix Bupleuri
生地	*shēng dì*	15 g	Radix Rehmanniae
赤芍	*chì sháo*	12 g	Radix Paeoniae Rubra
金银花	*jīn yín huā*	15 g	Flos Lonicerae Japonicae
蒲公英	*pú gōng yīng*	15 g	Herba Taraxaci

【Modifications】

➤ For cases with bowel fullness and constipation, add *xuán míng fěn* (玄明粉, Natrii Sulfas Exsiccatus) 10 g to relax the bowels and purge heat.

➤ For cases with pronounced pain and redness, add *shuǐ niú jiǎo* (水牛角, Cornu Bubali) 30 g and powdered *sān qī* (三七, Radix et Rhizoma Notoginseng) 3 g to clear heat, cool blood, invigorate blood, and stop pain.

➤ For cases with lots of yellow-green secretion, add *yě jú huā* (野菊花, Flos Chrysanthemi Indici) 10 g and *qiān lǐ guāng* (千里光, Herba Senecionis Scandentis) 10 g to clear heat and resolve toxin.

(4) Heathy Qi Deficiency and Enduring Pathogen

【 Syndrome Characteristics 】

Prolonged course, congealed-fat lesion that would not heal, slight ciliary congestion, mild eye pain and photophobia, pale tongue, weak pulse.

【 Treatment Principle 】

Reinforce healthy qi and eliminate pathogens

【 Representative Formula 】

For cases with qi deficiency, treat with *Tuō Lǐ Xiāo Dú Yǐn* (Internal Expulsion Toxin-Dispersing Decoction, 托里消毒饮); for cases with yin deficiency, treat with *Zī Yīn Tuì Yì Tāng* (Yin-Nourishing Nebula-Removing Decoction, 滋阴退翳汤)

【 Prescription 】

Internal Expulsion Toxin-Dispersing Decoction:

黄芪	*huáng qí*	15 g	Radix Astragali
皂角刺	*zào jiǎo cì*	10 g	Spina Gleditsiae
金银花	*jīn yín huā*	10 g	Flos Lonicerae Japonicae
桔梗	*jié gěng*	10 g	Radix Platycodonis
白芷	*bái zhǐ*	10 g	Radix Angelicae Dahuricae
川芎	*chuān xiōng*	6 g	Rhizoma Chuanxiong
当归	*dāng guī*	10 g	Radix Angelicae Sinensis
白术	*bái zhú*	10 g	Rhizoma Atractylodis Macrocephalae
茯苓	*fú líng*	15 g	Poria
太子参	*tài zǐ shēn*	10 g	Radix Pseudostellariae
蝉蜕	*chán tuì*	6 g	Periostracum Cicadae
木贼	*mù zéi*	10 g	Herba Equiseti Hiemalis

Yin-Nourishing Nebula-Removing Decoction:

知母	*zhī mǔ*	10 g	Rhizoma Anemarrhenae
生地	*shēng dì*	15 g	Radix Rehmanniae
玄参	*xuán shēn*	10 g	Radix Scrophulariae
麦冬	*mài dōng*	10 g	Radix Ophiopogonis
蒺藜	*jí lí*	10 g	Fructus Tribuli
菊花	*jú huā*	10 g	Flos Chrysanthemi
蝉蜕	*chán tuì*	6 g	Periostracum Cicadae
木贼	*mù zéi*	10 g	Herba Equiseti Hiemalis
青葙子	*qīng xiāng zǐ*	10 g	Semen Celosiae
菟丝子	*tù sī zǐ*	10 g	Semen Cuscutae
甘草	*gān cǎo*	3 g	Radix et Rhizoma Glycyrrhizae

【 Modifications 】

➤ For cases with prolonged ulcer that does not heal, add *huáng qí* (黄芪, Radix Astragali) 20 g to tonify qi, reinforce healthy qi, and express pathogen outward.

2. Acupuncture

Same as the treatment for herpes simplex keratitis.

3. Chinese Patent Medicines

(1) *Qīng Kāi Líng Zhù Shè Yè* (Heat-Removing Injection, 清开灵注射液)
20-40 ml, added into 250ml 0.9% Nacl solution; once a day. Applicable to patients with wind-heat, blazing fire in the liver and gallbladder, and intense heat toxin.

(2) *Qǐ Jú Dì Huáng Wán* (Lycium Berry, Chrysanthemum and Rehmannia Pill, 杞菊地黄丸) or *Míng Mù Dì Huáng Wán* (Brighten Eye and Rehmannia Root Granule, 明目地黄丸)
6 g, twice a day. Applicable to the pattern of healthy qi deficiency with lingering pathogen.

4. Simple and Proven Recipes

The coat of soybean is called "soybean skin", which has the function of clearing heat, resolving toxin, brightening the eyes, and removing nebula. It has been proven by modern pharmacology that soybean skin can inhibit staphylococci. In the clinic, the decoction of soybean skin is used to treat trauma and infection (abscess, sore and furuncle, burn, etc). To treat corneal nebula, use 1000 grams of soybean, a strip of snake slough, and 30 grams of white sugar. Wash the snake slough clean with licorice root water, then fry it with sesame oil until it turns yellow, add soybean and white sugar, and decoct it with water. Take one preparation batch a day.

5. External Treatment

(1) *Yú Xīng Cǎo Yǎn Yào Shuǐ* (Heartleaf Houttuynia Medicinal Eye Drop, 鱼腥草眼药水): Apply 1–2 drops every 2 hours.

(2) Apply *yě jú huā* (野菊花, Flos Chrysanthemi Indici) 30 g and *qiān lǐ guāng* (千里光, Herba Senecionis Scandentis) 30 g, decocted with water and dregs removed, as a fumigate or wet-compress on the affected eye.

6. Treatment with Western Medicine

(1) Antibiotic eye drops and ointments: Apply frequently in the acute stage, 1 drop

every 15–30 minutes. For very severe cases, use 1 drop every 5 minutes in the first 30 minutes. Apply ointment at bedtime. Subconjunctival injection can increase drug concentration in the cornea and the anterior chamber. Choose the effective antibiotic according to drug-sensitivity test.

(2) 1% Atropine eye drops or eye ointment: Mydriasis is mandatory if complicated with iridocyclitis.

(3) Corneal transplantation: If the medication doesn't work, corneal grafting may be necessary in cases of corneal perforation and protrusion of intraocular contents.

7. Dietary Therapy and Preventive Care

(1) For dietary therapy, refer to Section 1 (Herpes Simplex Keratitis).

(2) Eat a light diet and keep the bowels clear.

(3) Avoid wearing contact lens overnight. If the cornea is injured, apply antibiotic eye drops or heat-clearing and toxin-resolving drops promptly. If there is a foreign body in the cornea, see an ophthalmologist immediately to have it removed surgically. Treat dacryocystitis actively to reduce the risk factors.

Case Studies

Li, a 38-year-old male

【Chief Complaint】

Eye pain, photophobia, tearing, and blurred vision on the right eye for ten days

【Examination】

The patient presented with decreased visual acuity, conjunctival congestion, unsmooth corneal surface, gray-white opacity at the center of the cornea, hypopyon, and dilated pupil.

【Medical History】

The systemic signs included a crimson tongue with thick yellow coating, and a wiry and rapid pulse. The patient was fond of alcohol and meat, and had chronic constipation.

【Diagnosis】

Purulent keratitis complicated with hypopyon

【Prescription】

金银花	jīn yín huā	30 g	Flos Lonicerae Japonicae
蒲公英	pú gōng yīng	30 g	Herba Taraxaci
天花粉	tiān huā fěn	12 g	Radix Trichosanthis
黄芩	huáng qín	12 g	Radix Scutellariae
青皮	qīng pí	12 g	Pericarpium Citri Reticulatae Viride
龙胆草	lóng dǎn cǎo	12 g	Radix et Rhizoma Gentianae

黄连	huáng lián	12 g	Rhizoma Coptidis
蔓荆子	màn jīng zǐ	10 g	Fructus Viticis
生地	shēng dì	10 g	Radix Rehmanniae
知母	zhī mǔ	10 g	Rhizoma Anemarrhenae
大黄	dà huáng	10 g	Radix et Rhizoma Rhei
玄明粉	xuán míng fěn	15 g	Natrii Sulfas Exsiccatus
木通	mù tōng	5 g	Caulis Akebiae
甘草	gān cǎo	3 g	Radix et Rhizoma Glycyrrhizae

All the medicinals were decocted with water; the patient was given one batch a day.

【Follow-up】

After taking 6 batches, the patients visited our clinic for the second time. The physical examination showed that the visual acuity was CF/60 cm on the right eye, and both the conjunctival congestion and hypopyon had decreased. Systemic signs included a pale red tongue with yellow coating, and a wiry, rapid pulse. The patient was instructed to continue with the original formula for another 6 batches. On the third visit (two weeks later), the examination showed there was still mild conjunctival congestion, but the corneal ulcer had become flat and most of the hypopyon had been absorbed. The formula was modified by removing mù tōng (Caulis Akebiae) and changing the dosages of xuán míng fěn (Natrii Sulfas Exsiccatus) to 6 g and dà huáng (Radix et Rhizoma Rhei) to 5 g. At the patient's forth visit (3 weeks later), the examination results showed that the visual acuity was 20/100 on the right eye with no conjunctival congestion, no hypopyon, and only cloudy nebula remaining.

Classic Quotes

《目经大成·凝脂翳》：“此症初起目亦痛，多虬脉，畏光紧闭，强开则泪涌出。风轮上有点如星，色白，中有孔如锥刺伤，后渐渐长大，变为黄色，孔亦渐大，变为窟。有初起翳色便黄，大且厚，治依下法。”

“At the initial stage of the disease there will be eye pain, thready red vessels, photophobia and tightly closed eye, and tearing when trying to open the eye. Star-like white spot(s) can be seen in the cornea with a hole at the center, growing gradually and turning yellow. The hole gets bigger and bigger, and finally forms a cave. The nebula could also be yellow at the beginning, big and thick; treat it with the purgative method.”

The Great Compendium of Classics on Ophthalmology – Congealed-fat Nebula (Mù Jīng Dà Chéng – Níng Zhī Yì, 目经大成·凝脂翳)

Chapter 11
Uveitis

Section 1　Iridocyclitis

Iridocyclitis is an inflammation of the iris and ciliary body of the eye. In general, inflammation occurs in both the iris and the ciliary body. The disease also is named anterior uveitis, which is the most common form of uveitis and accounts for 50% of all uveitis cases. There are complex causes of the disease, which may be related to trauma, surgery, autoimmune conditions, and microbial infections. The vast majority of the causes are endogenous and related to immune response. HLA-B27 (human leukocyte antigen B27) is reported to have a close relationship with irydocyclitis. Iridocyclitis may be complicated by other systemic diseases such as rheumatoid disease, ulcerative colitis, and sarcoidosis.

The main clinical manifestations include impaired vision, eye pain, photophobia, excessive tearing, ciliary congestion, turbid aqueous humor, keratic precipitates, edema of the iris, and spasms and opisthosynechia of the pupil. This disease occurs most commonly in adolescents. Recurring symptoms can present themselves unilaterally or bilaterally, and can often lead to severe ocular complications. The objective treatment strategies in Western medicine are to remove inflammation, prevent opisthosynechia of the pupil, and reduce the potential risk for further complications.

In Chinese medicine, the disease is called *tóng shén jǐn xiǎo* (contracted pupils, 瞳神紧小) or *tóng shén gān quē* (pupil contraction, 瞳神干缺), because pupils of the patients appear contracted and there is opisthosynechia. The cause and pathogenesis of the disease is associated with pathogenic heat invading the eye, pathogenic fire of the liver and gallbladder invading upward through the channels, deficiency fire flaming upward, or wind-damp heat harassing the eye. Because the disease is mostly caused by the disorder of the *zang-fu* or pathogenic heat, the aim of treatment is to regulate the bowels and viscera, eliminate pathogens, and support healthy qi. With pattern identification as the basis for determining treatment and the flexible use of medicines, clinical symptoms can be relieved or even eradicated. Especially for the latter condition, the prognosis is very good in terms of improving vision and decreasing recurrent symptoms.

Clinical Manifestation

The clinical features of iridocyclitis include rapid onset, decreased vision, pain, photophobia, and excessive tearing.

Ocular examination: Ciliary or mixed hyperemia with turbid aqueous humor. In severe cases, hypopyon or floccular and colloid mass in the anterior chamber may be seen. Dust-like or pigmentary precipitates appear on the corneal endothelium, mostly in the bottom region of the cornea, showing the distribution in the form of a "base-down triangle". The iris is often unclear in the texture or a dark color because of congestion and edema. Due to bulging and exudation adhesion or for other reasons, the iris can move to attach to the cornea and form synechia iridis anterior peripherica. Some patients may present with nodules in the iris pigment epithelial surface of the pupillary margin, or near the central curling wheel. In the late stages, iris atrophy and a fibrinous membrane can form on the surface of the iris. Pupil cramps, sluggish or absence of papillary-light response may be present. The pigmentary epithelium of the pupillary margin may adhere to the anterior capsule of the lens, which is called the posterior synechia. Dilated pupil shows a "petal-shaped" edge. If the range of opisthosynechia is wide, the flow of aqueous humor may be obstructed, called "atresia of the pupil," which may lead to secondary glaucoma. If a large amount of inflammatory exudate covers the pupil area, it may cause occlusion of the pupil.

Treatment

1. Pattern Differentiation and Treatment

The disease is located on the iris and the pupil. In TCM, the pupil corresponds to the kidney, while the iris pertains to the liver, and the liver has an interior-exterior relationship with the gallbladder; therefore, the disease is closely associated to the liver, gallbladder, and kidney. This disease may be caused by intrusion of exogenous pathogenics, or visceral disorders. For cases caused by exogenous pathogenics, the main patterns are wind-heat or wind-damp-heat in the lung channel. The general treatment principles are to dispel wind, clear heat, and dispel dampness. For cases caused by viscera disorders, the main patterns are heat accumulating in the viscera or deficiency-fire flaming upward. General treatment principles are to quell fire, resolve toxin, cool blood, and nourish yin. At the later stages, because pathogenic qi has not yet been fully expelled and healthy qi has not been restored, it is important to nourish the liver and kidney and support healthy qi.

(1) Wind-Heat in the Liver Channel

[Syndrome Characteristics]

Rapid onset, blurred vision, eye pain, photophobia and excess tearing, circumcorneal congestion, turbid aqueous humor, dusty or punctiform keratic precipitate, unclear texture of the iris, contracted "frozen" pupils. Systemic symptoms include forehead pain, dry mouth, red tongue with thin white or yellow coating, floating rapid pulse.

【 Treatment Principle 】
Scatter wind and dissipate pathogens, clear liver heat

【 Representative Formula 】
Modified *Xīn Zhì Chái Lián Tāng* (New Bupleurum Coptis Decoction, 新制柴连汤)

【 Prescription 】

龙胆草	*lóng dǎn cǎo*	5 g	Radix et Rhizoma Gentianae
栀子	*zhī zǐ*	10 g	Fructus Gardeniae
黄芩	*huáng qín*	10 g	Radix Scutellariae
荆芥	*jīng jiè*	10 g	Herba Schizonepetae
防风	*fáng fēng*	10 g	Radix Saposhnikoviae
蔓荆子	*màn jīng zǐ*	10 g	Fructus Viticis
柴胡	*chái hú*	10 g	Radix Bupleuri
赤芍	*chì sháo*	12 g	Radix Paeoniae Rubra
通草	*tōng cǎo*	10 g	Medulla Tetrapanacis
生甘草	*shēng gān cǎo*	5 g	Radix et Rhizoma Glycyrrhizae

【 Modifications 】

➢ For cases with ciliary congestion, add *shēng dì* (生地, Radix Rehmanniae) 10 g, *dān pí* (丹皮 Cortex Moutan) 10 g, and *dì lóng* (地龙, Pheretima) 10 g to cool blood and abate redness.

➢ For cases with severe pain of the head and eye, add *jú huā* (菊花, Flos Chrysanthemi) 12 g, *sāng yè* (桑叶, Folium Mori) 12 g, *gé gēn* (葛根, Radix Puerariae Lobatae) 15 g, and *shēng má* (升麻, Rhizoma Cimicifugae) 8 g to scatter wind, clear heat, and alleviate pain.

(2) Intense Liver and Gallbladder Fire

【 Syndrome Characteristics 】
Rapid onset, acute vision decline or loss, eye pain that is worse with pressure, hyperdacryosis, congestion of conjunctiva, a great quantity of gray keratic precipitate, turbidity of the aqueous humor, hypopyon, swelling and textured iris, pupilary contraction. Systemic symptoms include heart vexation and irascibility, bitter mouth and dry pharynx, yellow urine and constipation, red tongue with yellow greasy coating, wiry rapid pulse.

【 Treatment Principle 】
Clear liver heat and drain the gallbladder

【 Representative Formula 】
Modified *Lóng Dǎn Xiè Gān Tāng* (Gentian Liver-Draining Decoction, 龙胆泻肝汤)

【 Prescription 】

龙胆草	lóng dǎn cǎo	5 g	Radix et Rhizoma Gentianae
栀子	zhī zǐ	10 g	Fructus Gardeniae
黄芩	huáng qín	10 g	Radix Scutellariae
黄连	huáng lián	5 g	Rhizoma Coptidis
车前草	chē qián cǎo	15 g	Herba Plantaginis
泽泻	zé xiè	10 g	Rhizoma Alismatis
通草	tōng cǎo	10 g	Medulla Tetrapanacis
柴胡	chái hú	10 g	Radix Bupleuri
生地	shēng dì	12 g	Radix Rehmanniae
当归	dāng guī	10 g	Radix Angelicae Sinensis

【 Modifications 】

➢ For cases with constipation, add *shú dà huáng* (熟大黄, Radix et Rhizoma Rhei) 6 g and *máng xiāo* (芒硝, Natrii Sulfas) 5 g to relieve constipation and drain heat.

➢ For cases with severe turbidity of the aqueous humor, or even upsurge of yellow humor, add *pú gōng yīng* (蒲公英, Herba Taraxaci) 15 g, *bài jiàng cǎo* (败酱草, Herba Patriniae) 15 g, *lián qiào* (连翘, Fructus Forsythiae) 10 g, *wěi jīng* (苇茎, Phragmitis Rhizoma) 30 g, *yì yǐ rén* (薏苡仁, Semen Coici) 15 g, *dōng guā rén* (冬瓜仁, Semen Benincasae) 20 g, and *táo rén* (桃仁, Semen Persicae) 5 g to resolve toxin, expel pus, and drain dampness.

➢ For cases with hyphema of the anterior chamber caused by exuberant heat damaging the collaterals, remove *dāng guī* (当归, Radix Angelicae Sinensis), add *dān pí* (丹皮, Cortex Moutan) 10 g, *chì sháo* (赤芍, Radix Paeoniae Rubra) 10 g, *shēng pú huáng* (生蒲黄, Pollen Typhae) 12 g to cool blood, stop bleeding and invigorate the blood.

(3) Wind-Heat with Dampness

【 Syndrome Characteristics 】

Rapid or slow onset, chronic, recurrent attacks, blurred vision or floaters in front of the eye, sagging pain of the eyeball, photophobia and excessive tearing, ciliary congestion, turbidity of the aqueous humor, gray-keratic precipitate, unclear textured iris, contracted pupils or aspheric pupil. Systemic symptoms include heavy head and dyspnea, decreased food intake and reduced appetite, vexing pain in the limb joints, inhibited bending and stretching, red tongue with yellow greasy thick coating, slippery rapid pulse.

【 Treatment Principle 】

Dispel wind and clear heat, remove dampness

【 Representative Formula 】

Modified *Yì Yáng Jiǔ Lián Sǎn* (Yang-Restraining Rhizoma Picrorhizae Powder, 抑阳酒连散)

【Prescription】

黄芩	huáng qín	10 g	Radix Scutellariae
黄连	huáng lián	5 g	Rhizoma Coptidis
黄柏	huáng bǎi	10 g	Cortex Phellodendri Chinensis
栀子	zhī zǐ	10 g	Fructus Gardeniae
生地	shēng dì	10 g	Radix Rehmanniae
知母	zhī mǔ	10 g	Rhizoma Anemarrhenae
寒水石	hán shuǐ shí	15 g	Glauberitum
羌活	qiāng huó	10 g	Radix et Rhizoma Notopterygii
防风	fáng fēng	10 g	Radix Saposhnikoviae
白芷	bái zhǐ	10 g	Radix Angelicae Dahuricae
独活	dú huó	10 g	Radix Angelicae Pubescentis
汉防己	hàn fáng jǐ	8 g	Radix Stephaniae Tetrandrae
蔓荆子	màn jīng zǐ	12 g	Fructus Viticis

【Modifications】
➢ For cases with predominant wind heat presenting with ciliary congestion, pain of the eyeball, remove *qiāng huó* (Radix et Rhizoma Notopterygii), *dú huó* (Radix Angelicae Pubescentis), and *bái zhǐ* (Radix Angelicae Dahuricae) to avoid internal wind caused by excessive usage of acrid warm medicinals; add *chōng wèi zǐ* (茺蔚子, Fructus Leonuri) 15 g, *qīng xiāng zǐ* (青葙子, Semen Celosiae) 10 g, and *chì sháo* (赤芍, Radix Paeoniae Rubra) 12 g to clear liver heat, cool blood, and relieve pain.

➢ For cases with predominant wind dampness presenting with turbidity of the aqueous humor and mild redness and pain of the eye, remove *zhī mǔ* (Rhizoma Anemarrhenae), *hán shuǐ shí* (Glauberitum), and *shēng dì* (Radix Rehmanniae) to avoid internal dampness caused by nourishing of yin, and add *bái kòu rén* (白蔻仁, Fructus Amomi Rotundus) 8 g, *fú líng* (茯苓, Poria) 15 g, and *hòu pò* (厚朴, Cortex Magnoliae Officinalis) 10 g to loosen the center and dispel dampness.

(4) Hyperactivity of Fire due to Yin Deficiency
【Syndrome Characteristics】
Disease appearing after the initial condition, varying intensity, dry eyes and clouded flowery vision, mild circumcorneal redness, turbidity of the aqueous humor, dusty keratic precipitate, withering of the iris, and pupil contraction. Systemic symptoms include deficiency vexation and agrypnia, heat in the center of the palms and soles, dry mouth and throat, red tongue with little coating, thready rapid pulse.
【Treatment Principle】
Supplement the liver and kidney, enrich yin and downbear fire

【Representative Formula】

Modified *Zhī Bǎi Dì Huáng Tāng* (Anemarrhena, Phellodendron and Rehmannia Decoction, 知柏地黄汤)

【Prescription】

知母	*zhī mǔ*	10 g	Rhizoma Anemarrhenae
黄柏	*huáng bǎi*	10 g	Cortex Phellodendri Chinensis
熟地黄	*shú dì huáng*	10 g	Radix Rehmanniae Praeparata
山茱萸	*shān zhū yú*	10 g	Fructus Corni
山药	*shān yào*	15 g	Rhizoma Dioscoreae
茯苓	*fú líng*	8 g	Poria
泽泻	*zé xiè*	8 g	Rhizoma Alismatis
牡丹皮	*mǔ dān pí*	10 g	Cortex Moutan
枸杞子	*gǒu qǐ zǐ*	15 g	Fructus Lycii
菊花	*jú huā*	10 g	Flos Chrysanthemi
茺蔚子	*chōng wèi zǐ*	12 g	Fructus Leonuri

【Modifications】

➢ For cases with dark redness of the circumcornea, add *dān shēn* (丹参, Radix et Rhizoma Salviae Miltiorrhizae) 10 g, *chì sháo* (赤芍, Radix Paeoniae Rubra) 10 g, and *zǐ cǎo* (紫草, Radix Arnebiae) 8 g to cool and invigorate blood and dispel stasis.

➢ For cases with deficiency vexation and agrypnia, add *suān zǎo rén* (酸枣仁, Semen Ziziphi Spinosae) 10 g, *bǎi zǐ rén* (柏子仁, Semen Platycladi) 12 g, and *yuǎn zhì* (远志, Radix Polygalae) 5 g to nourish the heart, quiet the spirit, and stabilize the mind. For cases with constipation, add *cǎo jué míng* (草决明, Semen Cassiae) 15 g, *huǒ má rén* (火麻仁, Fructus Cannabis) 15 g, and *sāng shèn* (桑椹, Fructus Mori) 15 g to enrich yin and moisten the intestines to relieve constipation.

➢ For cases with vexing heat in the five centers, add *dì gǔ pí* (地骨皮, Cortex Lycii) 12 g, *biē jiǎ* (鳖甲, Carapax Trionycis) 12 g, and *qīng hāo* (青蒿, Herba Artemisiae Annuae 10 g to nourish yin, clear heat, and eliminate heat vexation.

2. Acupuncture

BL 2 (*cuán zhú*)	*yú yāo* (鱼腰)	GB 1 (*tóng zǐ liáo*)
ST 2 (*sì bái*)	LI 4 (*hé gǔ*)	LU 7 (*liè quē*)
GB 20 (*fēng chí*)	*tài yáng* (太阳)	LV 3 (*tài chōng*)
LV 2 (*xíng jiān*)	ST 36 (*zú sān lǐ*)	SP 6 (*sān yīn jiāo*)

Using moderate needle stimulation, apply tonification for hyperactivity of fire due to yin deficiency, and reduction for other patterns. 3–5 acupoints are selected each time, retaining the needles for 20 minutes; treat once a day. Frequency of therapy is determined according to the patient's underlying condition.

3. Chinese Patent Medicines

(1) *Zhī Bǎi Dì Huáng Wán* (Anemarrhena, Phellodendron and Rehmannia Pill, 知柏地黄丸)

6 g, three times a day; applicable to deficiency-fire flaming upward.

(2) *Qǐ Jú Dì Huáng Wán* (Lycium Berry, Chrysanthemum and Rehmannia Pill, 杞菊地黄丸)

6 g, three times a day; applicable to liver-kidney depletion.

4. Treatment with Western Medicine

The patients may seek advice or treatment from conventional eye doctors of Western medicine. Common therapies may include:

(1) Mydriasis: Topical application of mydriatics is the main form of treatment in Western medicine. According to the patient's condition, one may use topical eye drops including atropine, homatropine, scopolamine, and subconjunctival injection with mydriasis mixtures when necessary.

(2) Glucocorticoids: 0.1% dexamethasone eye drops, 0.5% cortisone eye drops, or subconjunctival injection, intravenous drips, or oral glucocorticoids.

(3) Nonsteroid anti-inflammatory drugs: Eye drops or oral medication may include pranoprofen, diclofenac, or indomethacin.

(4) Etilogical treatment: Select corresponding etiological treatment for the identified underlying causes.

(5) Complication treatment: For cases with secondary glaucoma because of papillary closure, select peripheral iridectomy or YAG Laser Iridotomy after the inflammation has been controlled. For cases with severe cataract with accurate light projection, a cataract extraction may be performed when the inflammation is controlled and the condition becomes stable.

5. Dietary Therapy and Preventive Care

(1) During the period of the illness, get plenty of rest, use the eyes as little as possible, avoid glare and bright lights when indoors or outdoors, gradually increase physical exercise, and strengthen the body constitution over time.

(2) Eat less pungent, spicy, and greasy/fried foods because they can form dampness and heat, which could aggravate the condition and/or lead to recurrence.

Case Studies

Liu, a 21-year-old man

【Chief Complaint】

Redness, pain, and blurred vision in the left eye for three days

【Examination】

Visual acuity: OD 20/13; OS 20/66, obvious congestion of the circumcornea, 10 gray-white minute dots of keratic punctata, turbidity of the aqueous humor, pupilary contraction (2 mm), pain when directly pressing on the eyeball.

【Diagnosis】

Iridocyclitis of the left eye

【Pattern Differentiation】

Interior excess of the *jueyin* and *shaoyang* channels

【Treatment Principles】

Clear liver heat and drain the gallbladder.

【Prescription】

Modified *Lóng Dǎn Xiè Gān Tāng* (Gentian Liver-Draining Decoction, 龙胆泻肝汤)

龙胆草	lóng dǎn cǎo	6 g	Radix et Rhizoma Gentianae
栀子	zhī zǐ	10 g	Fructus Gardeniae
黄芩	huáng qín	10 g	Radix Scutellariae
黄连	huáng lián	5 g	Rhizoma Coptidis
柴胡	chái hú	10 g	Radix Bupleuri
生地	shēng dì	15 g	Radix Rehmanniae
当归	dāng guī	10 g	Radix Angelicae Sinensis
泽泻	zé xiè	10 g	Rhizoma Alismatis
车前子	chē qián zǐ	15 g	Semen Plantaginis
木通	mù tōng	6 g	Caulis Akebiae
甘草	gān cǎo	6 g	Radix et Rhizoma Glycyrrhizae

One batch per day, combined with 1% atropine drops three times per day.

【Follow-up】

After seven days, the patient's symptoms were alleviated. The formula was changed to *Shí Jué Míng Sǎn* (Concha Haliotidis Powder, 石决明散)

石决明	shí jué míng	25 g	Concha Haliotidis
草决明	cǎo jué míng	25 g	Semen Cassiae
赤芍	chì sháo	15 g	Radix Paeoniae Rubra
青葙子	qīng xiāng zǐ	18 g	Semen Celosiae

栀子	*zhī zǐ*	10 g	Fructus Gardeniae
荆芥	*jīng jiè*	10 g	Herba Schizonepetae
麦冬	*mài dōng*	15 g	Radix Ophiopogonis
木贼	*mù zéi*	15 g	Herba Equiseti Hiemalis

After taking five batches, the patient recovered. Visual acuity on the left eye was increased to 20/17.

(Excerpted from *Clinical Experience of Chen Da-fu's TCM Ophthalmology* [*Chén Dá Fú Zhōng Yī Yǎn Kē Lín Chuáng Jīng Yàn*])

Classic Quotes

《原机启微·强阳抟实阴之病》："强者，盛而有力也。实者，坚而内充也。故有力者，强而欲抟，内充者，实而自收。是以阴阳无两强，亦无两实，惟强与实，以扁则病，内抟于身，上见于虚窍也。足少阴肾为水，肾之精上为神水，手厥阴心包络为实火，火强抟水，水实而自收。其病神水紧小，渐小而又小，积渐之至，竟如菜子许。"

"Strong yang such as fire and heat is exuberant and powerful, while solid yin such as kidney water is firm and substantial inside the body. So, there is no strong yin and strong yang at the same time, nor solid yang and solid yin. When strong yang and solid yin tangle with each other, it will cause disease and attack the orifices. The kidney is ascribed to water; the essence of the kidney forms spirit water, while the envelope of the heart is ascribed to fire. When the fire flames upward burning spirit water, it causes the pupil to get tighter and tighter, smaller and smaller, finally like a rapeseed."

Enlightenment of Ophthalmology – Disease of Strong Yang Intermingling with Excess Yin (*Yuán Jī Qǐ Wēi – Qiáng Yáng Tuán Shí Yīn Zhī Bìng*, 原机启微·强阳抟实阴之病)

Section 2   Vogt-Koyanagi-Harada Syndrome

Vogt-Koyanagi-Harada Syndrome is a syndrome which displays diffuse exudative uveitis in both eyes and affects many organs and systems of the body. It is named Vogt-Koyanagi Syndrome if the major manifestation is presented as iridocyclitis, whereas it is named Harada Syndrome if it presents as exudative choroiditis.

Causes of the disease are still unknown. It may possibly be related to autoimmune diseases caused by viral infection, other immune responses to the retinal pigmentary epithelium, or associated with positive HLA antigens. Main clinical manifestations include decreased bilateral visual acuity, pupilary opisthosynechia, diffuse edema and exudates of the fundus, vitreous opacity, or even retinal detachment and other symptoms of severe uveitis, accompanied by systemic symptoms such as headache, palinacousia, and vitiligo.

This condition is commonly seen in both adolescents and adults, and usually attacks both eyes with a prolonged course and a high recurrence rate. Western medicine treats the disease with glucocorticoids in order to control inflammation, enlarging the pupil to prevent opisthosynechia, and other symptomatic treatments in an attempt to address the underlying causes.

The disease has no corresponding name in traditional Chinese medicine. According to various clinical manifestations, it may belong to the categories of *tóng shén jǐn xiǎo* (contracted pupils, 瞳神紧小), *tóng shén gān quē* (pupil contraction, 瞳神干缺), *yún wù yí jīng* (clouds and mist floating across the eye, 云雾移睛), and *shì zhān hūn miǎo* (blurred vision, 视瞻昏渺). The underlying causes are very complex, mostly associated with damp-heat brewing and binding, exuberant heat toxin, or deficiency-fire flaming upward. The main pathogen is heat brewing internally, harassing the channels of the eye, fumigating the iris, and burning the aqueous humor and the vitreous body, thus causing eye disease. Chinese medicine uses methods of regulating the *zang-fu* and eliminating the pathogen in order to support vital qi. We do this through pattern differentiation and treatment of the underlying pattern so as to control clinical symptoms, improve visual acuity, and decrease the rate of recurrence.

Clinical Manifestation

1. Systemic symptoms

Before the appearance of ocular symptoms, there are often systemic symptoms such as headache, tinnitus, hearing impairment, dizziness, nausea, vomiting, neck rigidity, and other meningisms. As the condition develops, the hair, eyebrow and eyelashes may whiten or fall off, and vitiligo may also appear on the skin.

2. Eye symptoms

(1) Vogt-koyanagi syndrome

Manifestations of the disease are similar to acute iridocyclitis, but some signs are more common, such as opisthosynechia or atresia of the pupil, secondary glaucoma, and cataract. General clinical presentations include ciliary congestion, turbidity of the aqueous humor, opisthosynechia of the pupil, and severe impaired vision. As the condition progresses, retinal edema and gray-white exudates of the choroid may develop.

(2) Harada syndrome

This disease has an acute onset beginning with severe signs of meningeal irritation and manifestation of posterior segment lesions. The patient's vision become distorted and visual acuity may be decreased. Examination of the fundus shows diffuse yellow-white exudative edema, hyperemia and unclear border of optic disc, exudative retinal detachment, and vitreous opacities. When inflammation develops to anterior segments, iridocyclitis may appear.

When the condition becomes stable, inflammation of anterior segments subside, and the destruction of the posterior retinal segments resolve; the fundus looks like "sunset-glow," an important diagnostic feature of the disease.

Treatment

1. Pattern Differentiation and Treatment

As this is a severe eye disease, it has a long course with potentially severe damage to the vision. The treatment principle should be determined under full consideration of the multiple underlying causes and complex pathogenesis. In the late stage, it is very important to supplement the *zang-fu*, support righteous qi, and secure the root in order to prevent recurrence of the disease.

(1) Damp-Heat Brewing and Binding

【Syndrome Characteristics】
Pressure and pain of the eyeball, photophobia and hyperdacryosis, impaired vision, turbidity of the aqueous humor, swelling of the iris, contracted pupils, possibly accompanied by vitreous opacity, and retinal edema. Systemic symptoms include headache and dizziness, tinnitus and palinacousia, dyspnea and nausea, red tongue with yellow greasy coating, and a slippery rapid pulse.

【Treatment Principle】
Clear heat and drain dampness

【Representative Formula】
Modified *Gān Lù Xiāo Dú Dān* (Sweet Dew Toxin-Removing Elixir, 甘露消毒丹)

【Prescription】

黄芩	*huáng qín*	10 g	Radix Scutellariae
连翘	*lián qiào*	10 g	Fructus Forsythiae
通草	*tōng cǎo*	8 g	Medulla Tetrapanacis
滑石	*huá shí*	20 g	Talcum
茵陈	*yīn chén*	20 g	Herba Artemisiae Scopariae
藿香	*huò xiāng*	8 g	Herba Agastachis
白蔻仁	*bái kòu rén*	8 g	Fructus Amomi Rotundus
石菖蒲	*shí chāng pú*	5 g	Rhizoma Acori Tatarinowii
射干	*shè gān*	10 g	Rhizoma Belamcandae
薄荷	*bò he*	5 g	Herba Menthae

| 茺蔚子 | *chōng wèi zǐ* | 12 g | Fructus Leonuri |
| 车前草 | *chē qián cǎo* | 15 g | Herba Plantaginis |

【 Modifications 】

➢ For cases with severe ciliary congestion or pronounced circuity and filling of the retinal vessels, add *dān shēn* (丹参, Radix et Rhizoma Salviae Miltiorrhizae) 15 g, *yù jīn* (郁金, Radix Curcumae) 10 g, and *chì sháo* (赤芍, Radix Paeoniae Rubra) 10 g to cool and invigorate the blood.

➢ For cases with marked swelling of the iris or edema of retina and papilla optica, add *yì yǐ rén* (薏苡仁, Semen Coicis) 15 g, *dōng guā pí* (冬瓜皮, Exocarpium Benincasae) 20 g, and *zé xiè* (泽泻, Rhizoma Alismatis) 10 g to drain water and disperse swelling.

(2) Blazing Liver Fire

【 Syndrome Characteristics 】

Eye pain that is worse with pressure, photophobia and hyperdacryosis, blurred vision, hyperemia of the bulbar conjunctiva, turbidity of the aqueous humor, abundance of gray-white punctiform keratic precipitate, contracted pupils, vitreous opacity, widespread yellow-white exudation in the fundus, retinal edema, or even retinal detachment. Systemic symptoms include headache and stiff neck, dizziness, tinnitus, vexation, agitation, and irascibility, dryness and bitterness of the mouth, red tongue with yellow coating, and wiry rapid pulse.

【 Treatment Principle 】

Clear liver heat and drain fire

【 Representative Formula 】

Modified *Lóng Dǎn Xiè Gān Tāng* (Gentian Liver-Draining Decoction, 龙胆泻肝汤)

【 Prescription 】

龙胆草	*lóng dǎn cǎo*	5 g	Radix et Rhizoma Gentianae
栀子	*zhī zǐ*	10 g	Fructus Gardeniae
黄芩	*huáng qín*	10 g	Radix Scutellariae
黄连	*huáng lián*	5 g	Rhizoma Coptidis
柴胡	*chái hú*	10 g	Radix Bupleuri
车前草	*chē qián cǎo*	12 g	Herba Plantaginis
通草	*tōng cǎo*	10 g	Medulla Tetrapanacis
生地	*shēng dì*	10 g	Radix Rehmanniae
赤芍	*chì sháo*	10 g	Radix Paeoniae Rubra
生甘草	*shēng gān cǎo*	5 g	Radix et Rhizoma Glycyrrhizae

【 Modifications 】

➢ For cases with headache and stiff neck, dizziness and tinnitus, add *bái sháo* (白芍,

Radix Paeoniae Alba) 15 g, *dì lóng* (地龙, Pheretima) 10 g, *shí jué míng* (石决明, Concha Haliotidis) 30 g, *gōu téng* (钩藤, Ramulus Uncariae Cum Uncis) 15 g, and *tiān má* (天麻, Rhizoma Gastrodiae) 10 g to calm the liver and extinguish wind.

➢ For cases with pronounced turbidity of the aqueous humor and blurred vision, add *jú huā* (菊花, Flos Chrysanthemi) 12 g, *xià kū cǎo* (夏枯草, Spica Prunellae) 10 g, *bái huā shé shé cǎo* (白花蛇舌草, Herba Hedyotis Diffusae) 20 g, and *chōng wèi zǐ* (茺蔚子, Fructus Leonuri) 12 g to drain fire, resolve toxin, and brighten the eyes.

(3) Intense Qi and Blood Heat

【 Syndrome Characteristics 】

Intense eye pain, hyperdacryosis, vision loss, hyperemia of the bulbar conjunctiva, turbidity of the aqueous humor and vitreous, contracted pupils, edema or punctiform and lamellar hemorrhage of the retina and papilla optica, and engorgement and filling of retinal vein. Systemic symptoms include intense splitting headache, stiff neck and back, nausea and vomiting, clouded spirit, vexation and agitation, dry pharynx and mouth, yellowish urine, red or crimson tongue with yellow dry coating, and surging rapid pulse.

【 Treatment Principle 】

Clear *ying* level heat and resolve toxin, outthrust heat and nourish yin

【 Representative Formula 】

Modified *Qīng Yíng Tāng* (*Ying* Heat-Clearing Decoction, 清营汤)

【 Prescription 】

生地	*shēng dì*	15 g	Radix Rehmanniae
丹皮	*dān pí*	12 g	Cortex Moutan
赤芍	*chì sháo*	10 g	Radix Paeoniae Rubra
玄参	*xuán shēn*	12 g	Radix Scrophulariae
麦冬	*mài dōng*	10 g	Radix Ophiopogonis
竹叶心	*zhú yè xīn*	5 g	Folium Pleioblasti
丹参	*dān shēn*	10 g	Radix et Rhizoma Salviae Miltiorrhizae
紫草	*zǐ cǎo*	10 g	Radix Arnebiae
黄连	*huáng lián*	5 g	Rhizoma Coptidis
金银花	*jīn yín huā*	12 g	Flos Lonicerae Japonicae
连翘	*lián qiào*	10 g	Fructus Forsythiae

【 Modifications 】

➢ For cases with retinal hemorrhage, remove *dān shēn* (丹参, Radix et Rhizoma Salviae Miltiorrhizae) and add *bái máo gēn* (白茅根, Rhizoma Imperatae) 20 g, *xiǎo jì* (小蓟, Herba Cirsii) 15 g, and *dà jì* (大蓟, Herba Cirsii Japonici) 15 g to cool blood and stop bleeding.

➢ For cases with generalized fever and thirst, add *zhī mǔ* (知母, Rhizoma Anemarrhenae, Rhizoma Anemarrhenae) 10 g, *shēng shí gāo* (生石膏, Gypsum Fibrosum)

30 g, and *lú gēn* (芦根, Rhizoma Phragmitis) 20 g to clear qi and blood heat.

(4) Hyperactivity of Fire due to Yin Deficiency

【 Syndrome Characteristics 】

Chronic tendency with recurrent attacks, dull pain of the eyeball, dryness and discomfort in the eye, clouded flowery vision, mild ciliary congestion, turbidity of the aqueous humor, pallor of the optic disc, and sunset-like fundus. Systemic symptoms include dull headache, vexing heat in the five centers, dry mouth and pharynx, red tongue with little coating, and thready rapid pulse.

【 Treatment Principle 】

Enrich yin and clear heat

【 Representative Formula 】

Modified *Qīng Shèn Yì Yáng Wán* (Kidney Heat-Clearing and Yang-Inhibiting Pill, 清肾抑阳丸)

【 Prescription 】

生地	*shēng dì*	12 g	Radix Rehmanniae
枸杞子	*gǒu qǐ zǐ*	15 g	Fructus Lycii
当归	*dāng guī*	10 g	Radix Angelicae Sinensis
白芍	*bái sháo*	12 g	Radix Paeoniae Alba
草决明	*cǎo jué míng*	12 g	Semen Cassiae
知母	*zhī mǔ*	10 g	Rhizoma Anemarrhenae
黄柏	*huáng bǎi*	10 g	Cortex Phellodendri Chinensis
黄连	*huáng lián*	5 g	Rhizoma Coptidis
寒水石	*hán shuǐ shí*	15 g	Glauberitum
茯苓	*fú líng*	10 g	Poria
独活	*dú huó*	5 g	Radix Angelicae Pubescentis
麦冬	*mài dōng*	10 g	Radix Ophiopogonis
葛根	*gé gēn*	10 g	Radix Puerariae Lobatae

【 Modifications 】

➢ For cases without severe heat symptoms, remove *hán shuǐ shí* (Glauberitum) and *huáng lián* (Rhizoma Coptidis) to prevent the excessive bitterness and cold from damaging healthy qi.

➢ For cases with marked blurred vision, add *jú huā* (菊花, Flos Chrysanthemi) 10 g, *chǔ shí zǐ* (楮实子, Fructus Broussonetiae) 15 g, and *shān zhū yú* (山茱萸, Fructus Corni) 10 g to nourish the liver and kidney and brighten the eyes.

➢ For cases with dry eyes, remove *dú huó* (Radix Angelicae Pubescentis) and *hán shuǐ shí* (Glauberitum), and add *mì méng huā* (密蒙花, Flos Buddlejae) 10 g and *shí hú* (石斛, Caulis Dendrobii) 15 g to nourish yin and moisten dryness.

➤ For cases with tidal heat, night sweating, deficiency vexation and insomnia, remove *dāng guī* (Radix Angelicae Sinensis) and *dú huó* (Radix Angelicae Pubescentis), and add *mǔ dān pí* (牡丹皮, Cortex Moutan) 10 g, *dì gǔ pí* (地骨皮, Cortex Lycii) 10 g, *biē jiǎ* (鳖甲, Carapax Trionycis) 15 g, *bǎi zǐ rén* (柏子仁, Semen Platycladi) 12 g, and *suān zǎo rén* (酸枣仁, Semen Ziziphi Spinosae) 15 g to clear deficiency heat, eliminate vexation, and quieten the spirit.

2. Chinese Patent Medicines

(1) *Zhī Bǎi Dì Huáng Wán* (Anemarrhena, Phellodendron and Rehmannia Pill, 知柏地黄丸)

Taken orally, 6 g, three times a day; applicable to hyperactivity of fire due to yin deficiency.

(2) *Qǐ Jú Dì Huáng Wán* (Lycium Berry, Chrysanthemum and Rehmannia Pill, 杞菊地黄丸)

Taken orally 6 g, three times a day; applicable to the last stage of the disease, or liver-kidney deficiency.

3. Treatment with Western Medicine

Patients may seek advice or treatment from a Western conventional ophthalmologist. Common therapies may include:

(1) Mydriasis: Prompt topical application of cycloplegics or mydriatic eye drops to release ciliary spasm and prevent pupil opisthosynechia.

(2) Glucocorticoids: Systemic (local-topical and oral) application of glucocorticoids is the main method of conventional treatment. It is important to gradually reduce the dosage over time in order to prevent recurrence due to early drug withdraw or a rebond effect.

(3) Immunosuppressant: For patients that are unable to tolerate the side effects of glucocorticoids, immunodepressants (such as chlorambucil, cyclophosphamide, and ciclosporin A) may be considered.

(4) Surgery: For cases with secondary glaucoma or complicated cataract, surgical intervention may be indicated after inflammation is stable.

4. Dietary Therapy and Preventive Care

(1) Eat a light and nutritious diet; eat less acrid, spicy, and greasy-fried foods.

(2) Keep good living habits, avoid staying up late or all night, and give up smoking and drinking alcohol.

(3) Engage in daily physical exercise in order to strengthen the constitution.

Case Study

Jiang, a 25-year-old male

First visit: April, 5, 1977

【 Chief Complaint & Medical History 】

Mr. Jiang presented with hyperpyrexia (abnormally high fever), headache, and tinnitus, and had been vomiting for 2 weeks. After four days, his fever abated but visual acuity in both eyes decreased. The doctor treated the disease with oral dexanethasone and intramuscular vitamin B12 injections.

Other signs and symptoms included a rapid, soft and weak pulse, red tongue with yellow thin coating, emaciation of the body, fatigued spirit and lack of strength, and desire to vomit.

【 Examination 】

Right visual acuity was 20/33, left visual acuity was 20/40, mild ciliary congestion, intensive thin punctiform keratitis punctata, marked edema and indistinct border of the optic papilla, physiological reflex in the macular region is absent, small hemorrhage of the retina. Left eye examination was similar to that of the right eye.

【 Diagnosis 】

Uveoencephalitis syndrome (Harada disease)

【 Pattern Differentiation 】

Correlation of the pulse and signs indicated that internal heat damaged both qi and yin. Therefore, symptoms manifested as weakness and fatigue, qi counterflow and desire to retch, and optic nerve congestion and retinal hemorrhage of both eyes, which correspond to the pattern of deficiency fire flaming upward.

【 Treatment Principles 】

Clear heat and engender liquid, sweep phlegm and stop vomitting

【 Prescription 】

竹叶	zhú yè	9 g	Folium Phyllostachydis Henonis
生石膏	shēng shí gāo	15 g	Gypsum Fibrosum
麦冬	mài dōng	6 g	Radix Ophiopogonis
制半夏	zhì bàn xià	6 g	Rhizoma Pinelliae (prepared)
炙甘草	zhì gān cǎo	4.5 g	Radix et Rhizoma Glycyrrhizae Praeparata cum Melle
党参	dǎng shēn	9 g	Radix Codonopsis
羚羊角粉	líng yáng jiǎo fěn	0.3 g	Cornu Saigae Tataricae (powder, taken separately)

The patient continued to use the medication prescribed by the Western doctor.

【 Follow-up 】

After four additional office visits, and modification of the medicinal formulas according to changes in pattern presentation, the patient gradually recovered. On September 30, visual acuity of both eyes was 20/13, and there was no report of recurrence. The patient stated that ten white hairs were found on the top of the head, but there were no changes in the eyebrows and eyelashes. In following up with the patient, he reported that the white hairs had disappeared.

(Excerpted from *Clinical Records of Ophthalmology* [*Yǎn Kē Lín Zhèng Lù,* 眼科临证录])

Question for Consideration

What are the clinical manifestations of Vogt-Koyanag Syndrome and Harada Syndrome?

Section 3   Behcet's Disease

Behcet's disease is a condition that affects many systems of the body, typically characterized by recurrent uveitis, oral ulcers, genital ulcers, and polymorphous skin lesions. Etiology of the disease is unknown, but may be related to viral and bacterial infections, autoimmune responses caused by self-antigens and immune and genetic factors. Basic pathological changes are occlusive vasculitis and tissue necrosis. It generally occurs to men in their 20s to 40s, and attacks both eyes. Western medicine mainly treats this with corticosteroids, immunosuppressive agents, and symptomatic treatment.

The disease has no corresponding name in TCM, but the clinical manifestations are similar to the "fox-creeper disease" (*hú huò bìng,* 狐惑病) described in *Essentials from the Golden Cabinet (Jīn Guì Yào Lüè,* 金匮要略). Therefore, it is called "red pigeon-like eyes" in some modern ophthalmology literature. Main pathogenesis are dysfunctions of the viscera, retention of damp-heat, pathogenic toxin transforming into fire and filling the *sanjiao,* stasis of the vessels and collaterals; heat steaming upward and dampness flowing down, scorching the iris, invading the oropharynx, disgorging the external genitalia, and invading the muscle and skin. As the disease includes both visceral depletion and excess of pathogenic toxins brewing and binding, it manifests clinically as signs of a deficiency-excess complex. The treatment principle is to regulate the whole body, dispel pathogens, and support healthy qi on the basis of pattern differentiation. Emphasis is placed on clearing heat, dispelling dampness, resolving toxins, and activating blood circulation to alleviate clinical symptoms, control the progression of the disease, increase and/or preserve vision, and, at the same time, decrease the risk of recurrence.

Clinical Manifestation

Behcet's disease is an autoimmune disease, involving multiple systems; it is of chronic, persistent, and inflammatory nature. In addition to some characteristic clinical manifestations of recurrent uveitis and oral and genital ulcers, it is often accompanied by damage to the skin, joints, and nervous system.

1. Ocular damage

Ocular damage is often seen after 2–3 years of the appearance of oral ulcers and skin lesions, mainly manifesting as uveitis. According to the location of inflammation, it can be divided into two types: iridocyclitis of the anterior segment, and posterior uveitis.

The main clinical manifestations of iridocyclitis include ciliary congestion, ophthalmalgia, photophobia, tearing, impaired vision, turbid aqueous humor, hypopyon, keratic precipitates, and opisthosynechia.

Posterior uveitis exhibits retinochoroiditis, retinal vasculitis, turbid aqueous humor, proliferate membrane of vitreous, retinal hemorrhage, yellow-white exudation or retinal edema, congestion and edema of the papilla, attenuation and expanding of retinal vessels, vascular white sheath, capillary, venous and arterial occlusion that appear as white lines, neovascularization, macular edema, hemorrhage, exudation, and even perforation; in severe cases, it is often associated with anterior uveitis.

As the disease progresses, retinal hemorrhage, edema, and exudate gradually become absorbed; residual or secondary changes may appear, such as retinal atrophy, optic nerve atrophy, arterio-venous vascular sheath, chorioretinal scars, and retinal pigmentary epithelial changes.

2. Oral Ulcers

Ulcers begin to appear and subsequently form round or oval ulcers, and often multiple lesions. The ulcers can integrate with each other into a large ulcer that is demarcated and surrounded by a hyperemic ring with marked pain.

3. Genital Ulcer

Genital ulcers are generally painful and sharply defined. The ulcers heal slowly and may leave scars. Ulcer pain in men is more pronounced than that in women, and ulcers in women mostly occurs premenstrually.

4. Other Damages

(1) Lesions of the skin: Skin lesions are common signs of this disease characterized by multiple forms and recurrence, of which erythema nodosum is the most common form. Others may include exudative erythema, ulcerative dermatitis, folliculitis, abscesses, or an

acne-like rash. In addition, allergic skin reactions are also a characteristic manifestation. After intramuscular or intravenous puncture, small papules and pustules often appear on the site of puncture.

(2) Lesions of the joints: Whereas knee joints are most vulnerable, lesions may also occur in the hands, feet, elbows and other joints, and show localized redness and pain. There is usually no occurrence of ankylosis, deformation, and migratory pain.

(3) The lesions of the digestive tract: Some patients may have gastrointestinal symptoms, such as nausea, vomiting, abdominal pain, diarrhea, constipation, bloody stool, or digestive tract ulcer, and even perforation.

(4) Lesions of the blood vessels: Arteries, veins, and small and large blood vessels can be involved, of which vein damage is the most common (mainly manifesting as thrombophlebitis). Severe vascular damage can lead to death.

(5) Lesions of the central nervous system: Some patients may show meningitis, intracranial hypertension, and symptoms and signs of injury to the cerebrum, cerebellum, or brain stem, of which the most common are mental abnormalities and centrokinetic disorders.

Treatment

Behcet's disease is a serious disease that is difficult to treat. The condition becomes chronic with recurrent attacks which can seriously damage the eyesight and in some cases can be life-threatening. Pathogenesis is very complex, possibly associated with damp-heat, toxins, and stasis. They combine together to cause the disease, but heat is the core issue. Therefore, clearing heat is the primary goal, and can be combined with strategies to drain dampness, resolve toxins, invigorate blood, and nourish yin. As the pathogenesis includes visceral deficiency and excess of pathogenic toxins, the clinical manifestations appear with a deficiency-excess complex. Therefore, it is very important to distinguish deficiency and excess as well as the degree of urgency and apply flexibility in selecting and using medicinals on the basis of pattern differentiation.

1. Pattern Differentiation and Treatment

(1) Damp-Heat in the Liver and Gallbladder
[Syndrome Characteristics]
Rapidly decreasing vision, congestion around the cornea, eye swelling and pain, photophobia, tears, contracted pupils, turbidity of the aqueous humor. Systemic symptoms may include redness, swelling, and sores of the mouth and tongue, desire to sleep, vexation and irascibility, fidgetiness whether lying down or standing up, rib-side distention and pain, poor appetite, erosion of the genitals, yellowish or reddish urine, dry stool, red tongue with yellow greasy coating, and slippery rapid pulse.

【 Treatment Principle 】
Clear liver heat and drain dampness
【 Representative Formula 】
Modified *Lóng Dǎn Xiè Gān Tāng* (Gentian Liver-Draining Decoction, 龙胆泻肝汤)
【 Prescription 】

龙胆草	*lóng dǎn cǎo*	5 g	Radix et Rhizoma Gentianae
栀子	*zhī zǐ*	12 g	Fructus Gardeniae
黄芩	*huáng qín*	10 g	Radix Scutellariae
柴胡	*chái hú*	10 g	Radix Bupleuri
车前草	*chē qián cǎo*	15 g	Herba Plantaginis
泽泻	*zé xiè*	10 g	Rhizoma Alismatis
通草	*tōng cǎo*	10 g	Medulla Tetrapanacis
生地	*shēng dì*	12 g	Radix Rehmanniae
蒲公英	*pú gōng yīng*	20 g	Herba Taraxaci
板蓝根	*bǎn lán gēn*	20 g	Radix Isatidis

【 Modifications 】

➢ For cases with severe ulcers and erythralgia of the mouth, skin or genitals, add *fú líng* (茯苓, Poria) 15 g, *jīn yín huā* (金银花, Flos Lonicerae Japonicae) 12 g, *lián qiào* (连翘, Fructus Forsythiae) 10 g, and *zǐ huā dì dīng* (紫花地丁, Herba Violae) 15 g to clear heat, drain fire, and resolve toxins to treat the sores.

➢ For cases with throat pain and erosion, add *shān dòu gēn* (山豆根, Radix et Rhizoma Sophorae Tonkinensis) 12 g, *jié gěng* (桔梗, Radix Platycodonis) 8 g, and *shè gān* (射干, Rhizoma Belamcandae) 10 g to drain fire, resolve toxins, and relieve sore-throat.

➢ For cases with red and turbid conjunctiva, and tortuosity and expanding of retinal vein, which are signs of exuberant heat causing stasis, add *chì sháo* (赤芍, Radix Paeoniae Rubra) 12 g, *mǔ dān pí* (牡丹皮, Cortex Moutan) 10 g, and *táo rén* (桃仁, Semen Persicae) 15 g to cool blood, activate blood circulation, and eliminate stasis.

➢ For cases with constipation, add *jué míng zǐ* (决明子, Semen Cassiae) 15 g and *shú dà huáng* (熟大黄, Radix et Rhizoma Rhei) 5 g to relieve constipation and drain heat.

(2) Damp-Heat Obstructing the Center
【 Syndrome Characteristics 】

Congestion of the conjunctiva and eye pain, photophobia, tearing, blurred vision, turbidity of the aqueous humor, dusty or punctiform keratic precipitate, edema of the iris, pupil contraction, even atresia of the pupil, vitreous opacities, edema and punctiform or lamellar exudation of the retina, plucked vessels, or white sheath. Systemic symptoms may include headache and dizziness, fever, aversion to the smell of food, glomus and fullness in the chest and stomach, sores on or in the mouth and tongue, erosion of anal and genital orifices, thirst but no desire to drink, heavy cumbersome limbs, or red sore joints, yellowish and scanty urine, sticky stools, red tongue with yellow greasy thick coating, and slippery rapid pulse.

【 Treatment Principle 】

Clear liver heat and drain dampness, resolve toxins and dissipate stasis

【 Representative Formula 】

Modified *Gān Lù Xiāo Dú Dān* (Sweet Dew Toxin-Removing Elixir, 甘露消毒丹)

【 Prescription 】

黄芩	*huáng qín*	15 g	Radix Scutellariae
茵陈	*yīn chén*	15 g	Herba Artemisiae Scopariae
滑石	*huá shí*	20 g	Talcum
连翘	*lián qiào*	10 g	Fructus Forsythiae
射干	*shè gān*	10 g	Rhizoma Belamcandae
石菖蒲	*shí chāng pú*	5 g	Rhizoma Acori Tatarinowii
通草	*tōng cǎo*	10 g	Medulla Tetrapanacis
藿香	*huò xiāng*	10 g	Herba Agastachis
白蔻仁	*bái kòu rén*	3 g	Fructus Amomi Rotundus
黄连	*huáng lián*	3 g	Rhizoma Coptidis
茯苓	*fú líng*	15 g	Poria
薏苡仁	*yì yǐ rén*	20 g	Semen Coicis

【 Modifications 】

➢ For cases with ungratifying defecation or tenesmus, remove *bái kòu rén* (白蔻仁, Fructus Amomi Rotundus) and add *dà fù pí* (大腹皮, Pericarpium Arecae) 10 g, *qín pí* (秦皮, Cortex Fraxini) 10 g, *bái tóu wēng* (白头翁, Radix Pulsatillae) 15 g, and *zhǐ shí* (枳实, Fructus Aurantii Immaturus) 10 g to move qi and free stagnation, clear heat, and remove dampness.

➢ For cases with severely painful and swollen joints, remove *shè gān* (射干, blackberry lily rhizome) and *bái kòu rén* (白蔻仁, Fructus Amomi Rotundus), and add *qín jiāo* (秦艽, Radix Gentianae Macrophyllae) 10 g, *xī xiān cǎo* (豨莶草, Herba Siegesbeckiae) 15 g, and *lù lù tōng* (路路通, Fructus Liquidambaris) 10 g to remove dampness, free the collaterals, and remove impediment.

➢ For cases with congestion of the conjunctiva and a red tongue with yellowish coating, remove *bái kòu rén* (白蔻仁, Fructus Amomi Rotundus) to prevent acridness and warmth from resulting in heat, and add *huáng bǎi* (黄柏, Cortex Phellodendri Chinensis) 8 g, *zhī zǐ* (栀子, Fructus Gardeniae Cape jasmine fruit) 10 g, and *xià kū cǎo* (夏枯草, Spica Prunellae) 15 g to clear heat and drain fire.

➢ For cases with edema of the retina, fullness and oppression in the chest and abdomen, and a greasy thick tongue coating, which are signs of dampness, add *dōng guā rén* (冬瓜仁, Semen Benincasae) 20 g, *zhū líng* (猪苓, Polyporus, Polyporus) 12 g, and *chì xiǎo dòu* (赤小豆, Semen Phaseoli) 15 g to drain dampness and clear heat.

(3) Accumulation and Stagnation of Warmth-Heat, with Toxin and Stasis Binding Together

【 Syndrome Characteristics 】

At the late stage of febrile disease, besides exhibiting signs in the eye caused by damp-heat obstructing the center, retinal vessels show partial occlusion or look like white thread. Systemic symptoms may include headache, fever, painful swollen joints, erythema nodosum or abscess of the limbs, ulcers of the lips and tongue, swelling and pain of the throat, ulcers of the external genitalia, pale red tongue or with stasis maculae, yellow thin tongue coating, and wiry rapid pulse.

【 Treatment Principle 】

Clear heat and outthrust pathogens, resolve toxins, and disperse swelling

【 Representative Formula 】

Modified *Huà Bān Tāng* (Macule-Transforming Decoction, 化斑汤)

【 Prescription 】

黄连	*huáng lián*	5 g	Rhizoma Picrorhizae
青黛	*qīng dài*	6 g	Indigo Naturalis
生石膏	*shēng shí gāo*	20 g	Gypsum Fibrosum
石决明	*shí jué míng*	20 g	Concha Haliotidis
生地	*shēng dì*	12 g	Radix Rehmanniae
玄参	*xuán shēn*	12 g	Radix Scrophulariae
知母	*zhī mǔ*	12 g	Rhizoma Anemarrhenae
山药	*shān yào*	15 g	Rhizoma Dioscoreae
牡丹皮	*mǔ dān pí*	12 g	Cortex Moutan
葛根	*gé gēn*	15 g	Radix Puerariae Lobatae
紫草	*zǐ cǎo*	10 g	Radix Arnebiae
生甘草	*shēng gān cǎo*	5 g	Radix et Rhizoma Glycyrrhizae

【 Modifications 】

➤ For cases with obvious skin abscess, remove *shān yào* (山药, Rhizoma Dioscoreae) and *zhī mǔ* (知母, Rhizoma Anemarrhenae) and add *hóng téng* (红藤, Caulis Sargentodoxae) 15 g, *bài jiàng cǎo* (败酱草, Herba Patriniae) 15 g, *pú gōng yīng* (蒲公英, Herba Taraxaci) 15 g, and *chuān xīn lián* (穿心莲, Herba Andrographis) 10 g to clear heat, resolve toxins, quicken the blood, and disperse swelling.

➤ For cases with retinal hemorrhage or obvious tortuosity and expansion of the retinal vessels, add *shēng pú huáng* (生蒲黄, Pollen Typhae) 10 g, *huā ruǐ shí* (花蕊石, Ophicalcitum) 15 g, and *dān shēn* (丹参, Radix et Rhizoma Salviae Miltiorrhizae) 10 g to dispel stasis and stop bleeding.

(4) Hyperactivity of Fire Due to Yin Deficiency with Residual Pathogen

【Syndrome Characteristics】

The pattern is commonly seen at the late stage or after recurrence, showing unclear eye pain, uncomfortable dry eyes, blurred vision and inability to see for a long time, mild ciliary congestion, turbid aqueous humor, iris thinner, pupillary metamorphosis, dirty retina, and a light-colored optic disc. Systemic symptoms include dizziness, tinnitus, red cheek, night sweating, vexing heat in the five centers, dry mouth and throat, frequent mouth sores, red tongue with little coating, and thready rapid pulse.

【Treatment Principle】

Nourish yin and clear heat, support healthy qi and secure the root

【Representative Formula】

Modified *Zhī Bǎi Dì Huáng Tāng* (Anemarrhena, Phellodendron and Rehmannia Decoction, 知柏地黄汤)

【Prescription】

知母	*zhī mǔ*	10 g	Rhizoma Anemarrhenae
黄柏	*huáng bǎi*	10 g	Cortex Phellodendri Chinensis
熟地黄	*shú dì huáng*	12 g	Radix Rehmanniae Praeparata
山茱萸	*shān zhū yú*	10 g	Fructus Corni
山药	*shān yào*	10 g	Rhizoma Dioscoreae
泽泻	*zé xiè*	8 g	Rhizoma Alismatis
牡丹皮	*mǔ dān pí*	10 g	Cortex Moutan
地骨皮	*dì gǔ pí*	8 g	Cortex Lycii
茯苓	*fú líng*	8 g	Poria

【Modifications】

➢ For cases with severe impaired vision, add *jú huā* (菊花, Flos Chrysanthemi) 10 g, *gǒu qǐ zǐ* (枸杞子, Fructus Lycii) 15 g, *chǔ shí zǐ* (楮实子, Fructus Broussonetiae) 15 g, and *sāng shèn* (桑椹, Fructus Mori) 12 g to nourish the liver and kidney and brighten the eyes.

➢ For cases with recurrent ulcers of the skin and external genitalia, add *shēng huáng qí* (生黄芪, Radix Astragali) 15 g, *bái zhú* (白术, Rhizoma Atractylodis Macrocephalae) 10 g, *rǔ xiāng* (乳香, Olibanum) 5 g, and *mò yào* (没药, Myrrha) 5 g to boost qi and support healthy qi, quicken the blood, and engender flesh.

➢ For cases with erythema nodosum of the limbs that do not heal, add *xuè jié* (血竭, Sanguis Draconis) 1.5 g for taking drenched, *yù jīn* (郁金, Radix Curcumae) 10g, *bái huā shé shé cǎo* (白花蛇舌草, Herba Hedyotis Diffusae) 12 g, and *bàn zhī lián* (半枝莲, Herba Scutellariae Barbatae) 10 g to invigorate blood, dispel stasis, resolve toxins, and dissipate mass.

2. Chinese Patent Medicines

(1) *Lóng Dǎn Xiè Gān Wán* (龙胆泻肝丸 , **Gentian Liver-Draining Pill**)
Taken orally, 6 g, two times a day; applicable to liver-gallbladder damp-heat.

(2) *Zhī Bǎi Dì Huáng Wán* (知 柏 地 黄 丸 , **Anemarrhena, Phellodendron and Rehmannia Pill**)
Taken orally, 6 g, three times a day; applicable to deficiency fire flaming upward.

(3) *Qǐ Jú Dì Huáng Wán* (**Lycium Berry, Chrysanthemum and Rehmannia Pill**, 杞菊地黄丸)
Taken orally, 6 g each time, three times a day; applicable to liver-kidney depletion, or later stage of disease course.

3. Simple and Proven Recipe

Chì Xiǎo Dòu Dāng Guī Sǎn (Rice Bean and Chinese Angelica Powder): *Chì xiǎo dòu* (赤小豆, Semen Phaseoli) 3 L (soak the beans in water for sprouting, then dry them in the sun) and *dāng guī* (当归, Radix Angelicae Sinensis); pound ingredients into a fine powder, and take 2 g, 3 times each day.

4. External Therapy

(1) *Kǔ Shēn Tāng* (Flavescent Sophora Decoction): To 60 g of *kǔ shēn* (苦参, Radix Sophorae Flavescentis), add 1000 ml of water, decoct it for 15 min; use the liquid to steam-wash the pudendal ulcer, three times a day.

(2) *Yín Huā Gān Cǎo Tāng* (Lonicera and Licorice Decoction): To 10 g of *yín huā* (银花, Flos Lonicerae Japonicae) and 5 g of *gān cǎo* (甘草, Radix et Rhizoma Glycyrrhizae), add 2 bowls of water and decoct it to 1 bowl; use the liquid to rinse the mouth, 5-6 times each day. Applicable to ulcer and pain of the mouth and throat.

(3) *Qīng Dài Sǎn* (Indigo Powder): Mix together pulverized *qīng dài* (青黛, Indigo Naturalis) 100 g, *shí gāo* (石膏, Gypsum Fibrosum) 100 g, *huá shí* (滑石, Talcum) 100 g, and *huáng bǎi* (黄柏, Cortex Phellodendri Chinensis) 50 g; apply topically to the affected area. Applicable to ulcer of the mouth and external genitalia.

5. Treatment with Western Medicine

Patients may seek advice or treatment from Western conventional eye doctors. Common therapies include:

(1) Topical therapy: Cycloplegics, glucocorticoids eye drops, or subconjunctival injection. These are mainly applicable to patients with problems in the anterior segment.

(2) Systemic therapy:

- Glucocorticoids (intravenous injection of hydrocortisone 200 mg), once daily, until the illness is relieved and symptoms are gone. An alternative may be to take 30 mg of prednisone orally, once every morning. When the illness controlled, slowly reduce the medication dosage in order to prevent recurrence.
- Colchicines, 0.5-1.0 mg orally, twice daily
- Cytotoxicdrugs and antimetabolites, such as Azathioprine, Chlorambucil, Cyclophosphamide
- Immunosuppressive agents, such as Cyclosprin

(3) Surgery may be indicated when inflammation is controlled and the condition is stable. Operative methods, such as retinal laser photocoagulation, complicated cataract extraction, or vitrectomy, may be indicated in severe cases.

6. Dietary Therapy and Preventive Care

(1) *Chì xiǎo dòu* (Semen Phaseoli) porridge: *Chì xiǎo dòu* (赤小豆, Semen Phaseoli) 20 g and *jīng mǐ* (粳米, polished round-grained non-glutinous rice) 100 g cooked together into porridge; applicable to damp-heat.

(2) The diet should be light and rich in nutrition. Avoid acrid, spicy, and greasy-fried foods as well.

(3) Develop healthy habits; quit smoking, excessive drinking of alcohol, and other bad habits.

(4) Get sufficient rest on a regular basis. Avoid staying up all night as this can damage the yin.

(5) Actively participate in daily physical exercise to increase overall physical fitness.

Case Studies

Qiu, a 43-year-old man

First visit: April, 25, 1958

[Chief Complaint & Medical History]

The patient presented with eye disease, sores of the mouth, and ulcer of the penis two years ago, along with gradually decreasing vision. Examination: right visual acuity was 20/200; left visual acuity was only able to identify the hand movement. He had a red tongue with white coating and a surging pulse.

[Pattern Differentiation]

Internal heat and dampness transforming into phlegm

【 Prescription 】

杏仁	xìng rén	12 g	Semen Armeniacae Amarum
生米仁	shēng mǐ rén	30 g	Semen Coicis
黄芩	huáng qín	30 g	Radix Scutellariae
生石膏	shēng shí gāo	20 g	Gypsum Fibrosum
桃仁	táo rén	9 g	Semen Persicae
百部	bǎi bù	12 g	Radix Stemonae
黄连	huáng lián	9 g	Rhizoma Coptidis
麻黄	má huáng	3 g	Herba Ephedrae
白蔻仁	bái kòu rén	6 g	Fructus Amomi Rotundus
车前草	chē qián cǎo	12 g	Herba Plantaginis
法半夏	fǎ bàn xià	9 g	Rhizoma Pinelliae Praeparatum
生甘草	shēng gān cǎo	5 g	Radix et Rhizoma Glycyrrhizae

1 batch per day; the formula was modified according to changes in symptoms.

【 Follow-up 】

After taking the medicinal decoctions for 40 days, the visual acuity on the right eye was increased to 20/60 and the left eye to 20/100. The patient's mental outlook was markedly improved. The treatment principle was changed to clear pathogenic toxin:

大腹皮	dà fù pí	9 g	Pericarpium Arecae
车前草	chē qián cǎo	9 g	Herba Plantaginis
生栀子	shēng zhī zǐ	6 g	Fructus Gardeniae
石斛	shí hú	15 g	Caulis Dendrobii
当归	dāng guī	15 g	Radix Angelicae Sinensis
生白术	shēng bái zhú	30 g	Rhizoma Atractylodis Macrocephalae
生米仁	shēng mǐ rén	30 g	Semen Coicis
赤小豆	chì xiǎo dòu	30 g	Semen Phaseoli
黄连	huáng lián	6 g	Rhizoma Coptidis
生甘草	shēng gān cǎo	15 g	Radix et Rhizoma Glycyrrhizae
猪苓	zhū líng	15 g	Polyporus

Since then, the patient visited several more times, and the formulas were modified with symptoms. On the last visit, visual acuity on the right eye was 20/25 and that of the left eye 20/40, with no indications of relapse or recurrence.

(Excerpted from Clinical Records of Ophthalmology by *Bo Zhong-ying* [*Bó Zhòng Yīng Yǎn Ké Yī Àn*, 伯仲英眼科医案])

Classic Quote

《金匮要略方论》:"狐惑之为病,状如伤寒,默默欲眠,目不得闭,卧起不安,蚀于喉为惑,蚀于阴为狐。""初得之三四日,目赤如鸠眼,七八日,目四眦黑。"

"Fox-creeper disease was a complex disease, the symptoms of which are likened to cold damage, with desire only to sleep, inability to close the eye, fidgetiness whether lying or standing, throat erosion known as 'creeper', and damage to the external genitals known as 'fox'. At the initial 3–4 days of illness, the eyes are red like pigeon's eyes; at 7–8 days, the four canthi appear dark."

Discusson on Formulas from Essentials from the Golden Cabinet (*Jīn Guì Yào Lüè Fāng Lùn*, 金匮要略方论)

Questions for Consideration

1. **What is the major pathogenesis of Behcet's disease?**
2. **What are the features of pattern identification of Behcet's disease?**

Chapter 12
Cataracts

Age-Related Cataract

Age-related cataract is the middle-aged onset of a lens opacification that typically occurs in people over age 50, the prevalence of which is significantly higher as age increases. As cataracts occurs mainly in elderly patients, it is commonly referred to as "senile cataract." The opacity may occur at any part of the lens, and some will not greatly affect visual acuity. Therefore, from the perspective of blindness suggested by the World Health Organization (WHO), it is called "clinical cataract" only if the visual acuity is lower than 20/40.

The disease is particularly prevalent in people over 50 years of age, and its incidence rate increases with age. Cataracts are the leading global cause for blindness. There are a total of 40 million to 50 million blind people worldwide, of which 46% are due to cataracts. As the aging population increases, the incidence of cataracts in the total population will continue to rise. Cataract development is directly related to pollution, nutrition, metabolism, genetics, and other factors. Oxidative stress can damage the lens and plays a major role in the formation of cataracts. The treatment of cataracts may include the use of medicinals at early stages, but when it becomes more developed to a certain extent and seriously impacts vision, surgical treatment is usually indicated.

In TCM, cataracts is called *yuán yì nèi zhàng* (round nebula internal oculopathy, 圓翳內障) Classification of cataracts is based on the location of turbidity spot, the shape, the degree, and the color; they are called floating nebula, sinking nebula, ice nebula, horizontal nebula, disperse nebula, jujube blossom nebula, *yàn yuè* binding moon nebula, yellow heart white nebula, black water congealed nebula, etc. This disease is more common in the elderly and people of feeble health. The disease is associated with liver and kidney deficiency, insufficiency of essence and blood, failure of qi to ascend to the eyes, or decline of spleen and stomach function, and the condition where the fluids of the *zang-fu* are not ascending to the eyes.

Cataractopiesis removal with a metal needle therapy is a surgical treatment method that originated in traditional Chinese medicine. This approach for treating the disease was documented in *Arcane Essentials from the Imperial Library* (*Wài Tái Mì Yào*, 外台秘

要) in the year AD 752. So far, there are no medicinals or medications that can prevent or treat cataracts. The amino acid N-Acytyl carnosine (NAC) is being researched, and NAC eye drops may be helpful. Pharmaceutical therapy for cataracts has been a hot topic of discussion for many years to explore.

Clinical Manifestation

According to the location of the opacities, age-related cataract is divided into 3 types, namely: cortical, nuclear, and subcapsular cataract. The classifications are based on location of the turbidity. Cortical cataract is the most common type, accounting for 65%–70%; followed by nuclear cataract, 25%–35%; subcapsular cataracts are relatively rare.

1. Age-related Cortical Cataract

Cortical cataract is the most common type, characterized by turbidity from the superficial cortex of the peripheral parts of the lens, and it gradually extends to the central parts, occupying most of the cortex. According to the clinical characteristics, cortical cataracts can be divided into four stages based on their development: early stage, advanced stage, mature stage, and postmature stage.

2. Nuclear Age-related Cataract

Nuclear cataract often co-exists with nuclear sclerosis. Initially, the turbidity starts from the fetus or adult nucleus (the center of the lens). Ats the cataract develops, the color of the nucleus changes gradually from yellow to deep yellow, brown, and even black. The condition gradually progresses over a period of several months, a few years, or longer. In early stages, patients present with lenticular myopathy; myopia may be present due to the increased refractive power of the nucleus.

3. Subcapsular cataract

The main feature of the subcapsular cataract is superficial cortex opacity under the capsule. Opacities are most often located under the posterior capsule, presenting as brown fine granules, or small vacuoles that make up a discoid turbidity. Sometimes, opacities can also occur under the anterior capsule. Lesions usually originate from the visual axis area of the posterior capsule. Therefore, it may cause severe visual impairments in the early stages; although the even lesions are less extensive, they may able to cause severe visual impairments.

Treatment

1. Pattern Differentiation and Treatment

(1) Liver Heat Harassing the Upper Body
【Syndrome Characteristics】
Blurred vision, gradual decline of visual acuity, lens opacities, headache, dry eyes, bitter taste in the mouth and dry throat, constipation, red tongue with thin yellow coating, wiry pulse.
【Treatment Principle】
Clear heat and calm the liver, brighten the eyes and remove nebula
【Representative Formula】
Modified *Shí Jué Míng Săn* (Concha Haliotidis, 石决明散)
【Prescription】

石决明	*shí jué míng*	20 g	Concha Haliotidis
草决明	*căo jué míng*	10 g	Semen Cassiae
羌活	*qiāng huó*	10 g	Radix et Rhizoma Notopterygii
栀子	*zhī zĭ*	10 g	Fructus Gardeniae
大黄	*dà huáng*	6 g	Radix et Rhizoma Rhei
熟地黄	*shú dì huáng*	10 g	Radix Rehmanniae Praeparata
荆芥	*jīng jiè*	10 g	Herba Schizonepetae
木贼	*mù zéi*	10 g	Herba Equiseti Hiemalis
青葙子	*qīng xiāng zĭ*	10 g	Semen Celosiae
芍药	*sháo yào*	10 g	Radix Paeoniae Alba
麦冬	*mài dōng*	10 g	Radix Ophiopogonis

【Modifications】
➢ For cases with slight liver heat, remove *zhī zĭ* (栀子, Fructus Gardeniae) and *dà huáng* (大黄, Radix et Rhizoma Rhei).
➢ For cases with liver heat with wind, add *gōu téng* (钩藤, Ramulus Uncariae Cum Uncis) 10 g, *bái jí lí* (白蒺藜, Fructus Tribuli) 10 g, and *jú huā* (菊花, Flos Chrysanthemi) 10 g to dispel wind, clear liver heat, and brighten the eyes.

(2) Liver and Kidney Insufficiency
【Syndrome Characteristics】
Blurred vision, gradual decline of visual acuity, lens opacities, dizziness and tinnitus, limp aching of the lumbus and knees, red tongue with little coating, thin thready pulse.
【Treatment Principle】
Supplement the liver and kidney

【Representative Formula】
Mmodified *Qǐ Jú Dì Huáng Wán* (Lycium Berry, Chrysanthemum and Rehmannia Pill, 杞菊地黄丸)

【Prescription】

枸杞子	*gǒu qǐ zǐ*	10 g	Fructus Lycii
菊花	*jú huā*	10 g	Flos Chrysanthemi
熟地	*shú dì*	20 g	Radix Rehmanniae Praeparata
山茱萸	*shān zhū yú*	10 g	Fructus Corni
山药	*shān yào*	15 g	Rhizoma Dioscoreae
茯苓	*fú líng*	15 g	Poria
泽泻	*zé xiè*	10 g	Rhizoma Alismatis
牡丹皮	*mǔ dān pí*	10 g	Cortex Moutan
女贞子	*nǚ zhēn zǐ*	10 g	Fructus Ligustri Lucidi
旱莲草	*hàn lián cǎo*	10 g	Herba Ecliptae

【Modifications】
➢ For cases with deficiency of liver blood, add *nǚ zhēn zǐ* (女贞子, Fructus Ligustri Lucidi) 15 g and *hàn lián cǎo* (旱莲草, Herba Ecliptae) 10 g to nourish liver blood.

➢ For cases with hyperactivity of fire due to yin deficiency, add *zhī mǔ* (知母, Rhizoma Anemarrhenae) 9 g, *huáng bǎi* (黄柏, Cortex Phellodendri Chinensis) 10 g, and *dì gǔ pí* (地骨皮, Cortex Lycii) 10 g to clear deficiency heat.

(3) Spleen Qi Deficiency
【Syndrome Characteristics】
Clouded flowery vision, gradual decline of visual acuity, lens opacities, fatigue, weak limbs, sallow yellow facial complexion, reduced eating with sloppy stool, poor appetite, loose stool, pale tongue with white coating, weak or thready pulse.

【Treatment Principle】
Fortify the spleen and boost qi, promote urination and drain dampness

【Representative Formula】
Mmodified *Bǔ Zhōng Yì Qì Tāng* (Center-Supplementing and Qi-Boosting Decoction, 补中益气汤)

【Prescription】

太子参	*tài zǐ shēn*	15 g	Radix Pseudostellariae
黄芪	*huáng qí*	10 g	Radix Astragali
白术	*bái zhú*	10 g	Rhizoma Atractylodis Macrocephalae
柴胡	*chái hú*	10 g	Radix Bupleuri
茯苓	*fú líng*	10 g	Poria

当归	*dāng guī*	15 g	Radix Angelicae Sinensis
熟地	*shú dì*	10 g	Radix Rehmanniae Praeparata
白芍	*bái sháo*	10 g	Radix Paeoniae Alba
川芎	*chuān xiōng*	10 g	Rhizoma Chuanxiong
甘草	*gān cǎo*	3 g	Radix et Rhizoma Glycyrrhizae

【Modifications】
➢ For cases with thin sloppy loose stool, add *yì yǐ rén* (薏苡仁, Semen Coicis) 15 g, *chǎo biǎn dòu* (炒扁豆, dry-fried Semen Lablab Album) 20 g, *chē qián zǐ* (车前子, Semen Plantaginis, wrapped) 20 g to invigorate the spleen, promote urination, and drain dampness.

2. Acupuncture

(1) Liver and Kidney Insufficiency

BL 18 (*gān shù*)	BL 23 (*shèn shù*)	KI 3 (*tài xī*)
LV 3 (*tài chōng*)	GB 20 (*fēng chí*)	GB 1 (*tóng zǐ liáo*)

BL 18 and BL 23, back-*shu* points, are combined with *yuan*-source points KI 3 and LV 3, to supplement the liver and kidney and nourish essence and blood. GB 20 and GB 1 together with SJ 23 (*sī zhú kōng*), all *shaoyang* channel points, can dredge channel qi in around the eye, achieve the effect of supplementing the liver and kidney, eliminating visual obstructions, and improving eyesight. Manipulation: Use tonifying method for BL 18, BL 23, KI 3, LV 3. For the others, use draining method. Retain the needle for 30 minutes, once every day. 10 sessions equal one course of treatment.

(2) Spleen Qi Deficiency

BL 20 (*pí shù*)	BL 21(*wèi shù*)	DU 20 (*bǎi huì*)
BL 1 (*jīng míng*)	ST 36 (*zú sān lǐ*)	GB 37 (*guāng míng*)
LI 4 (*hé gǔ*)		

BL 20 and BL 21 are used to fortify the spleen and stomach; DU 20 and ST 36 boost qi and stimulate clear yang qi to rise to the head and eyes; LI 4 dredges channel qi of the *yangming* channel; GB 37 and BL 1 are main points for eliminating visual screens and improving eyesight. Manipulation: Use tonifying method for all acupoints, selecting 32-gauge fine needles to puncture deeply for 1.5 *cùn*, with small-range twirling, not lifting and thrusting. Retain the needle for 30 minutes, and treat once every day. 10 treatments equal one course of treatment.

3. Chinese Patent Medicines

(1) *Shí Hú Yè Guāng Wán* (Dendrobium Night Vision Pill, 石斛夜光丸)

6–9 g each time, twice a day, to enrich yin, supplement the kidney, nourish the liver, and brighten the eyes; applicable to cataracts caused by liver and kidney insufficiency and fire hyperactivity due to yin deficiency.

(2) *Bō Yún Tuì Yì Wán* (Cloud-Removing and Nebula-Eliminating Pill, 拨云退翳丸)

6–9g each time, twice a day, to dispel wind, brighten the eyes, eliminate visual obstruction, and remove nebula; applicable to early-stage cataracts caused by wind-heat in the liver channel.

(3) *Qǐ Jú Dì Huáng Wán* (Lycium Berry, Chrysanthemum and Rehmannia Pill, 杞菊地黄丸)

6–9g each time, three times a day, to supplement the liver and kidney, nourish essence, and brighten the eyes; applicable for to cataracts caused by liver-kidney yin deficiency.

(4) *Zhàng Yǎn Míng Piàn* (Tiopronin Tablet, 障眼明片)

5 pieces, three times a day, to supplement the liver and kidney, remove nebula, and brighten the eyes. Applicable to cataracts caused by liver and kidney insufficiency.

4. Simple and Proven Recipe

Pearls in Chinese medicine have the action of calming the liver, brightening the eyes, and quieting the spirit. In the treatment of 65 cases (100 eyes) of cataracts with pearls, there was a 70% rate of efficacy.

5. External therapy

(1) *Shè Zhū Míng Mù Dī Yǎn Yè* (Musk and Pearl Eye-Brightening Drops, 麝珠明目滴眼液): Shake the mixture before use, 1–2 drops in each eye, 2–4 times a day. Used to disperse visual obstruction and brighten the eyes; applicable to senile cataracts at the early or middle stage.

(2) *Zhēn Zhū Míng Mù Yè* (Pearl Eye-Brightening Drops, 珍珠明目液): 1–2 drops in each eye, 3–4 times a day; applicable to senile cataract at the early stages.

6. Treatment with Western Medicine

(1) Medication: Drugs include anti-benzoquinone and sulfur preparation, aldose reductase inhibitors, vitamins and energy mixtures, and natural extracts (such as Glutathione, Vitamin C, Alginic Sodium Diester, Pirenoxine Sodium) for local or systemic treatment.

(2) Surgery: The most basic and effective method for treating cataracts is surgery. Currently, the main surgical method is phacoemulsification and intraocular lens implantation.

7. Dietary Therapy and Preventive Care

(1) Chamomile Seedlings Porridge: Seedlings ling of chamomile 30 g, *jīng mǐ* (粳米, Semen Oryza Sativa) 200 g, crystal sugar (to taste). Combine the ingredients in a pot, add some water and boil the mixture to make a porridge. Applicable to early- or middle-stage senile cataracts with an underlying cause of wind-heat in the liver channel.

(2) Mountain Yam and Chinese Date Porridge: *Shān yào* (山药, Rhizoma Dioscoreae) 60 g, *dà zǎo* (大枣, Fructus Jujubae) 30 g, *jīng mǐ* (粳米, Semen Oryza Sativa) 100 g, sugar (to taste). Cut the *shān yào* into pieces, combine it with the Chinese dates and rice in a pot, add 1000 ml water, and cook into a porridge; add sugar as desired. Applicable to early- or middle-stage senile cataract caused by weakness of the spleen and stomach.

(3) Steamed Wolfberry and Longan: *Gǒu qǐ zǐ* (枸杞子, Fructus Lycii) 30 g, *lóng yǎn ròu* (龙眼肉, Arillus Longan) 20 g. Place the ingredients in a bowl and steam it thoroughly until it becomes mush; applicable to senile cataracts in the early or middle stage with an underlying cause of liver and kidney deficiency.

Classic Quote

《针灸大成·卷九》：“怒气伤肝, 血不就舍, 肾水枯竭, 气血耗散, 临患之时, 不能节约, 恣意房事, 用心过多, 故得此症。”

"Anger damages the liver, blood failing to stay in the vessels, exhaustion of kidney yin, dissipation of qi and blood, inability to conserve [one's essence], sexual intemperance, and excessive mental work causes this disease (cataracts)."

The Great Compendium of Acupuncture and Moxibustion – Volume Nine (Zhēn Jiǔ Dà Chéng – Juàn Jiǔ, 针灸大成·卷九)

Chapter 13
Glaucoma

Section 1　Primary Angle-Closure Glaucoma

Primary angle-closure glaucoma is a form of glaucoma caused by an impaired outflow of aqueous fluid. This mechanism is the result of a blockage of the anterior chamber angle by the peripheral iris, causing a subsequent increase in IOP (intraocular pressure). The development of this condition varies according to location, race, gender, and age. It is more common in Asians, females, and people over the age of 40, especially people between 50–70 years of age. In China, the prevalence of primary angle-closure glaucoma is 1.79%, with 2.5% in people over 40. The ratio of primary open-angle glaucoma to closed-angle is about 3 : 1.

Angle-closure glaucoma has two primary groups of precipitating factors: one is an abnormal anatomic eye, such as a small eyeball, shallow anterior chamber, and big lens; the other group of causative factors includes overuse of the eyes, fatigue, agitation/stress, prolonged exposure to darkness, and so on. If both stress factors exist, the anterior chamber angle may close suddenly and subsequently block the aqueous drainage, thus increasing the IOP and causing glaucoma.

Primary angle-closure glaucoma is divided into acute and chronic categories. Both acute elevated IOP and chronic high IOP may cause compression and irreversible damage to the optic nerve, leading to impaired vision, constriction of visual field, and even total blindness. For this reason, elevated IOP must be detected and treated as early as possible.

In TCM, the disease pertains to *lù fēng nèi zhàng* (green wind glaucoma, 绿风内障), with the features of headache and distending pain in the eye, hardening of the eyeball, mydriasis, light green pupil, and severely decreased vision. It is also called *lù fēng* (green wind, 绿风), *lù máng* (green blindness, 绿盲), or *lù shuǐ guàn zhū* (green water perfusing eyeball, 绿水灌珠). The causes and pathogenesis may be associated with excessive fire of the liver and gallbladder; extreme heat producing wind, wind-fire attacking the orifices causing poor drainage; emotional stress causing the smooth flow of liver qi to congest; and stagnation of qi transforming into fire, disturbing the eyes and causing the spirit water (aqueous humor) to be blocked in the eye. Spleen dampness creates excess phlegm; stagnation of phlegm and fire attack upward towards the eyes, resulting in stagnation of the spirit water (aqueous humor), which may be yet another causative factor.

In the acute phase, patients are advised to visit Western medical doctors for emergency care in order to save the vision. If IOP is under control, Chinese medicine may be used as an assistant therapy for the purpose of relieving pain and improving other eye symptoms.

Clinical Manifestation

1. Acute angle-closure glaucoma:

It is divided into four phases based on the progression of the disease.

(1) Preclinical phase: The eye has an anatomical structural feature of angle-closure glaucoma but is free of symptoms.

(2) Period of onset: Caused by sudden partial or complete closure of the anterior chamber angle. Typical symptoms include marked distending eye pain, headache, nausea, vomiting, visual halos, blurred vision, ciliary flush or mixed congestion, fog-like edema of the cornea, mydriasis, and a fixed pupil commonly in upright-ellipse shape or deviating on one side. The anterior chamber is extremely shallow, and the IOP is usually higher than 50 mmHg.

(3) Remission stage: Among the cases of acute attack, whose symptoms disappeared by prompt treatment, this condition is only temporary; the possibility of acute attack may take place at any time. In this stage, scattered goniosynechia may be found in gonioscopic examination. IOP may be normal.

(4) Chronic aggressive-phase: Following long-term closure of the anterior chamber angle, the peripheral iris adheres to the trabecular meshwork permanently, which results in the continuous increase in IOP; the condition then turns into the chronic phase and progresses further.

2. Chronic angle-closure glaucoma:

The onset is undetectable and progresses slowly. Patients have no symptoms due to the slow and gradual elevation of the IOP. Over the course of the disease, adhesions of the anterior chamber angle and the increase of IOP progressively aggravate the condition. When there is a compression effect of the high IOP, the cup-disc ratio enlarges gradually and there will be glaucomatous optic nerve lesion resulting in a constricted visual field. If the disease progresses, it will cause visual deficits, blurred vision, or even a tubular visual field.

Treatment

Primary angle-closure glaucoma is an ophthalmic emergency. For patients in an acute episode, it is highly recommended to see an ophthalmologist for emergency care. If the

IOP cannot be controlled in time, this acute condition may cause permanent blindness.

1. Pattern Differentiation and Treatment

(1) Blazing Liver and Gallbladder Fire

【 Syndrome Characteristics 】

Acute onset, intense splitting headache. Pronounced distending pain in the eye, firm globe-like stone, acute vision loss, high IOP, conjunctival mixed congestion or ciliary flush, fog-like corneal edema, extreme shallow anterior chamber, and dilated pupil. Systemic symptoms and signs include nausea, vomiting, red urine, constipation, red tongue with thin yellow coating, and wiry-rapid pulse.

【 Treatment Principle 】

Clear heat and reduce fire, calm the liver and extinguish wind

【 Treatment Principle 】

Modified *Lǜ Fēng Líng Yáng Yǐn* (Green Wind Antelope Horn Decoction, 绿风羚羊饮)

【 Prescription 】

羚羊角	*líng yáng jiǎo*	6 g	Cornu Saigae Tataricae
黄芩	*huáng qín*	9 g	Radix Scutellariae
玄参	*xuán shēn*	10 g	Radix Scrophulariae
炒知母	*chǎo zhī mǔ*	15 g	Rhizoma Anemarrhenae (dry-fried)
大黄	*dà huáng*	6 g	Radix et Rhizoma Rhei
车前子	*chē qián zǐ*	10 g	Semen Plantaginis
茯苓	*fú líng*	10 g	Poria
防风	*fáng fēng*	10 g	Radix Saposhnikoviae
桔梗	*jié gěng*	10 g	Radix Platycodonis
细辛	*xì xīn*	3 g	Radix et Rhizoma Asari

【 Modifications 】

➢ Adding *gōu téng* (钩藤, Ramulus Uncariae Cum Uncis) 10 g, *lóng dǎn cǎo* (龙胆草, Radix et Rhizoma Gentianae) 10 g, and *huáng lián* (黄连, Rhizoma Coptidis) 6 g can enhance the function of clearing the liver and extinguishing wind.

➢ For cases with severe headache, add *chuān xiōng* (川芎,Rhizoma Chuanxiong) 10 g, *shí gāo* (石膏, Gypsum Fibrosum) 20 g, and *jú huā* (菊花, Flos Chrysanthemi) 10 g to clear heat and dissipate pathogen.

➢ For cases with nausea and vomiting, add *zhú rú* (竹茹, Caulis Bambusae in Taenia) 10 g and *fǎ bàn xià* (法半夏, Rhizoma Pinelliae Praeparatum) 10 g to direct adverse qi downward and arrest vomiting.

(2) Liver Constraint and Qi Stagnation

【 Syndrome Characteristics 】

Acute onset, marked distending pain of the eye, sudden vision loss, high IOP, dilated and fixed pupil, shallow anterior chamber, intense headache, dyspnea and belching, nausea, vomiting, bitter taste in the mouth, red tongue with yellow coating, and wiry-rapid pulse.

【 Treatment Principle 】

Clear heat and soothe the liver, harmonize the stomach and direct adverse qi downward

【 Representative Formula 】

Modified *Dān Zhī Xiāo Yáo Sǎn* (Free Wanderer Powder, 丹栀逍遥散) and *Zuǒ Jīn Wán* (Left Metal Pill, 左金丸)

【 Prescription 】

柴胡	*chái hú*	10 g	Radix Bupleuri
牡丹皮	*mǔ dān pí*	10 g	Cortex Moutan
栀子	*zhī zǐ*	10 g	Fructus Gardeniae
当归	*dāng guī*	10 g	Radix Angelicae Sinensis
白芍	*bái sháo*	10 g	Radix Paeoniae Alba
炒白术	*chǎo bái zhú*	15 g	Rhizoma Atractylodis Macrocephalae (dry-fried)
茯苓	*fú líng*	10 g	Poria
甘草	*gān cǎo*	10 g	Radix et Rhizoma Glycyrrhizae
生姜	*shēng jiāng*	10 g	Rhizoma Zingiberis Recens
薄荷(后下)	*bò he (hòu xià)*	6 g	Herba Menthae (added later)
黄连	*huáng lián*	10 g	Rhizoma Coptidis
吴茱萸	*wú zhū yú*	6 g	Fructus Evodiae

➢ For cases with dyspnea and distending pain in the chest and rib-side, add *yù jīn* (郁金, Radix Curcumae) 10 g and *xiāng fù* (香附, Rhizoma Cyperi) 10 g to soothe the liver, regulate qi, and relieve pain.

➢ For cases with distending pain and hardening of the eyeball, and corneal edema, add *zhū líng* (猪苓, Polyporus) 10 g and *tōng cǎo* (通草, Medulla Tetrapanacis) 10 g to promote urination and reduce heat.

(3) Phlegm-Fire Constraint

【 Syndrome Characteristics 】

Besides the symptoms above, systemic symptoms and signs include hot body, reddish complexion, dizziness on slight exertion, nausea and vomiting, dark urine and constipation, red tongue with greasy yellow coating, wiry-slippery-rapid pulse.

【 Treatment Principle 】

Reduce fire and clear up phlegm, pacify the liver and extinguish wind.

【 Representative Formula 】
Modified *Jiāng Jūn Dìng Tòng Wán* (General Pain-Stopping Pill, 将军定痛丸)
【 Prescription 】

大黄	*dà huáng*	15 g	Radix et Rhizoma Rhei
黄芩	*huáng qín*	10 g	Radix Scutellariae
礞石	*méng shí*	3 g	Chlorite-schist
陈皮	*chén pí*	10 g	Pericarpium Citri Reticulatae
半夏	*bàn xià*	10 g	Rhizoma Pinelliae
桔梗	*jié gěng*	15 g	Radix Platycodonis
白僵蚕	*bái jiāng cán*	10 g	Bombyx Batryticatus
天麻	*tiān má*	10 g	Rhizoma Gastrodiae
白芷	*bái zhǐ*	10 g	Radix Angelicae Dahuricae
薄荷 (后下)	*bò he* (*hòu xià*)	6 g	Herba Menthae (added later)

➢ For case with dizziness and vomiting frequently, add *zhú rú* (竹茹, Caulis Bambusae in Taenia) 10 g, and *tiān zhú huáng* (天竺黄, Concretio Silicea Bambusae) 10 g to clear fire and transform phlegm.

➢ For cases with markedly increased IOP, add *tōng cǎo* (通草, Medulla Tetrapanacis) 10g, *zé xiè* (泽泻, Rhizoma Alismatis) 15 g, and *zhū líng* (猪苓, Polyporus) 15 g to drain water and purge heat.

2. Acupuncture

(1) Needling Method

BL 1 (*jīng míng*)	BL 2 (*cuán zhú*)	GB 1 (*tóng zǐ liáo*)
GB 14 (*yáng bái*)	ST 2 (*sì bái*)	*tài yáng* (太阳)
GB 20 (*fēng chí*)	*yì míng* (翳明)	LI 4 (*hé gǔ*)
SJ 5 (*wài guān*)		

For cases with nausea and vomiting, add PC 6 (*nèi guān*) and ST 36 (*zú sān lǐ*).

(2) Ear Acupuncture: Includes *ěr jiān* (耳尖), *yǎn* (眼), etc.

3. Chinese Patent Medicines

(1) *Lóng Dǎn Xiè Gān Wán* (Gentian Liver-Draining Pill, 龙胆泻肝丸)
1 tablet, twice a day, applicable to the blazing liver-gallbladder fire.

(2) *Dān Zhī Xiāo Yáo Wán* (Moutan and Gardenia Free Wanderer Pill, 丹栀逍遥丸)
1 tablet, two times a day, applicable to liver constraint and qi stagnation.

(3) *Jiāng Jūn Dìng Tòng Wán* (General Pain-Stopping Pill, 将军定痛丸)
6 g, twice a day, applicable to the phlegm-fire constraint.

4. Other treatments

(1) Hyperosmolar dehydrant: 20% Mannitol 250 ml by intravenous drop can reduce IOP in as short as 30 minutes.

(2) 2% pilocarpine nitrate eye drops is a miotic that can reduce IOP. It should be administered frequently during the initial onset, and then decreased to 3–4 four times every day after pupilary constriction.

(3) Acetazolamide 500 mg and Sodium Bicarbonate 1000 mg, taken orally, and then decreased to Acetazolamide 250 mg, Sodium Bicarbonate 500 mg per 6 hours. It can reduce aqueous humor formation.

(4) If the IOP cannot be controlled by medication, surgery is indicated.

5. Simple and Proven Recipes

(1) *Lián zǐ* (莲子, Semen Nelumbinis) 30 g, *bǎi hé* (百合, Bulbus Lilii) 30 g. Add appropriate amount water and then mash into paste. One batch per day, take before sleep.

(2) *Yáng gān* (羊肝, Jecur Caprae) 60-90 g, both *gǔ jīng cǎo* (谷精草, Flos Eriocauli) and *bái jú huā* (白菊花, Flos Chrysanthemi) 12-15 g, decocted in water, one batch per day, take several batches.

(3) *Shā shēn* (沙参, Radix Glehniae) 15 g, *niú xī* (牛膝, Radix Achyranthis Bidentatae) 9 g, *gǒu qǐ zǐ* (枸杞子, Fructus Lycii) 15 g, and *jué míng zǐ* (决明子, Semen Cassiae) 9 g are decocted with water, remove the dregs, add appropriate amount honey for oral intake; one batch per day, take continually for several doses.

6. Dietary Therapy and Preventive Care

(1) Avoid tobacco, alcohol, and strong tea.

(2) Avoid or eat less pungent foods such as chilli, green onion, pepper, etc.

(3) Live a moderate lifestyle; do not harbor excessive stress from work or study. Especially avoid overuse of the eyes.

(4) Keep an open mind, do not mope, stay optimistic and in a positive mood, and avoid mental overstrain, which may induce IOP increase.

(5) Avoid excessive time spent in a dark environment in order to prevent IOP elevations. Prohibit the use of atropine, daturine, and belladonna.

(6) Always stay warm and avoid the cold.

Classic Quotes

Arcane Essentials from the Imperial Library – Eye Diseases (*Wài Tái Mì Yào - Yǎn Jí Pǐn Lèi Bù Tóng Hòu*, 外台秘要·眼疾品类不同候) states that the disease is caused by "obstruction of the eye orifice due to defect of the internal liver duct (内肝管缺，眼孔不通)". In the *Standards for Diagnosis and Treatment – Miscellaneous Disease – Seven Orifices Section* (*Zhèng Zhì Zhǔn Shéng – Zá Bìng – Qī Qiào Mén*, 证治准绳·杂病·七窍门), it states that the disease is caused by "phlegm-dampness due to fire constraint, anxiety and anger (痰湿所致，火郁、忧思、忿怒之过)." The treatment must be focused on contracting the pupil first during periods of onset, for if the pupil could be recovered, the eyesight could be saved (病既急者，以收瞳神为先。瞳神但得收复，目即有生意).

Questions for Consideration

What are the causes of acute angle-closure glaucoma? What is the treatment principle at the acute stage?

Section 2   Primary Open-Angle Glaucoma

Primary open-angle glaucoma, also called chronic simple glaucoma, is characterized by "open" anterior chamber angles, a glaucomatous optic disc change, visual field damage, and elevated intraocular pressure (IOP) over 21 mmHg. Glaucoma is the second leading cause of blindness, and the first irreversible leading cause. It usually attacks both eyes and develops slowly. According to the data published by the World Health Organization, there are 70 million glaucoma patients worldwide, and it is estimated to reach 80 million by the year 2020.

In traditional Chinese medicine, the disease pertains to bluish wind glaucoma (*qīng fēng nèi zhàng*, 青风内障). The common causes include qi constraint, phlegm-fire, overstrain, and yin deficiency. The emotional or physiological pathogenesis originates from excessive worry and anger, causing liver constraint and qi stagnation. The qi constraint either transforms into fire or liver dampness (producing phlegm). Stagnation of the phlegm transforms into fire; the phlegm-fire ascends upward and disturbs the eyes. Ascending fire (with underlying yin deficiency) due to exhaustion or excessive thinking results in disharmony of qi and blood, leading to disturbance of the vessels and collaterals and finally causing spirit water (aqueous humor) stasis. There are no obvious symptoms; therefore, the disease often goes undetected. Diagnosis usually occurs in the middle or later stages when patients typically go for an eye exam. Unfortunately, the best treatment opportunity has been missed and it is hard to save the damaged visual acuity and visual field-early detection and treatment yield the best results. Conventional Western treatment methods include topical application of ocular hypotensive agents, and laser or surgical treatment when necessary. Combined treatment of Chinese medicine and Western medicine can have a very good effect towards preventing optic neuropathy.

Clinical Manifestation

1. Subjective Symptoms

There are no symptoms reported in the early stages. A few patients may complain of mild dizziness and distending eye pain, blurred vision, and difficulty walking because of severe visual field damage in the advanced stage.

2. Examination of the Eyes

There are no abnormalities in the early stage. The intraocular pressure (IOP) fluctuates, and the highest IOP number can be detected by a 24-hour intraocular pressure monitoring. With the development of glaucoma, IOP gradually gets higher, but rarely surpasses 60 mmHg. At the same time, typical changes in the fundus can be found: depression of the optic disc, with progressive enlarging and deepening; displacement of blood vessels in the optic disc to the nasal quadrant; quick angulations in the course of the exiting blood vessels; and thinning of the neurosensory rim.

3. Visual Field

In the early stages, the most common change is the paracentral scotoma is less than ten degrees, often in supranasal visual field. With progression of the disease, the visual field defect may develop to nasal step scotoma, arcuate scotoma, ring scotoma, defect of peripheral fields, concentric contraction, tubular visual field, and finally total blindness.

Treatment

For primary open-angle glaucoma, the purpose of treatment is to prevent progression of the disease process and reduce the rate of loss of the retinal ganglion cells. One of the most important treatment methods is to stabilize the IOP, which will require the assistance of Western medical ophthalmology. Regulating the IOP may help but will not guarantee protection to the optic nerve. In conventional medicine most of the emphasis is placed on controlling the IOP, and there are most likely other factors that contribute to the degeneration of the optic nerve in glaucoma patients. Protecting the optic nerve in order to slow or arrest the neuro-degenerative process is the main objective in TCM ophthalmology.

1. Pattern Differentiation and Treatment

(1) Qi Constraint Transforming into Fire
【 Syndrome Characteristics 】

Distending pain in the head and the eyes, constrained emotions, sensation of fullness in the chest and rib-side, poor appetite and mental fatigue, vexation, bitter taste in the mouth, red tongue with yellow coating, and wiry-thready pulse.

【 Treatment Principle 】

Clear heat and soothe the liver

【 Representative Formula 】

Modified *Dān Zhī Xiāo Yáo Sǎn* (Peony Bark and Gardenia Free Wanderer Powder, 丹栀逍遥散)

【 Prescription 】

柴胡	*chái hú*	10 g	Radix Bupleuri
牡丹皮	*mǔ dān pí*	10 g	Cortex Moutan
栀子	*zhī zǐ*	10 g	Fructus Gardeniae
当归	*dāng guī*	10 g	Radix Angelicae Sinensis
白芍	*bái sháo*	10 g	Radix Paeoniae Alba
炒白术	*chǎo bái zhú*	15 g	Rhizoma Atractylodis Macrocephalae (dry-fried)
茯苓	*fú líng*	10 g	Poria
甘草	*gān cǎo*	10 g	Radix et Rhizoma Glycyrrhizae
郁金	*yù jīn*	10 g	Radix Curcumae
薄荷 (后下)	*bò he (hòu xià)*	6 g	Herba Menthae (added later)

【 Modifications 】

➢ For cases with severe yin-blood deficiency, add *shú dì huáng* (熟地黄, Radix Rehmanniae Praeparata) 15 g, *nǚ zhēn zǐ* (女贞子, Fructus Ligustri Lucidi) 15 g, and *sāng shèn* (桑椹, Fructus Mori) 10 g to nourish yin and blood.

➢ For cases with liver constraint transforming into fire and producing wind, add *xià kū cǎo* (夏枯草, Spica Prunellae) 10 g, *gōu téng* (钩藤, Ramulus Uncariae Cum Uncis) 10 g, and *jú huā* (菊花, Flos Chrysanthemi) to clear heat and pacify the liver and extinguish wind.

(2) Phlegm-Fire Flaring Up
【 Syndrome Characteristics 】

Distending eye pain, seeing unclearly, dizziness, poor appetite and excessive sputum, dyspnea and nausea, bitter taste in the mouth, red tongue with yellow coating, and wiry-slippery pulse.

【Treatment Principle】

Clear heat and dispel phlegm, harmonize the stomach and direct qi downward

【Representative Formula】

Modified *Huáng Lián Wēn Dǎn Tāng* (Rhizoma Coptidis Gallbladder-Warming Decoction, 黄连温胆汤)

【Prescription】

陈皮	chén pí	10 g	Pericarpium Citri Reticulatae
半夏	bàn xià	10 g	Rhizoma Pinelliae
茯苓	fú líng	10 g	Poria
甘草	gān cǎo	10 g	Radix et Rhizoma Glycyrrhizae
竹茹	zhú rú	10 g	Caulis Bambusae in Taenia
枳实	zhǐ shí	10 g	Fructus Aurantii Immaturus
黄连	huáng lián	10 g	Rhizoma Coptidis

【Prescription】

➢ For cases with pronounced headache, eye distention, add *chuān xiōng* (川芎, Rhizoma Chuanxiong) 10 g, *chē qián zǐ* (车前子, Semen Plantaginis) 10 g wrapped, and *tōng cǎo* (通草, Medulla Tetrapanacis) 10 g to promote urination, drain dampness, remove blood stasis, and relieve pain.

(3) Liver-Kidney Yin Deficiency

【Syndrome Characteristics】

Chronic cases, seeing unclearly, mydriasis, defect of visual field and optic atrophy, dizziness and tinnitus, weakness of the lumbus and knees, mental fatigue, pale tongue with thin white coating, and deep-thready pulse.

【Treatment Principle】

Supplement the liver and kidney

【Representative Formula】

Modified *Qǐ Jú Dì Huáng Wán* (杞菊地黄丸, Lycium Berry, Chrysanthemum and Rehmannia Pill)

【Prescription】

枸杞子	gǒu qǐ zǐ	10 g	Fructus Lycii
菊花	jú huā	10 g	Flos Chrysanthemi
牡丹皮	mǔ dān pí	10 g	Cortex Moutan
泽泻	zé xiè	10 g	Rhizoma Alismatis
茯苓	fú líng	10 g	Poria
熟地黄	shú dì huáng	10 g	Radix Rehmanniae Praeparata
山茱萸	shān zhū yú	10 g	Fructus Corni
淮山药	huái shān yào	15 g	Rhizoma Dioscoreae

女贞子	*nǚ zhēn zǐ*	15 g	Fructus Ligustri Lucidi
丹参	*dān shēn*	10 g	Radix et Rhizoma Salviae Miltiorrhizae
白芍	*bái sháo*	10 g	Radix Paeoniae Alba

【 Modifications 】

➢ For cases with bright white complexion, insomnia and amnesia, add *dǎng shēn* (党参, Radix Codonopsis) 15 g, *dāng guī* (当归, Radix Angelicae Sinensis) 15 g, *huáng qí* (黄芪, Radix Astragali) 30 g, and *chuān xiōng* (川芎, Rhizoma Chuanxiong) 10 g to tonify and nourish qi and blood.

2. Acupuncture

(1) Needling Method

BL 1 (*jīng míng*)	BL 2 (*cuán zhú*)	GB 1 (*tóng zǐ liáo*)
GB 14 (*yáng bái*)	ST 2 (*sì bái*)	*tài yáng* (太阳)
GB 20 (*fēng chí*)	*yì míng* (翳明)	LI 4 (*hé gǔ*)
SJ 5 (*wài guān*)		

For cases with nausea and vomiting, add PC 6 (*nèi guān*) and ST 36 (*zú sān lǐ*).

(2) Ear Acupuncture: Includes *ěr jiān* (耳尖), *yǎn* (眼), etc.

3. Chinese Patent Medicines

(1) *Dān Zhī Xiāo Yáo Wán* (Cortex Moutan and Fructus Gardeniae Free Wanderer Pill, 丹栀逍遥丸)

1 pill, two times a day, applicable to liver constraint and qi stagnation.

(2) *Míng Mù Dì Huáng Wán* (Eye Brightener Rehmannia Pill, 明目地黄丸)

9 g, two times per day; applicable to liver-kidney yin deficiency.

(3) *Zhī Bǎi Dì Huáng Wán* (Anemarrhena, Phellodendron and Rehmannia Pill, 知柏地黄丸)

Water pill, 10–15 tablets, two times per day; applicable to liver-kidney yin deficiency accompanied by deficiency fire flaming upward.

(4) *Shí Hú Yè Guáng Wán* (Dendrobium Night Vision Pill, 石斛夜光丸)

6 g, two times a day.

(5) *Yín Xìng Yè Piàn* (Ginggo Leaf Tablet, 银杏叶片)

1–2 tablets, three times a day; has protective effect on optic nerve.

(6) *Fù Míng Piàn* (Bright Recovery Tablet, 复明片)

5 tablets, three times a day; applicable to glaucoma patients with optic atrophy.

(7) Intravenous injection of Chinese medicinals, such as Breviscapine, extract

of ginkgo biloba leaf, ligustrazine, and puerarin, is another option when treating glaucomatous optic atrophy.

4. Treatment with Western Medicine

(1) Drug therapy to reduce IOP: The most commonly used topical drugs include Timolol Maleate Eye Drops, Brinzolamide Eye Drops, and Latanoprost Eye Drops. According to the patient's IOP level and systemic condition, choose the appropriate eye drops; in some cases a drug combination is needed.

(2) Surgery: Filtering surgery may be needed if IOP cannot be controlled by drugs.

(3) Optic nerve protection: Medication and supplements include a calcium ion antagonist such as Nimodipine and Betaxolol, adrenergic agonists such as Brimonidine, and antioxidants such as vitamin C and vitamin E.

5. Simple and Proven Recipes

(1) Walnut, date and sesame powder (*táo rén zǎo má fěn*, 桃仁枣麻粉): *Hé táo rén* (核桃仁, Semen Juglandis) 35 g, *suān zǎo rén* (酸枣仁, Semen Ziziphi Spinosae) 20 g, and *hēi zhī ma* (黑芝麻, Semen Sesami Nigrum) 30 g. Mix the ingredients together and fry it over low heat; remove from the stove when the mixture turns yellowish, then grind it into powder. Take one tablespoon per day, dry or with water.

(2) Plum blossom congee (*méi huā zhōu*, 梅花粥): *Jīng mǐ* (粳米, Semen Oryza Sativa, polished round-grained non-glutinous rice) 120 g, and fresh *méi huā* (梅花, Flos Mume, plum flower) 10 g. Wash *jīng mǐ* clean, add fresh *méi huā* and appropriate amount of water, and then cook into a congee. Take one bowl, twice per day; can be effective for patients with open-angle glaucoma that have blurred vision accompanied by dyspnea and abdominal distention.

(3) Walnut and honey egg drink (*táo rén mì dàn yǐn*, 桃仁蜜蛋饮): Milk 250 g, fried *hé táo rén* (核桃仁, Semen Juglandis, walnut) 35 g, *fēng mì* (蜂蜜, Mel, honey) 30 g, and one egg. Add the egg and ground walnut into the milk, blend it evenly and cook it until boiling, remove from the heat source, and add some honey into the milk after it cools down. Take once per day for a few weeks.

6. Dietary Therapy and Preventive Care

(1) Control fluid amount: Do not drink large amounts of any fluid at one time, generally no more than 500 ml each time, for it may severely dilute the blood, which will result in abnormally low osmotic pressure of plasma and then relatively high production of aqueous humor; this may increase IOP.

(2) Live a balanced lifestyle: Get enough sleep and proper exercise, avoid fatigue, and

keep up with your regular medication.

(3) Check IOP and visual fields regularly: The patient must follow the doctor's instruction to do regular follow-up examination and consistent treatment. The medication for controlling IOP may be a life-long requirement.

(4) Carry out screenings in high-risk groups of people, such as those with glaucoma in their family history, ocular hypertension, unknown causative impaired vision, and suspected abnormalities of the optic disc. This way, the patients may have an advantage by getting an early diagnosis and prompt treatment.

Case Study

Yuan, 25-year-old female

【 Chief Complaint 】

Distending pain of the right eye for the last two and a half years

【 Medical History 】

The patient had been diagnosed with glaucoma and treated by surgery. In the early postoperative days, her ocular pressure was stable. However, in the latter half year, her IOP fluctuated, accompanied by halo vision, headache, and distending eye pain and nausea, and all of the symptoms were aggravated with fatigue. Examination of the visual field showed a pathological change and progression as well. The left eye had similar symptoms but with more pronounced halo vision. The present treatment is application of 1% Pilocarpine Nitrate Eye Drops 6 times per day for the right eye and 2 times for the left eye, 2% Pilocarpine Eye Ointment for both eyes at night. The patient also suffered from a migraine recently. She was often irritable, and her stool was dry and hard with a frequency of once every four to five days. Her menstrual period came every 40 days with excessive bleeding.

【 Examination 】

Right vision: 20/60 (corrected to 20/25), near vision Jaeger 1; left vision: 20/20 (corrected to 20/16), near vision Jaeger 1. There is an iris boot defect located at 11:00–12:00, but no filtration follicle was found. Both pupils contract from the effect of the medicine.

IOP: Right eye at 35.76 mmHg, left eye at 25.81 mmHg. The optic disc of the right eye had a pathologically enlarged depression; other optic disc was normal. There was no obvious abnormality found in the left eye during examination of the fundus. The nasal visual field of the right eye was constricted by 25 to 30 degrees, and the bitemporal visual field was constricted to 60 degrees. Other signs include a slightly red tongue with thin-yellow coating and a wiry-thready pulse.

【 Diagnosis 】

Bluish wind glaucoma

【 Pattern Differentiation 】

Yin deficiency and hyperactivity of the liver; external wind complicated by internal wind invading the orifices

【 Treatment Principles 】

Enrich yin and calm the liver. Formula: Glaucoma Formula No.3 (a proven recipe composed by Wei Wen-gui)

【 Prescription 】

石决明	*shí jué míng*	24 g	Concha Haliotidis
白蒺藜	*bái jí lí*	10 g	Fructus Tribuli
决明子	*jué míng zǐ*	15 g	Semen Cassiae
防风	*fáng fēng*	6 g	Radix Saposhnikoviae
羌活	*qiāng huó*	6 g	Radix et Rhizoma Notopterygii
蝉蜕	*chán tuì*	6 g	Periostracum Cicadae
密蒙花	*mì méng huā*	6 g	Flos Buddlejae
白术	*bái zhú*	10 g	Rhizoma Atractylodis Macrocephalae
白芷	*bái zhǐ*	6 g	Radix Angelicae Dahuricae
细辛	*xì xīn*	3 g	Radix et Rhizoma Asari
生地	*shēng dì*	20 g	Radix Rehmanniae

All the ingredients were decocted with water and taken orally; fourteen batches in total. At the same time, she was administered *Shí Hú Yè Guáng Wán* (Dendrobium Night Vision Pill, 石斛夜光丸), one pill per day.

【 Follow-up 】

One month later, the IOP was almost normal. Then, she was told to stop using Pilocarpine eye ointment and change *Shí Hú Yè Guáng Wán* (Dendrobium Night Vision Pill, 石斛夜光丸) to *Míng Mù Dì Huáng Wán* (Eye Brightener Rehmannia Pill, 明目地黄丸), one pill, two times a day. The formula prescribed was the same as before. At her last visit (6 months later), her vision improved, IOP was reduced to normal, the headache, distending eye pain, and halo vision had disappeared. She had also stopped using her Pilocarpine Nitrate Eye Drops. The patient had normal urine and stool, thin pulse, and a slight red tongue with thin coating.

Examination of the eyes: The corrected vision of the right eye was 20/20, near vision Jaeger 1. The corrected vision of the left eye was 20/17, near vision Jaeger 1. IOP of both eyes: 5.5/5 = 17.30 mmHg, which is normal. Medicinal formulas were no longer needed but she remained under observation through routine follow-up evaluations.

Excerpted from Effective Cases of Dr. Wei Wen-gui (韦文贵验案)

Classic Quotes

《证治准绳·杂病·七窍门》：“青风内障证，视瞳神内有气色，昏蒙如晴山笼淡烟也。

然自视尚见，但比平时光华则昏蒙日进。"

"Bluish glaucoma presents with bluish discoloration of the pupil, like a light cloud covering the mountain. At the initial stages, the patient can see clearly; however, the vision will gradually become more and more blurred."

Standards for Diagnosis and Treatment – Miscellaneous Diseases – Seven Orifices Sect (*Zhèng Zhì Zhǔn Shéng – Zá Bìng – Qī Qiào Mén*, 证治准绳·杂病·七窍门)

Questions for Consideration

1. Which pattern is more common in bluish glaucoma, phlegm-fire flaring up or phlegm-fire stagnation?

2. What are the main syndrome characteristics, treatment principle, and representative formula?

Chapter 14
Fundus Ocular Diseases

Section 1   Retinal Artery Occlusion

Retinal artery occlusion is a blockage in the blood supply of the arteries to the retina resulting in acute vision loss or blindness. This condition may be caused by embolism, vasospasm, abnormalities of the vessel wall, or vessel compression from outside. The term "central retinal artery occlusion (CRAO)" is used if the blockage occurs in the stem of the artery. If the blockage occurs at the branch of the artery, it is called a branch retinal artery occlusion. The main clinical manifestations include acute and painless blindness or varied loss of vision, with shadow in the corresponding visual field. Fundus examination shows gray-white edema of the retina, red spot in the macular area, and marked narrowing and thinning of the arteries. This disease occurs more often in the elderly population. Occlusion can occur in both eyes, though most cases present with only one eye involved. In Western medicine, RAO is an ophthalmologic emergency, and the treatments include lowering intraocular pressure, dilating the blood vessels, antithrombotic therapy, and oxygen therapy.

In Chinese medicine, this disease pertains to *bào máng* (sudden blindness, 暴盲), also called *luò zǔ bào máng* (sudden blindness due to vessel obstruction, 络阻暴盲). The causes are associated with ascendant hyperactivity of liver yang, or counterflow of both qi and blood. Phlegm-dampness clouding the clear orifices due to overconsumption of fatty and sweet foods may be another cause. The main pathogenesis is obstruction of the vessels and inhibition of the orifices leading to visual dysfunction. Based on the theory of pattern differentiation and treatment, therapies of invigorating blood, dredging orifices, and opening blockages are helpful in saving and preserving the patient's vision.

Clinical Manifestation

Patient present with acute painless loss of monocular vision, and quadrant defects in the visual field, or tunnel vision. The funduscopic findings include a pale disc with a blurring margin, thread-like thinning of the artery, narrowing of the veins, segmentation of the blood column in some cases, diffuse gray-white edema of the retina especially in the posterior area, cherry-red spot or orange tongue-shaped area in the macular part or quadrant with gray-white edema. The funduscopic findings resolve gradually with the course of the disease, leaving a pale optic disc as optic atrophy.

Treatment

This condition is an ophthalmic emergency with an unfavorable prognosis, so treatment must be administered early on and as soon as possible. The main treatment principle is to remove the obstruction, invigorate the blood, dredge the collaterals, and open the orifices on the basis of pattern differentiation.

1. Pattern Differentiation and Treatment

(1) Qi and Blood Stasis and Obstruction
【 Syndrome Characteristics 】
Sudden vision loss with normal appearance of the affected eye, mydriasis, retinal edema, and narrowed and stagnant vessel of the eye. Systemic symptoms and signs may include irritability, dizziness, headache, fullness in the chest and rib-side, pale tongue with ecchymosis, and a wiry or rough pulse.
【 Treatment Principle 】
Invigorate blood and open the orifices
【 Representative Formula 】
Modified *Tōng Qiào Huó Xuè Tāng* (Orifice-Opening Blood-Activating Decoction, 通窍活血汤)
【 Prescription 】

桃仁	*táo rén*	8 g	Semen Persicae
红花	*hóng huā*	8 g	Flos Carthami
当归	*dāng guī*	12 g	Radix Angelicae Sinensis
川芎	*chuān xiōng*	12 g	Rhizoma Chuanxiong
赤芍	*chì sháo*	10 g	Radix Paeoniae Rubra
丹参	*dān shēn*	12 g	Radix et Rhizoma Salviae Miltiorrhizae
石菖蒲	*shí chāng pú*	5 g	Rhizoma Acori Tatarinowii
麝香（烊化）	*shè xiāng (yáng huà)*	10 g	Moschus (taken infused)

【 Modifications 】
➢ For cases with depressed emotions and marked fullness in the chest and rib-side, add *xiāng fù* (香附, Rhizoma Cyperi) 10 g, *chái hú* (柴胡, Radix Bupleuri) 10 g, and *qīng pí* (青皮, Pericarpium Citri Reticulatae Viride) 10 g to move qi, soothe the liver, and harmonize the movement of qi.

➤ For cases with severe retinal edema, add *yì mǔ cǎo* (益母草, Herba Leonuri) 10 g and *zé lán* (泽兰, Herba Lycopi) 8 g to invigorate blood and drain water to alleviate edema.

(2) Ascendant Hyperactivity of Liver Yang
【 Syndrome Characteristics 】

Sudden blindness or shadow in front of the affected eye. Fundus examination shows signs of RAO. The systemic symptoms and signs often include headache, dizziness, distending pain of the eye especially after anger or major emotional upset, redness and heat sensations in the face, insomnia and profuse dreams, impatience and irritability, bitter taste in the mouth and dry pharynx, red tongue with yellow coating, and wiry pulse.

【 Treatment Principle 】

Pacify the liver and subdue yang, invigorate blood and dredge the collaterals

【 Representative Formula 】

Modified *Tiān Má Gōu Téng Yǐn* (Gastrodia and Uncaria Decoction, 天麻钩藤饮)

【 Prescription 】

天麻	*tiān má*	10 g	Rhizoma Gastrodiae
钩藤（后下）	*gōu téng (hòu xià)*	15 g	Ramulus Uncariae cum Uncis (decocted later)
石决明	*shí jué míng*	30 g	Concha Haliotidis
黄芩	*huáng qín*	12 g	Radix Scutellariae
川牛膝	*chuān niú xī*	12 g	Radix Cyathulae
杜仲	*dù zhòng*	10 g	Cortex Eucommiae
桑寄生	*sāng jì shēng*	10 g	Herba Taxilli
川芎	*chuān xiōng*	10 g	Rhizoma Chuanxiong
红花	*hóng huā*	10 g	Flos Carthami

【 Modifications 】

➤ For cases with severe dizziness, add *guī bǎn* (龟板, Plastrum Testudinis) 15 g, *bái sháo* (白芍, Radix Paeoniae Alba) 12 g, *cí shí* (磁石, Magnetitum) 30 g, and *dì lóng* (地龙, Pheretima) 10 g to nourish yin and subdue yang and conduct blood downward.

➤ For cases with palpitations, forgetfulness, vexations, agitation, and insomnia, add *bǎi zǐ rén* (柏子仁, Semen Platycladi) 15 g, *yè jiāo téng* (夜交藤, Caulis Polygoni Multiflori) 15 g, and *hǔ pò* (琥珀, Succinum) 2 g to nourish the heart, tranquilize the mind, and calm fright.

(3) Phlegm-Heat Disturbing Upward
【 Syndrome Characteristics 】

Eye signs and symptoms are the same as above. Most of the patients are fat, and usually have dyspnea, excessive sputum, heavy-headedness and dizziness, red tongue with thick yellow and greasy coating, and slippery and rapid pulse.

【 Treatment Principle 】

Expel phlegm and open the orifices, invigorate blood and dredge the collaterals

【Representative Formula】
Modified *Dí Tán Tāng* (Phlegm-Expelling Decoction, 涤痰汤)
【Prescription】

陈皮	*chén pí*	10 g	Pericarpium Citri Reticulatae
法半夏	*fǎ bàn xià*	10 g	Rhizoma Pinelliae Praeparatum
茯苓	*fú líng*	12 g	Poria
枳实	*zhǐ shí*	10 g	Fructus Aurantii Immaturus
竹茹	*zhú rú*	15 g	Caulis Bambusae in Taenia
胆南星	*dǎn nán xīng*	8 g	Arisaema cum Bile
石菖蒲	*shí chāng pú*	5 g	Rhizoma Acori Tatarinowii
川芎	*chuān xiōng*	12 g	Rhizoma Chuanxiong
地龙	*dì lóng*	12 g	Pheretima
郁金	*yù jīn*	10 g	Radix Curcumae
甘草	*gān cǎo*	3 g	Radix et Rhizoma Glycyrrhizae

【Modifications】
➢ For cases with marked signs and symptoms of heat including yellow and thick phlegm, fever and rough breathing, flushing and conjunctival congestion, add *huáng qín* (黄芩, Radix Scutellariae) 12 g, *zhè bèi mǔ* (浙贝母, Bulbus Fritillariae Thunbergii) 12 g, and *hǎi fú shí* (海浮石, Pumex) 20 g to clear heat and expel phlegm.

➢ For cases with marked symptoms of excessive phlegm-dampness such as copious and clear sputum, a heavy and fatigued body, dyspnea, and vomitting, remove *zhú rú* (竹茹, Caulis Bambusae in Taenia) and *dǎn nán xīng* (胆南星, Arisaema cum Bile), and add *bái jiè zǐ* (白芥子, Semen Sinapis) 8 g, *xuán fù huā* (旋覆花, Flos Inulae) 10 g, and *cāng zhú* (苍术, Rhizoma Atractylodis) 12 g to dry dampness and transform phlegm.

(4) Qi Deficiency and Blood Stasis
【Syndrome Characteristics】
The eye looks normal, but cannot see clearly (if at all). The optic disc and retina is pale, and the vessels are thinner than normal. The systemic signs and symptoms may include a sallow yellow complexion, shortage of qi and no desire to talk, mental fatigue and lack of strength, dizziness and spontaneous sweating, a pale tongue with white coating, and a thin and weak pulse.
【Treatment Principle】
Replenish qi and invigorate blood, resolve stasis and dredge the collaterals
【Representative Formula】
Modified *Bǔ Yáng Huán Wǔ Tāng* (Yang-Supplementing and Five-Returning Decoction, 补阳还五汤)

【Prescription】

黄芪	*huáng qí*	30 g	Radix Astragali
当归	*dāng guī*	12 g	Radix Angelicae Sinensis
川芎	*chuān xiōng*	12 g	Rhizoma Chuanxiong
赤芍	*chì sháo*	10 g	Radix Paeoniae Rubra
桃仁	*táo rén*	8 g	Semen Persicae
红花	*hóng huā*	8 g	Flos Carthami
地龙	*dì lóng*	10 g	Pheretima
石菖蒲	*shí chāng pú*	5 g	Rhizoma Acori Tatarinowii
路路通	*lù lù tōng*	12 g	Fructus Liquidambaris

【Modifications】

➢ For cases with symptoms of qi deficiency, such as shortness of breath, fatigue, spontaneous sweating and fear of cold, remove *chuān xiōng* (川芎, Rhizoma Chuanxiong) and *shí chāng pú* (石菖蒲, Rhizoma Acori Tatarinowii), and add *dǎng shēn* (党参, Radix Codonopsis) 20 g, *bái zhú* (白术, Rhizoma Atractylodis Macrocephalae) 15 g, and *rén shēn* (人参, Radix et Rhizoma Ginseng) 10 g. If the condition is especially severe, supplement the middle and replenish qi.

➢ For cases with symptoms of blood deficiency, such as pale lips and tongue, severe palpitations, add *shú dì huáng* (熟地黄, Radix Rehmanniae Praeparata) 15 g, *sāng shèn* (桑椹, Fructus Mori) 15 g, and *gǒu qǐ zǐ* (枸杞子, Fructus Lycii) 15 g to nourish and invigorate blood.

➢ For cases with blurred vision and hyperplasia of the retinal pigment, add *gǒu qǐ zǐ* (Fructus Lycii) 15 g, *tù sī zǐ* (菟丝子, Semen Cuscutae) 12 g, *chǔ shí zǐ* (楮实子, Fructus Broussonetiae) 12 g, and *chōng wèi zǐ* (茺蔚子, Fructus Leonuri) 12 g to supplement the liver and kidney, invigorate blood, and brighten the eyes.

2. Acupuncture

In the early stage of the disease, use draining methods, while in the later stage, use mostly supplementation.

Main acupoints:

BL 1 (*jīng míng*)	*qiú hòu* (球后)	ST 1 (*chéng qì*)

Combination acupoints:

GB 20 (*fēng chí*)	BL 2 (*cuán zhú*)	*yú yāo* (鱼腰)
GB 1 (*tóng zǐ liáo*)	LI 4 (*hé gǔ*)	PC 6 (*nèi guān*)
ST 36 (*zú sān lǐ*)	SP 6 (*sān yīn jiāo*)	LV 3 (*tài chōng*)

Choose one local acupoint and three distal acupoints each time, alternating between groups of points. Retain the needles for 20-30 minutes each time, treating once each day. Since the main acupoints are located in the orbit, do not lift, thrust, rotate, or retain the needle when needling. Use caution so as to avoid pricking the eyeball and damaging the intraorbital vessels.

3. Chinese Patent Medicines

(1) *Bǔ Zhōng Yì Qì Wán* (**Center-Supplementing and Qi-Boosting Pill,** 补中益气丸)
9 g, three times a day; applicable to patterns of qi deficiency and blood stasis.

(2) *Qǐ Jú Dì Huáng Wán* (**Lycium Berry, Chrysanthemum and Rehmannia Pill,** 杞菊地黄丸)
6 g, three times a day; applicable to the later stages with recovery of retinal arterial blood and optic and retinal atrophy.

4. Simple and Proven Recipe

Rén shēn (人参,Radix et Rhizoma Ginseng) 30 g and *sū mù* (苏木, Lignum Sappan) 10 g, decocted with water and taken for many months.

5. Treatment by Western Medicine

RAO represents an ophthalmologic emergency and must be treated as early as possible. Common Western medical treatments include the following:

(1) **Dilate blood vessels**

A fast-acting, short-term vasodilator is preferred, such as nitroglycerin tablets (0.3–0.6 mg via sublingual administration), or amyl nitrite (0.2ml via inhalation), benzazoline (12.5–25 mg via retrobulbar injection) and nicacid (100 mg taken orally), three times a day.

(2) **Lower intraocular pressure**

Anterior chamber paracentesis, ocular massage, and oral medication or local application of ocular hypotensive agents.

(3) **Oxygen therapy**

Inhale a mixture of 5% carbon dioxide and 95% oxygen, for ten minutes every hour during the day, or once every four hours during the nighttime, in the initial stages.

(4) **Antithrombotic therapy**

According to the patient's condition, choose platelet-suppressant drug or cellosive.

6. Dietary Therapy and Preventive Care

(1) Take in a light and balanced diet; eat less spicy, fried, and sweet foods.

(2) Quit smoking and alcohol consumption.

(3) Stay optimistic and in a positive mood; avoid anger, frustration, and depression.

(4) At the initial onset, immediately see an ophthalmologist and get emergency treatment.

Classic Quote

《证治准绳·杂病·七窍门》："平日素无他病，外伤轮廓，内部损瞳神倏然盲而不见也""病致有三，曰阳寡，曰阴孤。曰神离，乃否塞关隔之病。"

"The patient is usually healthy, and nothing abnormal can be found from the outside of the eyeball"… "The causes include yang deficiency, yin deficiency, and absence of spirit. It is a kind of disease due to obstruction."

Standards for Diagnosis and Treatment – Miscellaneous Disease – Seven Orifices Section (Zhèng Zhì Zhǔn Shéng – Zá Bìng – Qī Qiào Mén, 证治准绳·杂病·七窍门)

Question for Consideration

What are the main syndrome characteristics, treatment principle, and representative formula for qi and blood stasis and obstruction in *bào máng* (sudden blindness, 暴盲)?

Section 2 Retinal Vein Occlusion

Retinal vein occlusion (RVO) is a common vascular disorder of the retina, with the characteristics of retinal hemorrhage, exudates, edema, and retinal vein enlargement. According to the sites of obstruction, RVO is divided into central retinal vein occlusion (CRVO) and branch retinal vein occlusion (BRVO) in the clinic. According to the severity of the condition, the disease is subdivided to ischemic and non-ischemic types. The underlying causes of the disease are complicated, and are mainly due to formation of intraluminal thrombosis, which can be associated with abnormalities of the vessel wall, lumen, and haemodynamics. RVO occurs with an acute onset, and effects are almost always residually chronic. RVO may lead to severe vision damage or even blindness due to macular edema, retinal neovascularization, and neovascular glaucoma. RVO occurs more commonly in the elderly population, and is distributed equally among both males and females. Most cases are unilateral. In Western medicine, it is mainly treated by anti-thrombus, anti-inflammatory, and retina laser photocoagulation methods.

In Chinese medicine, RVO belongs to *bào máng* (sudden blindness, 暴盲), and in recent years it is ascribed to *luò sǔn bào máng* (sudden blindness caused by vessel damage, 络损暴盲). It is most often caused by either ascendant hyperactivity of liver yang resulting in qi and blood ascending counterflow, or liver-kidney yin deficiency resulting in deficiency-fire scorching the collaterals. Phlegm-dampness obstruction and stagnation due to excessive consumption of fatty foods and sweet foods may be another causative factor. The main pathogenesis is blood spilling out of the vessels due to stasis and obstruction, which may result from various causes. Therefore, the treatment should focus on invigorating blood, dissolving stasis, and dredging collaterals on the basis of systemic pattern differentiation, which can promote the absorption of hemorrhage and exudates, reduce edema, and improve visual function.

Clinical Manifestation

The clinical manifestation is determined by the blockage sites and severity of the condition. It most often presents with acute onset and impaired vision to varying degrees. When the macula is involved, the central vision decreases. If the obstruction is at the stem of the retinal vein, there would be hyperemia of the optic disc with an unclear margin, turbid edema of the retina, extensive hemorrhage in flame-shape or radiating from the center of the optic disc, or can appear even as a boat-like preretinal hemorrhage. Other signs include retinal vessel tortuosity and engorgement in the shape of a sausage, yellow-white hard exudates, and "cotton-wool" spots. Furthermore, macular edema usually occurs at the late stages. If the obstruction occurs at the branch retinal vein, the symptoms are relatively mild. The pathological change is located in the area of where the affected branch vein distributes. If it is the ischemic type, the condition will be more severe. Besides more hemorrhage in the retina, the affected eye may develop rubeosis iris and neovascular glaucoma, which will lead to terminal blindness.

Treatment

1. Pattern Differentiation and Treatment

Blood spilling out of the vessels due to stasis and obstruction is the main pathogenesis of this disease. Therefore, invigorating blood, dissolving stasis, and dredging collaterals is the vital treatment principle and must be applied all throughout the process. Based on the point of "fluid and blood come from the same source" and "disturbance of blood leads to excessive water", it is advisable to treat retinal or macular edema by methods of invigorating blood and draining water, or by strengthening the spleen and expelling dampness, which can usually improve the therapeutic effect. According to the theories of "qi being the commander of blood, and blood being the mother of qi", and "qi flow promotes blood transportation, while qi stagnation leading to blood stasis", one must seriously consider using qi-regulating medicinals in the treatment.

(1) Qi Stagnation and Blood Stasis

【Syndrome Characteristics】

The eye looks normal, but the visual acuity drops sharply. On fundus examination, optic disc edema may be present with a blurred margin, scattered spots, and a sheeted hemorrhage as well as vein engorgement. The systemic signs and symptoms may include headache and distending eye pain, fullness and discomfort in the chest and rib-side, repressed emotions, poor appetite and belching, pale tongue with thin-white coating, and wiry pulse.

【Treatment Principle】

Soothe the liver and resolve constraint, regulate qi and invigorate blood

【Representative Formula】

Modified *Xuè Fǔ Zhú Yū Tāng* (Blood Stasis-Expelling Decoction, 血府逐瘀汤)

【Prescription】

柴胡	*chái hú*	10 g	Radix Bupleuri
枳壳	*zhǐ qiào*	12 g	Fructus Aurantii
香附	*xiāng fù*	10 g	Rhizoma Cyperi
当归	*dāng guī*	12 g	Radix Angelicae Sinensis
川芎	*chuān xiōng*	12 g	Rhizoma Chuanxiong
赤芍	*chì sháo*	12 g	Radix Paeoniae Rubra
桃仁	*táo rén*	10 g	Semen Persicae
红花	*hóng huā*	8 g	Flos Carthami
牡丹皮	*mǔ dān pí*	10 g	Cortex Moutan
蒲黄 (包煎)	*pú huáng (bāo jiān)*	15 g	Pollen Typhae (wrap)

【Modifications】

➢ For cases with severe hemorrhage with bright red color, remove *chuān xiōng* (川芎, Rhizoma Chuanxiong), *hóng huā* (红花, Flos Carthami), and *táo rén* (桃仁, Semen Persicae); in cases of excessive bleeding, add *bái máo gēn* (白茅根, Rhizoma Imperatae) 30 g, *jīng jiè tàn* (荆芥炭, Herba Schizonepetae Carbonisatum) 12 g, and *dà jì* (大蓟, Herba Cirsii Japonici) 12 g to cool the blood and stop bleeding.

➢ For cases with marked disc hyperemia and swelling, or combined with retinal edema, add *yì mǔ cǎo* (益母草, Herba Leonuri) 12 g, *zé lán* (泽兰, Herba Lycopi) 10 g, and *chē qián cǎo* (车前草, Herba Plantaginis) 12 g to invigorate blood and drain water.

(2) Yin Deficiency with Yang Hyperactivity

【Syndrome Characteristics】

The eye looks normal, but the visual acuity drops sharply. On fundus examination, there is extensive hemorrhage with bright red coloring. Systemic signs and symptoms may include dizziness and tinnitus, reddish complexion and hot flashes, night sweats, insomnia and profuse dreams, vexation and irritability, red tongue with thin coating, and wiry, thready and rapid pulse.

【Treatment Principle】
Nourish yin and subdue yang, cool and invigorate blood
【Representative Formula】
Modified *Biē Jiǎ Yǎng Yīn Jiān* (Turtle Shell Yin-Nourishing Decoction, 鳖甲养阴煎)
【Prescription】

鳖甲	*biē jiǎ*	15 g	Carapax Trionycis
龟板	*guī bǎn*	15 g	Plastrum Testudinis
枸杞子	*gǒu qǐ zǐ*	15 g	Fructus Lycii
白芍	*bái sháo*	15 g	Radix Paeoniae Alba
地骨皮	*dì gǔ pí*	10 g	Cortex Lycii
生地	*shēng dì*	15 g	Radix Rehmanniae
牡丹皮	*mǔ dān pí*	10 g	Cortex Moutan
赤芍	*chì sháo*	10 g	Radix Paeoniae Rubra
玄参	*xuán shēn*	15 g	Radix Scrophulariae
蒲黄	*pú huáng*	15 g	Pollen Typhae

【Modifications】
➢ For cases with vexing heat in the five centers, pronounced red face and lips, add *zhī mǔ* (知母, Rhizoma Anemarrhenae) 10 g and *huáng bǎi* (黄柏, Cortex Phellodendri Chinensis) 10 g to nourish yin and reduce fire.

➢ For cases with dizziness, add *tiān má* (天麻, Rhizoma Gastrodiae) 12 g, *gōu téng* (钩藤, Ramulus Uncariae Cum Uncis) 15 g, and *shí jué míng* (石决明, Concha Haliotidis) 30 g to pacify the liver and extinguish wind.

(3) Combined Phlegm and Stasis
【Syndrome Characteristics】
Symptoms occur at the late stage of the disease, blurred vision, retinal vein tortuosity and engorgement, marked retinal turbidity and edema, extensive exudates; may be accompanied by cystoid macular edema, obesity, heaviness of the head and dizziness, dyspnea and stuffiness, pale tongue or with stasis spots and glossy coating, and slippery or wiry-rough pulse.
【Treatment Principle】
Invigorate blood and dredge collaterals
【Representative Formula】
Modified *Huó Xuè Sàn Jié Tāng* (Blood-Invigorating and Stasis-Removing Decoction, 活血散结汤)
【Prescription】

陈皮	*chén pí*	10 g	Pericarpium Citri Reticulatae
法半夏	*fǎ bàn xià*	10 g	Rhizoma Pinelliae Praeparatum

茯苓	*fú líng*	15 g	Poria
浙贝母	*zhè bèi mǔ*	10 g	Bulbus Fritillariae Thunbergii
玄参	*xuán shēn*	10 g	Radix Scrophulariae
牡蛎	*mǔ lì*	30 g	Concha Ostreae
夏枯草	*xià kū cǎo*	15 g	Spica Prunellae
海藻	*hǎi zǎo*	15 g	Sargassum
丹参	*dān shēn*	15 g	Spica Prunellae
郁金	*yù jīn*	15 g	Radix Curcumae
当归	*dāng guī*	10 g	Radix Angelicae Sinensis
胆南星	*dǎn nán xīng*	10 g	Arisaema cum Bile

【Modifications】

➢ For cases with abdominal fullness and loose stool, add *bái zhú* (白术, Rhizoma Atractylodis Macrocephalae) 12 g, *zhǐ qiào* (枳壳, Fructus Aurantii) 10 g, and *hòu pò* (厚朴, Cortex Magnoliae Officinalis) 10 g to move qi and invigorate the spleen.

➢ For cases with qi deficiency and no desire to talk and weak limbs, remove *xuán shēn* (玄参, Radix Scrophulariae) and *zhè bèi mǔ* (浙贝母, Bulbus Fritillariae Thunbergii), and add *zhì huáng qí* (炙黄芪, Radix Astragali Praeparata cum Melle) 30 g, *bái zhú* (白术, Rhizoma Atractylodis Macrocephalae) 12 g, *táo rén* (桃仁, Semen Persicae) 10 g, and *hóng huā* (红花, Flos Carthami) 8 g to replenish qi and invigorate blood.

➢ For cases with retinal edema and turbidity, extensive hard exudates, and cotton wool spots, add *wǎ léng zǐ* (瓦楞子, Concha Arcae) 20 g and *hǎi gé qiào* (海蛤壳, Concha Meretricis seu Cyclinae) 15 g to soften hardness and dissipate masses.

2. Acupuncture

Acupuncture has the function of smoothing channels and collaterals, moving qi, and invigorating blood. Clinical practice indicates that appropriate use of acupuncture can promote the absorption of retinal hemorrhage and edema, and preserve and improve visual function. However, it must be noted that lifting, thrusting, or twirling should not be used when puncturing intraorbital acupoints, to avoid bleeding caused by damage to the vessels behind the eyeball. Be especially cautious with depth and angle of needling insertion to avoid pricking the eyeball and optic nerve. It is suggested to use gauge 32, 1 *cun* or 1.5 *cun* needles when puncturing intraorbital acupoints; for the other points, choose gauge 30, 1.5 *cun* or 2.5 *cun* needles.

Manipulation and treatment course: When puncturing at BL 1 (*jīng míng*), slowly insert the needle to the depth of 1 *cun*, and withdraw the needle after the arrival of qi. When puncturing at *qiú hòu* (球后), insert the needle to a depth of 1.5 *cun* using the same method as that of BL 1. Treat once per day; 10 sessions is one treatment course. Unless stated otherwise, 3–4 courses may be needed.

(1) Qi Stagnation And Blood Stasis

BL 1 (*jīng míng*)	*qiú hòu* (球后)	BL 2 (*cuán zhú*)
tài yáng (太阳)	LI 4 (*hé gǔ*)	LV 3 (*tài chōng*)

For other acupoints besides BL 1 and *qiú hòu*, use drainage method and withdraw the needle after the arrival of qi.

(2) Yin Deficiency with Yang Hyperactivity

BL 1 (*jīng míng*)	*qiú hòu* (球后)	*tài yáng* (太阳)
SP 6 (*sān yīn jiāo*)	BL 18 (*gān shù*)	BL23 (*shèn shù*)

2-3 treatment courses may be needed.

(3) Phlegm and Stasis Binding Together

BL 1 (*jīng míng*)	*qiú hòu* (球后)	BL 2 (*cuán zhú*)
SP 10 (*xuè hǎi*)	SP 8 (*dì jī*)	ST 36 (*zú sān lǐ*)
LI 4 (*hé gǔ*)	RN 9 (*shuǐ fēn*)	

For points other than BL 1 and *qiú hòu*, use even supplementation and drainage method.

3. Chinese Patent Medicines

(1) *Yún Nán Bái Yào Jiāo Náng* (Yun Nan Bai Yao Capsule, 云南白药胶囊)

500 mg (2 capsules), three times a day; applicable to qi stagnation and blood stasis, and yin deficiency and yang hyperactivity.

(2) *Fù Fāng Xuè Shuān Tōng Jiāo Náng* (Compound Thrombus-Clearing Capsule, 复方血栓通胶囊)

3 capsules, three times per day; applicable to qi deficiency and blood stasis and/or qi deficiency.

4. Treatment by Western Medicine

Common treatment methods include the following:

(1) Etiological treatment: Find out the causes of the disease, and treat the primary diseases such as high blood pressure and diabetes mellitus.

(2) Medication: For the early stage without obvious hemorrhagic tendency, it is applicable to use fibrinolysis drugs such as urokinase, defibrase, etc. Blood viscosity-reducing drugs can be considered, including low molecular dextran, while taking a small

dose of aspirin and persantine is helpful to lessen platelet aggregation. For young patients, it is recommended to treat with antibiotics and glucocorticoids according to systemic condition.

(3) Laser therapy: Use laser therapy for patients with retinal capillary nonperfusion, marked retinal hemorrhage, or severe macular edema.

5. Dietary Therapy and Preventive Care

(1) The disease has a long course. So, it is important to encourage patients to build confidence, overcome impatience, and insist on a relatively lengthy treatment over many months.

(2) Take in light foods and a highly nutritious diet. Avoid sweet, greasy-fried, and spicy foods.

(3) Quit smoking and drinking alcohol.

Case Studies

Fan, 58-year-old female

[Chief Complaint]

Sudden vision loss of the right eye two months ago.

[Medical History]

The patient had a history of arteriosclerosis for fifty years. The vision in the right eye decreased suddenly without any inducing factors two months ago. She was diagnosed with "retinal vein occlusion" and was treated with Western medicine at a local hospital. Because she had no response to the therapy, she came to our clinic for further treatment.

[Examination]

The visual acuity was 20/100 on the right eye and 20/13 on the left eye. Nothing abnormal was found on the anterior segment of the right eye.

Fundus examination after mydriasis: The color and border of the right optic disc was normal. The temporal-superior branch vein was tortuous and appeared to be dilated and bead-like. There were spots, clot-like hemorrhaging, and exudates along the affected vein. Arteries were thinner than normal with a ratio 1 : 2 to the caliber of the vein. The cross-compression sign was positive. Macular pigment was deranged and the fovea centralis reflection had disappeared. Nothing abnormal was found in the left eye during fundus examination. She had a dark red tongue with thin white coating and a deep pulse.

IOP: Tn. BP: 130/80 mmHg.

[Diagnosis]

Sudden blindness (branch retinal vein occlusion of the right eye)

[Pattern Differentiation]

Frenetic movement of blood due to heat; damage to vessels and collaterals

【 Treatment Principles 】
Clear heat, cool blood, and stop bleeding
【 Prescription 】
Modified *Táo Hóng Sì Wù Tāng* (桃红四物汤, Peach Kernel and Carthamus Four Substances Decoction)

桃仁	*táo rén*	6 g	Semen Persicae
红花	*hóng huā*	6 g	Flos Carthami
栀子	*zhī zǐ*	10 g	Fructus Gardeniae
生地	*shēng dì*	10 g	Radix Rehmanniae
赤芍	*chì sháo*	10 g	Radix Paeoniae Rubra
丹参	*dān shēn*	10 g	Radix et Rhizoma Salviae Miltiorrhizae
葛根	*gé gēn*	10 g	Radix Puerariae Lobatae
白茅根	*bái máo gēn*	15 g	Rhizoma Imperatae
大蓟	*dà jì*	15 g	Herba Cirsii Japonici
小蓟	*xiǎo jì*	15 g	Herba Cirsii

One batch per day of the above formula was administered.

【 Follow-up 】
The formula was modified according to the patient's pattern change on her return visit. On her last visit, the visual acuity of the right eye was increased to 20/16 and the hemorrhage was mostly absorbed. She was prescribed with the initial formula, adding *huáng qí* (黄芪, Radix Astragali) 10 g and *gǒu qǐ zǐ* (枸杞子, Fructus Lycii) 15 g to strengthen the curative effects.

Question for Consideration

Retinal hemorrhage is one of the main manifestations of retinal vein occlusion; why do we still want to emphasize "invigorating blood" in treatment?

Section 3   Diabetic Retinopathy

Diabetic retinopathy is a common complication of diabetes mellitus and one of the most common leading causes of blindness. The incidence is related to the course of diabetes mellitus and blood sugar level. With the improvement of living standards and medical conditions, the mortality of diabetics has decreased markedly, but the course has been prolonged; thus, the incidence of diabetic retinopathy has an obvious trend of growing progressively year by year. It has been shown by epidemiological data that the incidence of diabetic retinopathy is 8% in the patients who have had diabetes for three years, 25%

in the patients with history of 5 years of diabetes, and 60% with history of 10 years, while it can reach up to 80% in the patients with a history of 25 years.

This primary characteristic of diabetic microangiopathy in the eyes has a special fundus presentation. It may attack both eyes or each eye individually. Diabetic retinopathy usually has a prolonged course with progressive degenerative vision loss. In Western medicine, treatment includes retinal laser photocoagulation and vitrectomy when necessary to save the vision. It should be noted that controlling blood sugar levels in order to treat the primary underlying condition is very important as a means of preventing and treating diabetic retinopathy.

In traditional Chinese medicine, it pertains to *xiāo kě bìng mù bìng* (dispersion-thirst eye disease, 消渴病目病). This disease often occurs at the middle or late stages of dispersion-thirst disease. It is a severe ophthalmic complication of dispersion-thirst. The main pathogenesis is associated with yin deficiency and dryness heat, or deficiency of both the spleen and liver. From yin deficiency and internal heat to dual qi and yin deficiency, and finally to both yin and yang deficiency and blood stasis are the main pathologic features. In TCM, pattern differentiation is based on the systemic syndrome combined with the retinal condition. Generally, the treatment principles include moistening the lung, strengthening the spleen, and nourishing the kidney, along with the methods to stop bleeding, resolve stasis, drain water, and dissipate stagnation so as to promote absorption of an existing hemorrhage, exudation and swelling, thus to improve visual function and decrease the risk of blindness.

Clinical Manifestation

Often there are no symptoms in the early stages. Varied vision loss may occur when the macula is involved. If vitreous hemorrhage or retinal detachment occurs, it will cause severe vision loss and even total blindness.

The main changes of the fundus include aneurysms, hemorrhage, hard exudate, cotton wool spots, macular swelling, blood vessel changes, and vitreous change described as the following:

- Aneurysms: Tiny red spot with clear boundary, varied in number and located at one position for a long time.
- Hemorrhage: At the early stage, there is often hemorrhage in the shape of a small dot. Following development of the disease, hemorrhage increases and may occur in the retinal nerve fiber layer in the shape of a feather, flame, or even big sheets in severe cases.
- Hard exudate: Scattered or close-up waxy yellow spots with clear boundaries in different sizes and shapes.
- Cotton wool spot: Ⅲ-defined gray-white cotton spot near the retina arteries.
- Pathological changes of retinal vessels: Changes are similar to vessel changes caused by

hypertension, characterized by sclerosis and occlusion of the retinal artery, tortuosity, and engorgement and ectasia of the retina vein. In the late stages, the vein may appear bead-like.

- Macular edema: Retinal thickening with loss of foveal light reflex.
- Changes in the vitreous humor: In the late stage, there is massive hemorrhage and proliferation in the vitreous humor and retina, and finally it may cause traction retinal detachment and neovascular glaucoma, leading to blindness. When the hemorrhage is minor, dust or flocculent turbidity may be seen in the vitreous humor. If there is a lot of blood spill into the vitreous humor, nothing or only weak red reflections may be seen in the fundus examination. In slit lamp microscope examination, red blood clot or floating yellow-brown dust can be found in the vitreous humor.

For the convenience of exchange and consensus, the International Ophthalmology Council drew up a new international classification standard for diabetic retinopathy and macular edema as the following:

International Clinical Classification of Diabetic Retinopathy:

1. No apparent retinopathy: No abnormities of fundus.
2. Mild non-proliferative diabetic retinopathy (NDPR): Microaneurysm only.
3. Moderate non-proliferative diabetic retinopathy: More than just microaneurysm but less than severe NDPR.
4. Severe non-proliferative diabetic retinopathy: Any of the following but no sign of proliferative retinopathy:
   a) Extensive (>20) intraretinal hemorrhage in each of 4 quadrants
   b) Definite venous beading in 2 or more quadrants
   c) Prominent intraretinal microvascular abnormities in 1 or more quadrants
5. Proliferative diabetic retinopathy: Include 1 or more of the pathologic changes:
   a) Neovascularization
   b) Vitreous hemorrhage
   c) Preretinal hemorrhage

International Clinical Classification of Diabetic Macular Edema:

1. Diabetic macular edema absent: No retinal thickening or hard exudates in posterior pole
2. Mild diabetic macular edema: Some retinal thickening or hard exudates in posterior pole, but distant from the macula.
3. Moderate diabetic macular edema: Retinal thickening or hard exudates approaching the center of the macula but not involving the center.
4. Severe diabetic macular edema: Retinal thickening or hard exudates involving the center of the macula.

Treatment

1. Pattern Differentiation and Treatment

This is an ocular complication of diabetes mellitus, and therefore both the eye condition and the underlying pattern should be carefully diagnosed. Because blood stasis is an important pathogenesis, and recurring hemorrhage is the main symptom, the principle of "stop bleeding without causing blood stasis and regulate blood without damaging the healthy qi" should be highly noted when selecting medicinal formulas. Both vitreous proliferation and hard exudation are concrete pathological products; therefore, adding some hardness-softening mass-dissipating medicinals may improve the curative effect. Macular edema is a treatment nodus of the disease, and the pathogenesis is associated with a "blood disorder that may lead to swelling"; thus, combining some blood-regulating medicinals or spleen-strengthening and dampness-expelling medicinals within the formula is very helpful in improving the clinical symptoms.

(1) Yin Deficiency and Dry Heat
【Syndrome Characteristics】
Blurred vision, retinal micrangium, spot hemorrhage, thirst and polydipsia, polyuria, vexation and insomnia, red tongue with white coating or scant coating, and thready and rapid pulse.
【Treatment Principle】
Nourish yin and clear heat; cool blood
【Representative Formula】
Modified *Yù Quán Wán* (Jade Spring Pill, 玉泉丸)
【Prescription】

麦冬	*mài dōng*	12 g	Radix Ophiopogonis
北沙参	*běi shā shēn*	12 g	Radix Glehniae
茯苓	*fú líng*	10 g	Poria
乌梅	*wū méi*	10 g	Fructus Mume
天花粉	*tiān huā fěn*	10 g	Radix Trichosanthis
葛根	*gé gēn*	10 g	Radix Puerariae Lobatae
甘草	*gān cǎo*	10 g	Radix et Rhizoma Glycyrrhizae

【Modifications】
➤ For cases with marked thirst, add *tiān mén dōng* (天门冬, Radix Asparagi) 10 g and *xuán shēn* (玄参, Radix Scrophulariae) 10 g to nourish yin, engender fluid, and moisten dryness.

➢ For cases with massive retinal hemorrhage of bright red color, add *pú huáng* (蒲黄, Pollen Typhae) 10 g, *bái máo gēn* (白茅根, Rhizoma Imperatae) 10 g, *dà jì* (大蓟, Herba Cirsii Japonici) 15 g and *xiǎo jì* (小蓟, Herba Cirsii) 10 g to cool blood, stop bleeding, and regulate blood.

(2) Qi And Yin Deficiency

【 Syndrome Characteristics 】

Blurred vision, floating shadows in the visual field, retinal hemorrhage, macular edema, scattered hard exudates, lusterless complexion, mental fatigue and lack of strength, dry mouth, vexation heat in the chest, palms and soles, pale tongue with thick white coating, and a deep, thready and weak pulse.

【 Treatment Principle 】

Benefit qi and nourish yin; cool blood

【 Representative Formula 】

Modified *Yù Nǚ Jiān* (Jade Lady Decoction, 玉女煎) combined with *Shēng Mài Sǎn* (Pulse-Engendering Powder, 生脉散)

【 Prescription 】

熟地黄	shú dì huáng	12 g	Radix Rehmanniae Praeparata
麦冬	mài dōng	12 g	Radix Ophiopogonis
知母	zhī mǔ	10 g	Rhizoma Anemarrhenae
牛膝	niú xī	10 g	Radix Achyranthis Bidentatae
党参	dǎng shēn	15 g	Radix Codonopsis
五味子	wǔ wèi zǐ	10 g	Fructus Schisandrae Chinensis
炙黄芪	zhì huáng qí	15 g	Radix Astragali Praeparata cum Melle
玄参	xuán shēn	10 g	Radix Scrophulariae
牡丹皮	mǔ dān pí	10 g	Cortex Moutan
赤芍	chì sháo	10 g	Radix Paeoniae Rubra

【 Modifications 】

➢ For cases with profuse retinal hemorrhage, add *pú huáng* (蒲黄, Pollen Typhae) 10 g, *bái máo gēn* (白茅根, Rhizoma Imperatae) 15 g, and *mò hàn lián* (墨旱莲, Herba Ecliptae) 15 g to cool blood and stop bleeding.

➢ For cases with marked macular edema, add *yì mǔ cǎo* (益母草, Herba Leonuri) 10 g and *zé lán* (泽兰, Herba Lycopi) 10 g to regulate blood and drain water.

➢ For cases with widespread hard exudates, add *biē jiǎ* (鳖甲, Carapax Trionycis) 12 g and *mǔ lì* (牡蛎, Concha Ostreae) 15 g to soften hardness and dissipate stagnation.

(3) Yin and Yang Deficiency

【 Syndrome Characteristics 】

Severe vision damage, widespread retinal hemorrhage and hard exudation, wool-cotton spot, diffuse macular edema, tortuosity and extension of the retinal vessels or beadlike changes of retinal vessels, usually accompanied by pale, white, or sallow-yellow complexion, emaciation or obesity, dizziness and tinnitus, mental fatigue and lack of strength, shortage of qi and reluctance to talk, cold body and limbs, frequency of nocturia, pale enlarged tongue with white slippery coating, and a deep thready pulse.

【 Treatment Principle 】

Warm yang and promote qi transportation

【 Representative Formula 】

Modified *Jì Shēng Shèn Qì Wán* (Life-Saving Kidney Qi Pill, 济生肾气丸)

【 Prescription 】

熟地黄	*shú dì huáng*	15 g	Radix Rehmanniae Praeparata
山茱萸	*shān zhū yú*	15 g	Fructus Corni
干山药	*gān shān yào*	15 g	Rhizoma Dioscoreae
泽泻	*zé xiè*	15 g	Rhizoma Alismatis
茯苓	*fú líng*	15 g	Poria
牡丹皮	*mǔ dān pí*	15 g	Cortex Moutan
肉桂	*ròu guì*	5 g	Cortex Cinnamomi
制附片 (先煎)	*zhì fù piàn (xiān jiān)*	5 g	Radix Aconiti Coreani Praeparata (decocted for long time)
蒲黄	*pú huáng*	12 g	Pollen Typhae
三七	*sān qī*	3 g	Radix et Rhizoma Notoginseng
花蕊石	*huā ruǐ shí*	20 g	Ophicalcitum

【 Modifications 】

➤ For cases with pronounced macular edema, add *yì mǔ cǎo* (益母草, Herba Leonuri) 12 g, *chē qián zǐ* (车前子, Semen Plantaginis) 12 g, and *zhū líng* (猪苓, Polyporus) 12 g to regulate blood, drain water, and alleviate edema.

➤ For cases with profuse hard exudates and wool-cotton spots, add *shān zhā* (山楂, Fructus Crataegi) 12 g, *jī nèi jīn* (鸡内金, Endothelium Corneum Gigeriae Galli) 10 g, and *bèi mǔ* (贝母, Bulbus Fritillaria) 10 g to disperse accumulation and eliminate stagnation.

➤ For cases with massive retinal hemorrhage or recurrent bleeding due to neovascularization, add *xiān hè cǎo* (仙鹤草, Herba Agrimoniaehairy) 12 g, *jīng jiè tàn* (荆芥炭, Herba Schizonepetae Carbonisatum) 12 g, and *ǒu jié* (藕节, Nodus Nelumbinis Rhizomatis) 15 g to astringe and stop bleeding.

(4) Phlegm and Static Blood Binding Together

【 Syndrome Characteristics 】

Severe vision damage, dark shadows floating in front of the eye, retinal edema, diffused hard exudates and wool-cotton spots, neovascularization and recurrent hemorrhage, vitreous and retinal proliferation, vitreous hemorrhage, and fundus that cannot be seen or with just a weak red reflex. The systemic manifestations include a puffy or swollen figure, heavy body, no desire to talk, dyspnea and anorexia, dark purple tongue with stasis maculae, thick and greasy coating, and a deep and thready pulse.

【Treatment Principle】

Invigorate blood and disperse stasis, dispel phlegm and eliminate stagnation

【Representative Formula】

Modified *Huó Xuè Sàn Jié Tāng* (Blood-Invigorating and Stagnation-Eliminating Decoction, 活血散结汤)

【Prescription】

陈皮	*chén pí*	10 g	Pericarpium Citri Reticulatae
法半夏	*fǎ bàn xià*	10 g	Rhizoma Pinelliae Praeparatum
茯苓	*fú líng*	15 g	Poria
玄参	*xuán shēn*	10 g	Radix Scrophulariae
牡蛎	*mǔ lì*	20 g	Concha Ostreae
浙贝母	*zhè bèi mǔ*	8 g	Bulbus Fritillariae Thunbergii
丹参	*dān shēn*	8 g	Radix et Rhizoma Salviae Miltiorrhizae
当归	*dāng guī*	5 g	Radix Angelicae Sinensis
郁金	*yù jīn*	8 g	Radix Curcumae
海藻	*hǎi zǎo*	15 g	Sargassum
夏枯草	*xià kū cǎo*	15 g	Spica Prunellae
茜草根	*qiàn cǎo gēn*	8 g	Radix et Rhizoma Rubiae
生蒲黄	*shēng pú huáng*	12 g	Pollen Typhae

【Modifications】

➢ For cases with severe hemorrhage, remove *dāng guī* (当归, Radix Angelicae Sinensis) and *dān shēn* (丹参, Radix et Rhizoma Salviae Miltiorrhizae) to avoid the risk of recurrent bleeding due to invigorating blood, and add *dà jì* (大蓟, Herba Cirsii Japonici) 10 g, *sān qī* (三七, Radix et Rhizoma Notoginseng) 3 g, and *huā ruǐ shí* (花蕊石, Ophicalcitum) 15 g to dispel stasis and stop bleeding.

➢ For cases with vitreous hemorrhage and proliferation, which is a manifestation of phlegm and stasis binding together, add *fú shí* (浮石, Pumex pumice) 10 g, *wǎ léng zǐ* (瓦楞子, Concha Arcae) 15 g, and *kūn bù* (昆布, Thallus Laminariae) 10 g to disperse blood stasis and eliminate stagnation.

2. Acupuncture

Acupuncture is helpful to improve systemic symptoms and decrease the level of blood sugar; at the same time, it can also promote the absorption of the retinal hemorrhage and improve vision. However, because diabetics have poor resistance, great cautions should be taken in order to prevent infection when needling. Do not lift, thrust, or rotate when puncturing intraorbital acupoints so as to not damage the vessels behind the eyeball and cause bleeding. In addition, the depth and angle of needling insertion should be applied carefully in order to avoid pricking the eyeball and optic nerve. For intraocular acupoints, we suggest to use 1 *cun*, gauge 32 needles, and for the other acupoints, use 1.5 – 2.5 *cun*, 30-gauge needles.

(1) Yin Deficiency with Dry Heat

BL 2 (*cuán zhú*)	BL 1 (*jīng míng*)	ST 36 (*zú sān lǐ*)
LV 3 (*tài chōng*)	BL 17 (*gé shù*)	BL 23 (*shèn shù*)

Manipulation and treatment course: When puncturing at BL 1 (*jīng míng*), slowly insert the needle for 0.5 *cun* and withdraw the needle after arriving of qi. Use drainage methods when puncturing the other points, and retain the needles for 15 minutes. Treat once each day; 10 sessions is one treatment course. According to patient's condition, 2–4 treatment courses may be needed with a 3-day interval after two treatment courses.

(2) Qi and Yin Deficiency

BL 2 (*cuán zhú*)	GB 1 (*tóng zǐ liáo*)	BL 1 (*jīng míng*)
LU 5 (*chǐ zé*)	SP 8 (*dì jī*)	SP 6 (*sān yīn jiāo*)
RN 6 (*qì hǎi*)		

Manipulation and treatment course: The manipulation for BL 1 (*jīng míng*) is the same as above; for other acupoints, use even supplementation and drainage methods. Retain the needles for 15 minutes, and treat once each day; 10 sessions is a treatment course. 3–4 courses in total are suggested.

(3) yin and yang deficiency

qiú hòu (球后)	SJ 23 (*sī zhú kōng*)	LU 5 (*chǐ zé*)
SP 6 (*sān yīn jiāo*)	RN 12 (*zhōng wǎn*)	RN 6 (*qì hǎi*)

Manipulation and treatment course: When puncturing *qiú hòu* (球后), slowly insert the needle for 1.5 *cun*, and withdraw the needle after arriving of qi. For the other aucupoints, use a tonification method. Retain the needles for 20 minutes, and you may manipulate the needles in order to enhance the needling sensation during retention. Treat once per day; 10 sessions is a treatment course. 3–4 courses in total is suggested.

(4) Phlegm and Stasis Binding Together

BL 2 (*cuán zhú*)	GB 1 (*tóng zǐ liáo*)	SP 10 (*xuè hǎi*)
SP 8 (*dì jī*)	ST 36 (*zú sān lǐ*)	LI 4 (*hé gǔ*)

Manipulation and treatment course: Use even tonification and drainage methods, retain the needles for 20 minutes, and perform needle manipulation during retention. Treat once each day; 10 sessions is treatment course. 3–4 course in total is suggested.

If the patient has a yin and yang deficiency with marked yang deficiency signs and symptoms such as physical cold and cold limbs, frequent nocturia, pale and enlarged tongue, it is applicable to use suspended moxibustion on RN 4 (*guān yuán*), RN 6 (*qì hǎi*), ST 36 (*zú sān lǐ*), and Bl 23 (*shèn shù*). Choose 2 acupoints for each treatment; moxa each point until the skin of the points turns slightly red; this usually occurs after 10 minutes. Treat once per day; 10 sessions is a treatment course. The total number of courses depends on the patient's condition and rate of response.

3. Chinese Patent Medicines

(1) *Zhī Bǎi Dì Huáng Wán* (知柏地黄丸 , **Anemarrhena, Phellodendron and Rehmannia Pill)**

6 g, three times a day; applicable to yin deficiency and dryness heat.

(2) *Fù Fāng Xuè Shuān Tōng Jiāo Náng* (**Compound Thrombus-Clearing Capsule,** 复方血栓通胶囊)

3 pieces, three times a day; applicable to qi and yin deficiency.

(3) *Jīn Guì Shèn Qì Wán* (**Golden Cabinet's Kidney Qi Pill,** 金匮肾气丸)

6 g, three times a day; applicable to yin and yang deficiency.

4. Treatment with Western Medicine

Common conventional treatments include several aspects:

(1) Treatment of the primary disease: Control levels of blood sugar, blood pressure, and blood fat.

(2) Laser treatment: Take fundus fluorescence angiography examination first to decide whether laser treatment is needed.

(3) Vitrectomy: For cases with prolonged vitreous hemorrhage, especially accompanied by proliferative vitreous retinopathy or traction detachment of retina, vitrectomy is the preferred method and must be taken promptly to save the visual acuity.

5. Dietary Therapy and Preventive Health Care

(1) Patients may choose one of the following therapies according to his/her own condition.

Bitter gourd cooked with tofu, bitter gourd cooked with water chestnut, wax gourd and Job's tears congee, or wax gourd and red bean soup.

(2) Medically diagnosed diabetics should have a regular eye exam, and receive corresponding treatments if there is any indication of retinopathy.

(3) Adopt healthy living habits; quit bad habits such as poor diet, smoking, and alcohol.

(4) Engage in daily physical exercise, which is very helpful in strengthening the overall constitution.

(5) Control blood sugar.

Case Studies

Jin, a 52-year-old female

【 Chief Complaint 】

Blurred vision over the last three months. She had a 10-year history of diabetes.

【 Examination 】

Her visual acuity was 20/100 on the right eye and 20/400 on the left eye.

Fundus examination: The optic disc is normal, while the vessels of the retina are dilated and tortuous. Microaneurysms and gray-white exudates are found at the end of vessels. The reflex of central fovea of the macula is diffused. The left fundus was unclear because of severe vitreous opacity.

【 Diagnosis 】

Dispersion-thirst eye disease (*xiāo kě bìng mù bìng*, 消渴病目病)

【 Pattern Differentiation 】

Dry heat obstructing the collaterals

【 Treatment Principles 】

Nourish yin and moisten dryness, cool blood and dissipate stasis

【 Prescription 】

Modified *Yù Yīn Liáng Sàn Tāng* (Yin-Nourishing, Blood-Cooling and Stasis-Dissipating Decoction, 育阴凉散汤)

熟地黄	*shú dì huáng*	12 g	Radix Rehmanniae Praeparata
山茱萸	*shān zhū yú*	10 g	Fructus Corni
干山药	*gān shān yào*	12 g	Rhizoma Dioscoreae
牡丹皮	*mǔ dān pí*	6 g	Cortex Moutan
苍术	*cāng zhú*	10 g	Rhizoma Atractylodis
玉竹	*yù zhú*	12 g	Rhizoma Polygonati Odorati
花粉	*huā fěn*	12 g	Radix Trichosanthis
黄连	*huáng lián*	6 g	Rhizoma Coptidis
茜草	*qiàn cǎo*	9 g	Radix et Rhizoma Rubiae
白茅根	*bái máo gēn*	10 g	Rhizoma Imperatae
藕节	*ǒu jié*	10 g	Nodus Nelumbinis Rhizomatis
大蓟	*dà jì*	10 g	Herba Cirsii Japonici
小蓟	*xiǎo jì*	10 g	Herba Cirsii

Decocted with water and taken orally; 1 batch a day.

【 Follow-up 】

The patient visited our clinic again after taking 14 batches, 2 weeks of treatment. Her visual acuity was 20/60 in both eyes. She was administered the same formula for another 14 batches. At her third visit, the patient said she could see more clearly than before, but she had weak limbs and numbness of the extremities. She was treated with the same formula; after taking 80 batches, her visual acuity was improved to 20/30 in both eyes, and the overall retinopathy was improved as well.

Excerpted from *Treatment for Fundus Diseases by TCM* (中医治疗眼底病)

Classic Quotes

《黄帝素问宣明论方燥门》:"又如周身热燥怫郁,故变为雀目或内障,痈疽疮疡……为肾消也。此为三消病也。"

"Again, like heat, dryness, anger and depression of the whole body causing night blindness or any other internal oculopathy, swelling or sores…all are the syndromes of kidney dispersion. It is the disease of the three dispersion-thirsts."

Formulas from the Discussion Illuminating the Yellow Emperor's Basic Questions–Dryness Section (Huáng Dì Sù Wèn Xuān Míng Lùn Fāng Zào Mén, 黄帝素问宣明论方燥门)

《秘传证治要诀及类方三消》,"三消久之,精血即亏,或目无见,或手足偏废如风疾非,然此症消肾得之为多。"

"A prolonged course of the three dispersion-thirsts will damage essence and blood, and then may cause blindness or disability of the hand and foot as the kind that wind pathogen causes, but it is usually due to kidney dispersion."

The Secret Transmission of Principle for Diagnosis and Treatment and Three Dispersion-thirsts (Mì Chuán Zhèng Zhì Yào Jué Jí Lèi Fāng Sān Xiāo, 秘传证治要诀及类方三消)

Questions for Consideration

1. Why it is important to emphasize "stop bleeding without causing stasis, regulate blood without damaging healthy qi" when treating diabetic retinopathy?

2. What should be noted when doing suspended moxibustion on RN 4 (*guān yuán*), RN 6 (*qì hǎi*), etc. on patients with pronounced yang deficiency?

Section 4   Retinal Periphlebitis

Periphlebitis of the retina, also known as Eales disease, is a retinal vascular disease commonly seen in the clinic. It is one of the most serious ophthalmology diseases that leads to vision loss in young people. It was once associated with TB infection or the result of an autoimmune response. However, the underlying pathogen is still unclear. The disease presents that obstructive disorder mainly arises in the peripheral retinal vein with dead cell perfusion, white sheath of the perivasculature, neovascularization, and recurrent retinal vitreous hemorrhages. It was originally called youth recurrent retinal vitreous hemorrhage. It is more common in young males, with the most common onset occurring from age twenty to thirty. The lesion often occurs bilaterally in varying periods and to varying degrees. Western medicine treatment includes laser, vitrectomy, and symptomatic treatment (such as blood-stanching and anti-inflammatory medications).

In traditional Chinese medicine, this condition is classified into various syndromes based on different manifestations. It is called "vitreous opacity" when the macula is not involved, minimal bleeding in the vitreous body with less vision impairment, feeling of a fog moving before the eyes; "sudden blindness" occurs when a large amount of blood flows from the fundus into the vitreous body leading to a sudden decrease in vision. It is also has been described as "blood passing through the posterior aspect of the pupil" in modern literature of Chinese ophthalmology.

The cause of the disease is associated with accumulated heat in the *zang-fu*, deficiency fire flaming upward, and qi deficiency with inability to control the blood. The main mechanism is pathogenic heat scorching the collaterals of the eyes, in addition to qi deficiency causing a loss of control of the blood that leads to collateral external bleeding, and may leak into the vitreous humor, which obstructs shining of the vitreous light. The disease is associated with disharmony of the *zang-fu*, obstruction, and stasis. It can be treated by regulating the *zang-fu*, dispelling stasis, and dissipating masses so as to help the stasis dissolve. The goal is to promote the vision, decrease proliferation of the retina and vitreous body, control recurrence, and cure stubborn cases.

Clinical Manifestation

At an early age, there is blurred vision with the perception of "fog moving". As the disease develops, massive hemorrhage flushes into the vitreous body, the patient will present with a sudden decrease in vision without pain to the degree of limited light perception. Recovery may occur when the stasis has dissolved; however, it may easily become recurrent and finally lead to blindness because of a tractional detachment of the retina. Fundus examination shows tortuosity, extension or helical shape of the peripheral retinal vein with white sheaths along the surroundings of the veins, and superficial hemorrhage in the lesion retina; hemorrhagic vitreous opacity is seen when the bleeding flushes into the vitreous body. Proliferative membrane and traps may be seen in the cases with recurrent hemorrhage; tractional detachment of the retina may also occur.

Treatment

This hemorrhagic fundus disease is rooted in a *zang-fu* disharmony. Recurrence of hemorrhage and binding of phlegm and stasis are considered characteristic of the turbid vitreous humor. The treatment strategy is to stop the bleeding and invigorate blood combined with dispersing phlegm, softening hardness, and dissipating masses.

1. Pattern Differentiation and Treatment

(1) Intense Liver Fire
【 Syndrome Characteristics 】
Normal appearance of the eyes, sudden occurrence of flying shadows before eyes, blindness, massive internal bleeding of the eyes; generalized symptoms presents as headache, distention of the eyes, dizziness, tinnitus, red complexion, vexation and irritation, distending pain in the chest and rib-side, bitter taste in the mouth, dryness of the pharynx, red tongue with yellow coating, and wiry and rapid pulse.
【 Treatment Principle 】
Clear liver heat and drain fire, cool blood and resolve stasis
【 Representative Formula 】
Modified *Fēn Zhū Sǎn* (Eye-Calming Powder, 分珠散)
【 Prescription 】

生蒲黄	shēng pú huáng	15 g	Pollen Typhae (raw)
花蕊石	huā ruǐ shí	20 g	Ophicalcitum
槐花	huái huā	10 g	Flos Sophorae
生地黄	shēng dì huáng	10 g	Radix Rehmanniae
赤芍	chì sháo	10 g	Radix Paeoniae Rubra
栀子	zhī zǐ	12 g	Fructus Arctii
黄芩	huáng qín	12 g	Radix Scutellariae
龙胆草	lóng dǎn cǎo	6 g	Radix et Rhizoma Gentianae
荆芥	jīng jiè	8 g	Herba Schizonepetae
生甘草	shēng gān cǎo	5 g	Radix et Rhizoma Glycyrrhizae (raw)

【 Modifications 】
➢ When dry stool is seen, *shēng dà huáng* (生大黄, raw Radix et Rhizoma Rhei) is

administered in a dose of 6 g, and *máng xiāo* (芒硝, Natrii Sulfas) 8 g added to relax the bowels, discharge heat, and remove pathogens; when gum bleeding persists along with thirst with a desire to drink cold drinks, *zhī mǔ* (知母, Rhizoma Anemarrhenae) 10 g, *shí gāo* (石膏, Gypsum Fibrosum) 30 g, and *xuán shēn* (玄参, Radix Scrophulariae) 12 g are added to clear stomach fire and promote fluid production to quench thirst.

➢ When depression with, chest stuffiness and sighing is seen; *chái hú* (柴胡, Radix Bupleuri) 6 g, *zhǐ qiào* (枳壳, Fructus Aurantii) 10 g, and *xiāng fù* (香附, Rhizoma Cyperi) 12 g are added to soothe the liver and relieve constraint.

➢ When bleeding is prolonged for a long time without resolving, *shēng dì* (生地, Radix Rehmanniae) and *lóng dǎn cǎo* (龙胆草, Radix et Rhizoma Gentianae) are removed, with *mǔ lì* (牡蛎, Concha Ostreae) 30 g, *wǎ léng zǐ* (瓦楞子, Concha Arcae) 20 g, and *xià kū cǎo* (夏枯草, Spica Prunellae) 15 g added to resolve stasis and dissipate masses.

(2) Deficiency-Fire Scorching the Collaterals

【Syndrome Characteristics】

Recurrent bleeding, alternating normal and abnormal vision, vitreous humor turbidity, or fundus periphery blood vessels uneven in calibre, perception of foggy vision, retinal hemorrhage; generalized symptoms such as flushed cheek bones and lips, vexing heat in chest, palms and soles, dry throat and mouth, red tongue with little coating, a thready and rapid pulse.

【Treatment Principle】

Nourish yin and reduce fire, cool the blood and stop bleeding.

【Representative Formula】

Modified *Shēng Pú Huáng Tāng* (Raw Cattail Pollen Decoction, 生蒲黄汤)

【Prescription】

生地黄	*shēng dì huáng*	15 g	Radix Rehmanniae
牡丹皮	*mǔ dān pí*	10 g	Cortex Moutan
生蒲黄	*shēng pú huáng*	15 g	Pollen Typhae (raw)
生三七粉	*shēng sān qī fěn*	5 g	Radix et Rhizoma Notoginseng (raw, powdered)
墨旱莲	*mò hàn lián*	20 g	Herba Ecliptae
荆芥炭	*jīng jiè tàn*	10 g	Herba Schizonepetae Carbonisatum
郁金	*yù jīn*	10 g	Radix Curcumae
丹参	*dān shēn*	8 g	Radix et Rhizoma Salviae Miltiorrhizae
知母	*zhī mǔ*	8 g	Rhizoma Anemarrhenae
黄柏	*huáng bǎi*	10 g	Cortex Phellodendri Chine
龟板	*guī bǎn*	15 g	Plastrum Testudinis
鳖甲	*biē jiǎ*	15 g	Carapax Trionycis

【Modifications】

➤ With dry cough and scanty sputum, tidal fever with night sweat is seen, *tiān mén dōng* (天门冬, Radix Asparagi) 12 g, *wǔ wèi zǐ* (五味子, Fructus Schisandrae Chinensis) 15 g, *bái jí* (白及, Rhizoma Bletillae) 12 g added to astringe yin and moisten lung.

➤ When vexation, insomnia, dreamfulness is seen, *suān zǎo rén* (酸枣仁, Semen Ziziphi Spinosae) 15 g, *bǎi zǐ rén* (柏子仁, Semen Platycladi) 12 g, and *shǒu wū téng* (首乌藤, Caulis Polygoni Multiflori) 15 g added to nourish heart and tranquilize mind.

➤ When tidal fever and flushed cheeks gets severe in the afternoon, *qīng hāo* (青蒿, Herba Artemisiae Annuae) 8 g, *yín chái hú* (银柴胡, Radix Stellariae) 8 g, and *dì gǔ pí* (地骨皮, Cortex Lycii) 10 g is added to clear deficiency-heat.

(3) Deficiency of Both Heart and Spleen

【Syndrome Characteristics】

Chronic, recurrent bleeding of internal eyes; generalized symptoms such as shallow yellow complexion, mental fatigue, physical overstrain, palpitations, shortage of qi, anorexia, loose stool, light tongue with white coating, a deep thready pulse with weakness.

【Treatment Principle】

Nourish the heart and invigorate the spleen, replenish the qi and controlling blood.

【Representative Formula】

Modified *Guī Pí Tāng* (Spleen-Restoring Decoction, 归脾汤)

【Prescription】

党参	dǎng shēn	15 g	Radix Codonopsis
黄芪	huáng qí	15 g	Radix Astragali
白术	bái zhú	15 g	Rhizoma Atractylodis Macrocephalae
茯苓	fú líng	10 g	Poria
龙眼肉	lóng yǎn ròu	10 g	Arillus Longan
酸枣仁	suān zǎo rén	10 g	Semen Ziziphi Spinosae
远志	yuǎn zhì	5 g	Radix Polygalae
木香	mù xiāng	8 g	Radix Aucklandiae
白茅根	bái máo gēn	30 g	Rhizoma Imperatae
仙鹤草	xiān hè cǎo	12 g	Herba Agrimoniae
生三七粉	shēng sān qī fěn	5 g	Radix et Rhizoma Notoginseng (powder)
大枣	dà zǎo	10 g	Fructus Jujubae

【Modifications】

➤ For cases with poor appetite, abdominal distention after food, and loose stool, remove *lóng yǎn ròu* (龙眼肉, Arillus Longan), *suān zǎo rén* (酸枣仁, Semen Ziziphi Spinosae), *dà zǎo* (大枣, Fructus Jujubae), add *yì yǐ rén* (薏苡仁, Semen Coicis) 15 g, *shān yào* (山药, Rhizoma Dioscoreae) 15 g, *jī nèi jīn* (鸡内金, Endothelium Corneum

Gigeriae Galli) 10 g, and *shén qū* (神曲, Massa Medicata Fermentata) 10 g to invigorate the spleen and remove food stagnation.

➢ For cases with edema in the retina and macular area, add *zé lán* (泽兰, Herba Lycopi) 10 g and *chē qián zǐ* (车前子, Semen Plantaginis) 10 g to activate blood and drain water.

➢ For cases with proliferation and organization in the retina and vitreous body, remove *xiān hè cǎo* (仙鹤草, Herba Agrimoniae), *gān cǎo* (甘草, Radix et Rhizoma Glycyrrhizae), add *hǎi zǎo* (海藻, Sargassum) 15 g, *kūn bù* (昆布, Thallus Laminariae; Thallus Eckloniae) 15 g, and *mǔ lì* (牡蛎, Concha Ostreae) 30 g to soften hardness and dissipate masses.

➢ For cases with recurrent bleeding in retina of light color, symptoms of qi deficiency such as shortage of qi, spontaneous sweating and weakness, increase the dosage of *dǎng shēn* (党参, Radix Codonopsis) and *huáng qí* (黄芪, Radix Astragali) to 30 g respectively, or change *dǎng shēn* (党参, Radix Codonopsis) into *hóng shēn* (红参, Radix et Rhizoma Ginseng Rubra) 10 g with an increased dosage of *huáng qí* (黄芪, Radix Astragali) 50 g to replenish qi and control blood.

2. Chinese Patent Medicines

(1) *Yún Nán Bái Yào Jiāo Náng* (Yun Nan Bai Yao Capsule, 云南白药胶囊)
250 mg (one tablet), three times a day, applicable to every prophase bleeding syndromes.

(2) *Zhī Bǎi Dì Huáng Wán* (Anemarrhena, Phellodendron and Rehmannia Pill, 知柏地黄丸)
6 g, two times a day, applicable to yin deficiency and effulgent fire.

(3) *Guī Pí Wán* (Spleen-Restoring Decoction, 归脾丸)
6 g, three times a day, applicable to deficiency of both heart and spleen.

3. Treatment with Western Medicine

Please consult a western specialist or ophthalmologists for medical treatment. Common therapies may include:

(1) General treatment: Intense activity should be avoided to decrease the hemorrhage in the acute bleeding stage. Semi reclining position should be taken. Moreover, suitable amounts of Vitamin C, Rutin, Calcium agent, hemostatics involving carbazochrome, dicynone can be used to take the bleeding under control.

(2) Glucocorticoids: Application of suitable glucocorticoids in the initial stages of the disease can decrease the inflammatory reaction of the retina.

(3) Treatment of laser photocoagulation: Fundus laser photocoagulation should be done during early metaphase in order to preserve better vision. It is better to get laser treatment as early as possible, especially when comparatively large amount of capillary

nonperfusion area is seen in retina.

(4) Surgical care: It needs to get vitrectomy for severe vitreous hemorrhage with prolonged non-absorbed bleeding, or one with obvious proliferative vitreoretinopathy.

4. Dietary Therapy and Preventive Care

(1) It is better to take a nourishing and bland diet-stay away from spicy and grilled foods.

(2) Give up smoking or drinking. It is forbidden to drink alcohol during the bleeding stage to avoid increasing of bleeding.

(3) It is better to take a semi reclining position when resting during bleeding stage in order to promote hemostasis.

(4) Keep calm and reduce irritable tendencies or pessimism to avoid depressed emotions as it can transform into fire.

Case Studies

Xing, 38-year-old male

【Chief Complaint】

Continued floating of butterfly shaped shadows in front of both eyes, accompanied by decreased vision of his left eye.

【Medical History】

The patient went to the hospital when a great deal of shadowing appeared before his eyes three years ago. He was diagnosed with periphlebitis of retina on both eyes, and vitreous hemorrhage on both eyes. He had improved after treatment. Recurrent bleeding happened for four times after the first year. It was the fifth occurrence before he came to our clinic. The vision on the left eye was severely destroyed. The patient asked for TCM treatment because of the failed attempts to keep the bleeding under control.

【Examination】

Right vision: 20/16, left vision: 20/300. Right eye: slight vitreous opacity, normal discus optic, circuitous veins on bitamporal side plucked as beads, with sheet of gray-white material located from the posterior pole to the ambitus, white sheath is along side the venous tributary, no reflection on foveomacular. Left eye: sheet of cloud flocculation filling in the vitreous body, reflected schillerization, venous engorgement and tortuosity may be seen indistinctly, with white sheath along side, large amount of bleeding and gray material on bitamporal side. There were no abnormal signs of the four examinations, except for the thready, slight slow pulse and light enlarged tongue with teeth marks.

【Diagnosis】

Bilateral fog moving before the eyes.

【Pattern Differentiation】

Deficiency of both qi and yin, deficiency of liver and kidney, qi deficiency and blood stasis.

【 Treatment Principles 】

Nourish yin and replenish qi, invigorate blood and move stasis, pacify the liver to improve vision.

【 Prescription 】

Modified *Yǎn Dǐ Chū Xuè Sān Fāng* (Fundus-Bleeding Third Formula, 眼底出血三方加味)

炒荆芥	*chǎo jīng jiè*	9 g	Herba Schizonepetae (stir-fried)
三七粉	*sān qī fěn*	3 g	Radix et Rhizoma Notoginseng (powdered, wrapped separately to be taken together with decoction)
茺蔚子	*chōng wèi zǐ*	9 g	Fructus Leonuri
珍珠母	*zhēn zhū mǔ*	25 g	Concha Margaritiferae Usta
生地	*shēng dì*	15 g	Radix Rehmanniae
焦白术	*jiāo bái zhú*	9 g	Rhizoma Atractylodis Macrocephalae (stir-fried to brown)
玄参	*xuán shēn*	12 g	Radix Scrophulariae
薄荷	*bò he*	5 g	Herba Menthae
青葙子	*qīng xiāng zǐ*	9 g	Semen Celosiae
党参	*dǎng shēn*	12 g	Radix Codonopsis
白蒺藜	*bái jí lí*	10 g	Fructus Tribuli
火麻仁	*huǒ má rén*	15 g	Fructus Cannabis
黑芝麻	*hēi zhī ma*	12 g	Semen Sesami Nigrum
桑叶	*sāng yè*	10 g	Folium Mori
槐花	*huái huā*	10 g	Flos Sophorae

All were prescribed for 14 days.

【 Follow-up 】

The vision was improved with less shadows on the second consultation. Three packages of *Liù Yī Sǎn* (Six-to-One Powder) were added to the previous prescription in order to clear heat and eliminate the dampness (given for seven days). On his last visit, the right vision was 20/13 and left vision was 20/25. Ophthalmic examination of the right eye showed slight vitreous opacity, normal color of discus opticus, plumped veins on bitamporal side. Venous white sheath had vanished, the reflection of foveomacular was evident. The fundus examination of the left eye showed flocculation opacity in the vitreous body, slightly plumped retina veins, sheet of material on the bitamporal side, sheets of gray-white material and yellow-white hardness effusion combined together in the macula area. All the bleeding had been absorbed. Foveal reflex could be seen indistinctly. The condition came to be stable. Another 7-day prescription was administered to the patient to strengthen the effects.

Classic Quotes

《杂病证治准绳·目·血灌瞳神证》："谓视瞳神不见其墨莹，但见其一点鲜红，甚则紫浊色也。病至此，亦甚危，且急也，初起一二日尚可救，迟则救亦不愈。"

"It is critical when a bright red spot is seen in the pupil instead of black, even if it is a dark purple color. It can be cured in the first two days, and will be irreversible if delayed."

Standards for the Diagnosis and Treatment of Miscellaneous Diseases – Eyes - Blood Passing through the Pupil (Zá Bìng Zhèng Zhì Zhǔn Shéng – Mù – Xuě Guàn Tóng Shén Zhèng, 杂病证治准绳·目·血灌瞳神证)

Question for Consideration

Briefly describe the cause and pathogenesis of retinal periphlebitis.

Section 5   Central Serous Chorioretinopathy

Central serous chorioretinopathy (CSC), is a common retinal disorder characterized by a local serous detachment of the retina in the macula and surrounding area. Patients usually present with a distortion in central vision as if a mesh curtain is in front of the eye. Some patients complain distorted vision, however upon visual exam, the eye looks normal. The cause of CSC is still unclear, but the most popular theory is that CSC is caused by damage to the retinal pigment epithelium (RPE) and neuroepithelium. Risk factors include cold, fatigue, stress, mental strain, lack of sleep, excessive smoking and alcohol, etc. Generally, most CSC occurs in men aged 20-55, with 40 having the peak age of incidence. Men are more often affected than women with the rate of 5:1 - 10:1, and about 90% patients are affected in one eye. CSC is a self-limited disease with a good overall prognosis, where most cases resolve spontaneously within 3-6 months. However, recurrence is common and likely if the underlying factors are addressed. After multiple relapses, irreversible damage of vision may occur. In Western medicine, CSC may be treated by medication and laser photocoagulation.

CSC pertains to *shì zhān yǒu sè* (tinted vision, 视瞻有色) in traditional chinese medicine, also called as *shì zhí rú qū* (seeing straight things as crooked, 视直如曲) or *shì xiǎo wéi dà* (seeing small things as big, 视小为大). The cause and pathology is due to a dysfunction of the spleen's transformation function resulting in the failure transformation of *jing* (essence), thus the eyes fail to be nourished. Other patterns may be associated with the accumulation of phlegm-dampness obstructing in the middle burner, steaming upwards and clouding the sensory orifices, sweat-pore obstruction due to qi stagnation and blood stasis caused by emotional depression, or lack of nourishment due to insufficiency of the liver and the kidney, depletion of essence and blood, and loss of heart essence. Overuse of the eyes may be another causative factor, for it may consume qi and blood thus leading to collapse of spirit light (*shen*). According to pattern differentiation, Chinese Medicine can shorten the course of disease; accelerate the regression of edema and the absorption of exudates, thus to improve vision.

Clinical Manifestation

Symptoms: blurred vision, central amblyopia, central blister, distorted vision and abnormal colored vision, blind spots and distorted curve can be found in the Amsler Grid examination.

Fundus findings: There is a round or oval shape of slight edema presenting in the macula area with an annular reflective ring. The reflection of macula fovea centralis disappears. Subsequently, there are some yellow-white exudate spots in the edema area. After repeated attacks, residual gray-yellow hard exudates as well as pigment abnormity or depletion may be present. Generally, the fovea reflection will appear gradually in most cases.

Fluorescein angiography (FFA) findings: Fluorescein leakage can be seen at the early phase of angiography and in active cases. The following two types are the common patterns:

Spurting pattern (Smokestack phenomenon): There is one or several needlepoint size leakage spots in the arterial phase or early vein phase, which occurs in the defect area of pigmentary epithelium. Immediately, the leakage points enlarge quickly and spurts upward like smoke in shape of umbrella or mushroom. The dye then diffuses in the subretinal area, outlining the whole area of detachment.

Dispersion pattern (Inkblot diffusion): It is also known as a dispersion pattern if the leakage area rapidly scatters to the surrounding region. Sometime the small fluorescent dots may be located peripherally outside of the central area, and most often appears in the superior retina.

Treatment

1. Pattern Differentiation and Treatment

(1) Water-Damp Invading Upward
[Syndrome Characteristics]
Blurred vision, central amblyopia, distorted vision, abnormal colored vision, relatively

severe macular edema, disappearance of the foveal reflex, shortness of breath, no appetite to talk, lack of strength in the four limbs, reduced desire for food intake, loose stool, pale tongue with white greasy coating, soggy and slippery pulse.

【Treatment Principle】

Tonify qi and invigorate the spleen, drain water and dampness

【Representative Formula】

Modified *Shēn Líng Bái Zhú Sǎn* (Ginseng, Poria and Atractylodes Macrocephalae Powder, 参苓白术散)

【Prescription】

太子参	*tài zǐ shēn*	15 g	Radix Pseudostellariae
白术	*bái zhú*	15 g	Rhizoma Atractylodis Macrocephalae
山药	*shān yào*	15 g	Rhizoma Dioscoreae
白扁豆	*bái biǎn dòu*	10 g	Semen Lablab Album
砂仁	*shā rén*	10 g	Fructus Amomi
薏苡仁	*yì yǐ rén*	15 g	Semen Coicis
茯苓	*fú líng*	15 g	Poria
陈皮	*chén pí*	10 g	Pericarpium Citri Reticulatae
当归	*dāng guī*	10 g	Radix Angelicae Sinensis
白芍	*bái sháo*	10 g	Radix Paeoniae Alba
桃仁	*táo rén*	10 g	Semen Persicae
川芎	*chuān xiōng*	10 g	Rhizoma Chuanxiong
桂枝	*guì zhī*	10 g	Ramulus Cinnamomi

【Modifications】

➤ For cases with severe macular edema, add *chē qián zǐ* (车前子, Semen Plantaginis) 30 g and *zé xiè* (泽泻, Rhizoma Alismatis) 10 g to drain water and dampness.

(2) Depression of Liver Qi

【Syndrome Characteristics】

Blurred vision, central blistering, distorted vision and abnormal color vision, macular edema with yellow-white exudative spots, dizziness, hypochondriac pain, bitter mouth and dry throat, red tongue with thin yellow coating, thready and wiry pulse.

【Treatment Principle】

Soothe the liver and resolve constraint, move qi and invigorate blood.

【Representative Formula】

Modified *Xiāo Yáo Sǎn* (Free Wanderer Powder, 逍遥散)

【Prescription】

柴胡	*chái hú*	15 g	Radix Bupleuri
当归	*dāng guī*	10 g	Radix Angelicae Sinensis

赤芍	chì sháo	15 g	Radix Paeoniae Rubra
川芎	chuān xiōng	10 g	Rhizoma Chuanxiong
茺蔚子	chōng wèi zǐ	15 g	Fructus Leonuri
丹参	dān shēn	15 g	Radix et Rhizoma Salviae Miltiorrhizae
菊花	jú huā	15 g	Flos Chrysanthemi
白芍	bái sháo	10 g	Radix Paeoniae Alba
生地	shēng dì	15 g	Radix Rehmanniae
白术	bái zhú	10 g	Rhizoma Atractylodis Macrocephalae
茯苓	fú líng	15 g	Poria
炙甘草	zhì gān cǎo	5 g	Radix et Rhizoma Glycyrrhizae Praeparata cum Melle
丹皮	dān pí	10 g	Cortex Moutan

【 Modifications 】

➢ For cases with more exudates in macular area, increase *dān shēn* (丹参, danshen root) to 15 g, and add *yù jīn* (郁金, Radix Curcumae) 10 g and *shān zhā* (山楂, Fructus Crataegi) 10 g to rectify qi, invigorate blood and dissipate mass.

(3) Deficiency of the Liver and the Kidney

【 Syndrome Characteristics 】

Dry eyes, blurred vision, visual distortion and discoloration, pigment disorders on macular area, disappearance of foveal light reflex, yellow white exudative dots, dizziness, tinnitus, seminal emission and aching lumbus, red tongue with thin coating, thready and rapidly pulse.

【 Treatment Principle 】

Nourish the liver and the kidney

【 Representative Formula 】

Modified *Sì Wù Wǔ Zǐ Wán* (Four Agents and Five-Seed Pill, 四物五子丸)

【 Prescription 】

熟地	shú dì	20 g	Radix Rehmanniae Praeparata
当归	dāng guī	10 g	Radix Angelicae Sinensis
赤芍	chì sháo	10 g	Radix Paeoniae Rubra
川芎	chuān xiōng	10 g	Rhizoma Chuanxiong
菟丝子	tù sī zǐ	10 g	Semen Cuscutae
车前子	chē qián zǐ	20 g	Semen Plantaginis
枸杞子	gǒu qǐ zǐ	10 g	Fructus Lycii
覆盆子	fù pén zǐ	10 g	Fructus Rubi

【 Modifications 】

➢ For cases with more exudates in macular area, add *shān zhā* (山楂, Fructus Crataegi) 10 g, *hǎi zǎo* (海藻, Sargassum) 10 g, and *kūn bù* (昆布, Thallus Laminariae) 10 g to soften hardness and dissipate mass.

2. Acupuncture

(1) Needling acupuncture

BL 1 (*jīng míng*)	ST 1 (*chéng qì*)	*qiú hòu* (球后)
LI 4 (*hé gǔ*)	KI 3 (*tài xī*)	LV 3 (*tài chōng*)
GB 37 (*guāng míng*)		

Use 1.5 inch, 32 gauge needles, and puncture quickly subcutaneously, then slowly insert the needle along the space between eyeball and orbital inner wall about 1 *cun* depth, twist the needle gently with small amplitude and low frequency (DO NOT lift and thrust). After the patient feels a fairly intensive needling sensation, retain the needles for 30 min. During the needle retention period, manipulate needles 2–3 times. Choose a combination of acupoints based on the underlying pattern. For LI 4 (*hé gǔ*) and GB 37 (*guāng míng*) acupoints, use even supplementation and drainage method. For KI 3 (*tài xī*), use the supplementation method. For LV 3 (*tài chōng*), use a drainage method. Treat once every day, 10 treatments is a full course. It is suggested to take 3–5 days interval between 2 courses of treatment and then resume.

(2) Qi Gong Acupuncture

The points are divided into 3 groups:

① BL 1 (*jīng míng*), 太阳 (*tài yáng*), 球后 (*qiú hòu*), ST 1 (*chéng qì*).

② *Yì míng* (翳明), *Xin Ming* I , ST 36 (*zú sān lǐ*), LI 4 (*hé gǔ*).

③ *Xin Ming* II , *yìn táng* (印堂), LI 11(*qū chí*), LV 2, GB 37 (*guāng míng*).

Manipulation: Choose one of the three groups each time and alternate with each session. Set the patient in supine position, ask the patient to touch their tongue to the roof of their mouth; recite the words "*Jing*" and "*Song*", close the eyes lightly, relax the body, eliminate distracting thoughts, visualize the lower *dān tián* (3 fingers below the navel and 2 inches inside), keep the attention at this area for about 10 minutes before starting the acupuncture treatment. When needling, the doctor should move qi to fingertips, and transport qi into the points through the needle, ask the patient to transfer thought from *dān tián* to the acupoints. Retain the needles for 5–6 min for each acupoint. After this time withdraw the needles, ask the patient take 3 deep breaths, and then puncture the second series of acupoints. Generally, needle the acupoints in the head and face first, then needle distal points, do not choose more than 6 acupoints each time.

(3) Ear Acupuncture:

Ear acupoints include eye1, eye 2, liver and sebaceous glands of the affected side. Once every 2–3 days, retain the needle for 30–60 minutes. Or once everyday, puncture both ears in turn.

3. Chinese Patent Medicines

(1) *Chén Xià Liù Jūn Wán* (Tangerine Peel and Pinellia Six-gentlemen Pill, 陈夏六君丸)

Take orally, 6–9 g, 2–3 times everyday to supply the spleen and the stomach, rectify qi and transform phlegm, applicable to the deficiency of the spleen and the stomach, and water-dampness invading upward.

(2) *Xiāo Yáo Wán* (Free Wanderer Pill, 逍遥丸)

Take orally, 6–9g, 2–3 times everyday, to soothe the liver and strengthen the spleen, nourish the blood and regulate menstruation, applicable to binding depression of liver qi.

(3) *Qǐ Jú Dì Huáng Wán* (Lycium Berry, Chrysanthemum and Rehmannia Pill, 杞菊地黄丸)

6–9g, twice a day to nourish the liver and kidney, replenish essence and brighten the eyes; applicable to liver-kidney yin deficiency.

4. Simple and Proven Recipes

Modified *Zhù Jǐng Wán* (Long Vistas Pill, 驻景丸)

楮实子	*chǔ shí zǐ*	25 g	Fructus Broussonetiae
菟丝子	*tù sī zǐ*	25 g	Semen Cuscutae
茺蔚子	*chōng wèi zǐ*	18 g	Fructus Leonuri
木瓜	*mù guā*	10 g	Fructus Chaenomelis
薏苡仁	*yì yǐ rén*	30 g	Semen Coicis
三七粉	*sān qī fěn*	3 g	Radix et Rhizoma Notoginseng
炒鸡内金	*chǎo jī nèi jīn*	10 g	Endothelium Corneum Gigeriae Galli (dry-fried)
炒谷芽	*chǎo gǔ yá*	30 g	Fructus Setariae Germinatus (dry-fried)
炒麦芽	*chǎo mài yá*	30 g	Fructus Hordei Germinatus (dry-fried)
枸杞子	*gǒu qǐ zǐ*	10 g	Fructus Lycii
山药	*shān yào*	15 g	Rhizoma Dioscoreae

Modification: For cases with macular edema at the early stage, add *huáng dòu juǎn* (黄豆卷, soya bean roll) 20 g, *fú líng* (茯苓, Poria) 15 g, *bì xiè* (萆薢, Rhizoma Dioscoreae Hypoglaucae) 10 g, and *qiàn shí* (芡实, Semen Euryales) 10 g to drain water and dampness.

5. External therapy

Drug iontophoresis: *Dān Shēn Zhù Shè Yè* (Select Salviae Miltiorrhiza Injection, 丹参注射液), *Sān Qī Zhù Shè Yè* (Pseudoginseng Root Injection, 三七注射液), etc. for iontophoresis, 15 minutes each time; treat once every day, 10 treatments are needed for a treatment course. Take a 3–5 day interval after a treatment course.

6. Western Medical Treatment

(1) Medication treatment: Vitamin C, Vitamin E and Rutoside can reduce permeability of the capillary. For cases with insomnia, an oral sedative may be indicated.

(2) Laser Treatment

For cases with marked serous detachment, severe fluorescence leakage, and the leakage points located outside the papilla-macula fibers area above 250 μm distance from the fovea centralis, laser photocoagulation is indicated. Of course, treatment must be done by an ophthalmologist.

7. Dietary Therapy and Preventive Care

(1) Heat-clearing and dampness-dispelling porridge: *Chì xiǎo dòu* (赤小豆, Semen Phaseoli) 30 g, *bái biǎn dòu* (白扁豆, Semen Lablab Album) 20 g, *yì yǐ rén* (薏苡仁, Semen Coicis)20 g, *qiàn shí* (芡实, Semen Euryales) 20 g, *bì xiè* (萆薢, Rhizoma Dioscoreae Hypoglaucae) 10 g, *chì fú líng* (赤茯苓, Poria Rubra) 15 g, *mù mián huā* (木棉花, Cortex Bombacis Malabaricir) 20 g, *dēng xīn huā* (灯心花, Medulla Junci) 10 g.

First, decoct *bì xiè* (Rhizoma Dioscoreae Hypoglaucae) 10 g, *chì fú líng* (Poria Rubra) 15 g, *mù mián huā* (Cortex Bombacis Malabarici) 20 g, *dēng xīn huā* (Medulla Junci) and then put *chì xiǎo dòu* (Semen Phaseoli) 30 g, *bái biǎn dòu* (Semen Lablab Album) 20 g, *yì yǐ rén* (Semen Coicis) 20 g, and *qiàn shí* (Semen Euryales) 20 g into the decoction and cook it into porridge; applicable to the dampness due to spleen deficiency.

(2) Flastem Milkvetch Seed Chrysanthemum Tea: *shā yuàn zǐ* (沙苑子, Semen Astragali Complanati) 30 g, *bái jú huā* (白菊花, Flos Chrysanthemi) 10 g. Drink as tea, warm the decoction before taking. The tea has the function of supplying the liver and the kidney, brightening the eye; applicable to the insufficiency of the liver and the kidney presenting with symptoms like dizziness, low back pain, urinary frequency.

(3) *Kūn bù* (昆布, Thallus Laminariae) 30 g, *hǎi zǎo* (海藻, Thallus Sargassi Pallidi) 30 g, *huáng dòu* (黄豆, Soybeans) 60–90 g. Add appropriate amount water to cook into mush, then add a little salt or sugar, take orally, applicable to cases in the later stage with exudates in the retina.

(4) Prevention and early treatment is very important. In daily life, arrange work and rest reasonably, and try to identify and reduce risk factors such as excessive mental stress, poor sleep, fatigue, cold and microbial infections. During the course of treatment, it is highly recommended that the patient get adequate rest, avoid excessive mental work and manual labor, and restrict TV, computer and reading time.

(5) Avoid extreme emotional stimuli, excessive use of the eyes, over-exertion and

staying up late (past 11pm), regulate daily diet in a healthy way — eat less spicy, greasy-fried, refined and processed foods, and ensure enough sleep. All of the above are helpful to reduce the incidence of recurrence.

Case Studies

Mr. Lee, male, 36 years old

【 Chief Complaint 】

Blurred vision of the right eye explained, "like a shadow covering the eyes," for more than two weeks.

【 Medical History 】

The symptoms occurred soon after he was frightened in an accident. Before he came to our clinic, he had been treated with western medicine which had been ineffective.

【 Examination 】

Conscious mind and good physical health, language fluency, bilateral examination of the pupils revealed them to be the same size and symmetrically round, there was reflection of light present.

Visual acuity: Right eye, 20/40; left eye, 20/13. Moderate macular edema, foveal light reflex had disappeared in the right eye, no abnormity found in the left eye, pink tongue with thin white coating, a thready and wiry pulse.

【 Diagnosis 】

Central serous chorioretinopathy.

【 Treatment Principles 】

Nourish the liver and the kidney, tonify blood and brighten the eyes.

【 Acupoint selection 】

GB 20 (fēng chí)	BL 2 (cuán zhú)	qiú hòu (球后)
LV 3 (tài chōng)	KI 3 (tài xī)	

Method: Except GB 20 (fēng chí) and 球后 (qiú hòu), all the acupoints were needled and retained for 30 min after the arrival of de qi. When puncturing GB 20 (fēng chí), needle sensation ought to be facilitated towards the forehead. For qiú hòu (球后), insert the needle about 1.5 cun, withdraw the needle when the patient felt soreness and a distending ache. The patient's right eye felt better after the first acupuncture treatment was completed. After the second treatment, the visual acuity of the right eye improved to 20/30. After 10 treatments, the visual acuity on the right eye was improved to 20/20, the macular edema significantly subsided, foveal light reflex appeared. The same treatment was continued for 5 additional sessions after 3-day interval. Then the visual acuity was 20/13 on the right eye, and the macular edema disappeared. To consolidate the curative effect, the patient was treated with acupuncture for another 5 additional sessions. 3 months later, follow-up observation showed that visual acuities were 20/13 on both eyes.

(*Yin Ke-jing Medical Records*, 殷克敬医案)

Classic Quotes

《证治准绳·杂病·七窍门》: "视瞻有色证，非若萤星、云雾二证之细点长条也，乃目凡视物有大片甚则通行。"

Symptom of tinted vision is not like the symptoms of fog moving in front of the eyes or a flying firefly in front of the eyes, but large fixed shades in front of the eyes which block the light.

Standards for Diagnosis and Treatment–Miscellaneous disease–Seven Orifices Section (*Zhèng Zhì Zhǔn Shéng–Zá Bìng–Qī Qiào Mén*, 证治准绳·杂病·七窍门)

Questions for Consideration

1. According to "inner five-wheel differentiation", which viscera does the macula belong to?

2. In Western medicine, which disease pertains to "tinted vision"? What is the pathomechanism of the disease according to Chinese medicine theory?

Section 6   Age-Related Macular Degenaration

Age-related macular degeneration (AMD), also named as senile macular degeneration (SMD), is the leading cause of legal blindness in the developed world among people aged over 65. It typically begins at age 50, and the prevalence increases with age. There is no sexual predilection to developing AMD. The disease attacks both eyes simultaneously or one after the other. Based on clinical and pathological features, AMD is classified into two types: atrophic (dry form or nonexudative) and exudative (wet form), the former is more common.

In Traditional Chinese Medicine, the disease is belonged to *shì zhān hūn miǎo* (blurring vision, 视瞻昏渺) or *shì zhí rú qū* (metamorphopsia, 视直如曲).

Clinical Manifestation

1. Atrophic AMD

Progressive atrophy of the retinal pigmentary epithelium leads to the degeneration of photoreceptor cells and a decline of central vision. Occurrence is in adults over age 45, and the visual decline is slow affecting one or both eyes.

Visual acuity: Nothing is perceived in the early stages, only a few of patients have visual blur, visual distortion or reading trouble. With the developing course of the disease, the central vision deteriorates to varying degrees.

Fundus examination: In the early stages, irregular pigment disperses among the macular area, light reflection of the central fovea is weak or missing, drusen is scattered. In late stage AMD, drusen increases in number and coalesces, retinal pigment epithelium atrophys, atrophic and merged choroidal capillary vessels change into geographic atrophy.

Visual field: At the early stage, 5 to 10 degrees of relative central scotoma may be present, with time, absolute central scotoma appearing in the visual field. Amsler grid testing is always abnormal.

Fluorescein angiography: Hyperfluorescence appears as transmitted fluorescence (window defect) in the early stages with clear drusen and hypopigmented areas, which enhances, attenuates and subsidises with background fluorescence. Hypofluorescence may appear in hyperpigmented areas. In some cases, fluorescence dots may be seen in the late stages because of drusen staining. In advanced cases of the disease, choroidal capillaries atrophy and occlude in atrophic area of macular pigment epithelium, in where hypofluorescence could be seen with vestigial large choroidal blood vessels.

2. Exudative AMD

Choroidal (subretinal) neovascularization leads to leaking fluid, hemorrhage and scarring etc. It typically happens over age 45 in one eye after the other. The visual decline is sharp and severe.

Visual acuity: Visual blur and distortion happen at the early stages, where after central vision rapidly decreases.

Fundus examination: In the early stages, drusen coalesces, pigment disperses among macula area, light reflection of the central fovea is weak or missing. Later, choroidal (subretinal) neovascularization membrane appears in the macula, typical manifestation reveals an off white or dark irregular round focus of the macula. Hemorrhaging could be around or on the surface of the focus, subretinal hematoma, retinal bleeding or vitreous hemorrhage could also be seen. Yellow-white hard drusens are always found around hemorrhage and fluid area. In the late stages, exudation and hemorrhage are gradually absorbed, irregular clumping or round-like yellow or yellow-white scarring with ecchymosis form around the macula. In some cases, new vessels may be found around former scar tissue and enlargement may be caused as a result of fluid leaking or bleeding being absorbed and cicatrized.

Visual field: Central scotoma appears corresponding to the lesion, and Amsler grid testing is abnormal.

Fluorescein angiography: Subretinal neovascularization appears in the early stages with a clear boundary of a lace-like, wheel-like, granulo-like or patching-like form. In the late stages, dye may leak out as hyperfluorescence after the background fluorescence subsides. Dye-stained edema fluid originates from a retinal neuroepithelial detachment area and the hemorrhage area may be shielded.

Treatment

1. Pattern Differentiation and Treatment

(1) Internal Blockage of Phlegm-dampness

【Syndrome Characteristics】

Visual activity decreases and vision distorts, yellow-white drusen are scattered throughout the macula with exudation, bleeding and scarring are present in the fundus examination. Chest distress, anorexia and thirst without drinking desire could appear with red tongue, a yellow-greasy coating and a wiry-slippery pulse.

【Treatment Principle】

Remove dampness and transform phlegm, clear heat and improve vision.

【Representative Formula】

Modified *Sān Rén Tāng* (Three Kernels Decoction, 三仁汤)

【Prescription】

杏仁	*xìng rén*	9 g	Semen Armeniacae Amarum
滑石	*huá shí*	12 g	Talcum
通草	*tōng cǎo*	9 g	Medulla Tetrapanacis
竹叶	*zhú yè*	6 g	Folium Phyllostachydis Henonis
白蔻仁	*bái kòu rén*	6 g	Fructus Amomi Rotundus
厚朴	*hòu pò*	9 g	Cortex Magnoliae Officinalis
薏苡仁	*yì yǐ rén*	12 g	Semen Coicis
半夏	*bàn xià*	9 g	Rhizoma Pinelliae

【Modifications】

➤ For cases with spleen qi deficiency, add *fú líng* (茯苓, Poria) 15 g, *bái zhú* (白术, Rhizoma Atractylodis Macrocephalae) 9 g and *huáng qí* (黄芪, Radix Astragali) 15 g to tonify qi and invigorate the spleen.

➤ For cases with heat, add *zhī zǐ* (栀子, Fructus Gardeniae) 9 g, *huáng qín* (黄芩, Radix Scutellariae) 9 g, and *lóng dǎn cǎo* (龙胆草, Radix et Rhizoma Gentianae) 12 g to clear qi.

➤ For cases with retinal hemorrhage, add *chì sháo* (赤芍, Radix Paeoniae Rubra) 15 g, *dāng guī* (当归, Radix Angelicae Sinensis) 9 g and *sān qī* powder (三七, Radix et Rhizoma Notoginseng, infused) 3 g to cool blood and dispel stasis.

(2) Qi Stagnation and Blood Stasis

【Syndrome Characteristics】

Visual activity decreases and the vision becomes distorted. In a fundus examination, there could be pigmentary disorder, drusen, irregular round-like focus with off-white or dark gray color, exudation, bleeding or scar, etc. Vertigo and dizziness prickle in rib-side, bitter mouth and dry throat could be checked out with dark-purple tongue and wiry-unsmooth pulse.

【 Treatment Principle 】

Sooth the liver and relieve depression, activate blood and resolve stasis.

【 Representative Formula 】

Modified *Xiāo Yáo Săn* (Free Wanderer Powder, 逍遥散)

【 Prescription 】

牡丹皮	*mŭ dān pí*	9 g	Cortex Moutan
炒栀子	*chăo zhī zǐ*	9 g	Fructus Gardeniae (dry-fried)
当归	*dāng guī*	12 g	Radix Angelicae Sinensis
白芍	*bái sháo*	15 g	Radix Paeoniae Alba
柴胡	*chái hú*	9 g	Radix Bupleuri
茯苓	*fú líng*	12 g	Poria
白术	*bái zhú*	6 g	Rhizoma Atractylodis Macrocephalae
薄荷 (后下)	*bò he (hòu xià)*	6 g	Herba Menthae (decocted later)
生姜	*shēng jiāng*	6 g	Rhizoma Zingiberis Recens

【 Modifications 】

➢ For cases with qi-depression manifesting with emotional upset, sighing and wiry pulse, add *qīng pí* (青皮, Pericarpium Citri Reticulatae Viride) 15 g, *xiāng fù* (香附, Rhizoma Cyperi) 9 g to sooth liver.

For cases with acute bleeding, add *bái máo gēn* (白茅根, Rhizoma Imperatae) 20 g, *cè bǎi yè* (侧柏叶, Cacumen Platycladi) 10 g, and *xiǎo jì* (小蓟, Herba Cirsii) 10 g to cool the blood and stop bleeding.

➢ For cases with blood-stasis with dark-purple hemorrhaging, narrow or circuitous blood vessels, add *dān shēn* (丹参, Radix et Rhizoma Salviae Miltiorrhizae) 15 g, *dì lóng* (地龙, Pheretima) 12 g and *hóng huā* (红花, Flos Carthami) 9 g to resolve blood stasis.

(3) Liver-Kidney Depletion

【 Syndrome Characteristics 】

Visual activity decreases and vision distorts. The fundus examination is similar to the former pattern. In long-term, chronic cases, low back pain (sore or weakness), impotence, weak knees, vertigo and tinnitus, poor memory, red tongue, thin tongue coating and a thready-weak pulse could be checked out.

【 Treatment Principle 】

Nourish the liver and kidney.

【 Representative Formula 】

Modified *Zhù Jǐng Wán* (Long Vistas Pill, 驻景丸)

【 Prescription 】

熟地黄	*shú dì huáng*	15 g	Radix Rehmanniae Praeparata
楮实子	*chǔ shí zǐ*	10 g	Fructus Broussonetiae
枸杞子	*gǒu qǐ zǐ*	10 g	Fructus Lycii
车前子	*chē qián zǐ*	9 g	Semen Plantaginis
五味子	*wǔ wèi zǐ*	15 g	Fructus Schisandrae Chinensis
当归	*dāng guī*	9 g	Radix Angelicae Sinensis
花椒	*huā jiāo*	6 g	Pericarpium Zanthoxyli

【 Modifications 】

➢ For cases with heat, substract *huā jiāo* (Pericarpium Zanthoxyli).

➢ For cases with yin deficiency with effulgent fire, including dry mouth and dry throat, heat vexation and restlessness, red tongue with thin coating, and a thready-rapid pulse, add *zhī mǔ* (知母, Rhizoma Anemarrhenae) 9 g, *huáng bǎi* (黄柏, Cortex Phellodendri Chinensis) 9 g, *tiān huā fěn* (天花粉, Radix Trichosanthis) 12 g and *shí hú* (石斛, Caulis Dendrobii) 10 g, change *shú dì huáng* (Radix Rehmanniae Praeparata) into *shēng dì* (生地, Radix Rehmanniae) to nourish yin and clear heat.

➢ For cases with yang hyperactivity including vertigo and a wiry pulse, substract *huā jiāo* (Pericarpium Zanthoxyli), add *tiān má* (天麻, Rhizoma Gastrodiae) 15 g, *jú huā* (菊花, Flos Chrysanthemi) 9 g, and *gōu téng* (钩藤, Ramulus Uncariae Cum Uncis) 15 g to subdue yang and descend counterflow of qi.

2. Acupuncture

In cases with non-bleeding, choose:

qiú hòu (球后)	GB 15 (*tóu lín qì*)	BL 1 (*jīng míng*),
GB 20 (*fēng chí*)	LI 4 (*hé gǔ*)	GB 37 (*guāng míng*)
SP 6 (*sān yīn jiāo*)	BL 23 (*shèn shù*)	BL 2 (*cuán zhú*)
yú yāo (鱼腰)	ST 2 (*sì bái*)	

Choose both distal and proximal 2 to 3 points each time, and use even supplementation and drainage. *Jīng míng* and *qiú hòu* points should NOT be manipulated. After aching and bloating feeling appear in local area, retain the needles for 30 to 40 minutes, once everyday; 10 days is a course of treatment.

3. Chinese Patent Medicines

(1) *Qǐ Jú Dì Huáng Wán* (Lycium Berry, Chrysanthemum and Rehmannia Pill, 杞菊地黄丸)

1 pill each time, twice a day, applicable to liver-kidney yin deficiency.

(2) *Fù Fāng Xuè Shuān Tōng Jiāo Náng* (**Compound Formula of Thrombus Cleared Capsule, 复方血栓通胶囊**)

4 to 6 pieces each time, three times a day; applicable to qi deficiency and blood stasis.

4. Treatment with Western Medicine

Please consult your ophthalmologist for the treatment, common therapies for wet-AMD may include: retinal laser photocoagulation, photodynamic therapy (PDT), transpupillary thermal therapy (TTT), etc.

5. Dietary Therapy and Preventive Care

(1) Reactively light diet, avoid spicy food or fatty-fried food, and inhibit smoking and drinking.

(2) Wear UV protected sunglasses when outdoors.

(3) Rest during periods of retinal bleeding, avoid extreme emotional fluctuations and excessive use of the eyes.

(4) Treat general underlying diseases actively, such as hypertension, hyperlipemia, diabetes, etc.

Case Studies

Meng, a 67-year-old male.

[Chief Complaint]

Reduced visual ability and distorted vision on his left eye in the last 2 weeks. The vision in his right eye was bad due to his suffering with AMD for the last three years.

[Examination]

Visual acuity was 20/200 on the right eye and 20/67 on the left eye. Amsler grid was showed distortions in the left eye. Both eyes appeared normal externally, the lens cortexes were slightly opaque. In a fundus examination of the right eye, the edge of the optic disc was clear and the color appeared to be normal. The reflection of arteries was enhanced and the veins showed angioplerosis. Sheeted off-white scarring and pigmentation was observed in the posterior pole of retina. In the left eye fundus examination, the optic disc and retinal vessels were similar to the right eye, slight edema of retina was seen in macula region, with a purple red color, clear boundary, 2 PD size of deep layer hemorrhage.

[Medical History]

The patient had a medical history of hypertension, his blood pressure usually fluctuated between 140–160/80–100mmHg due to irregular treatment of his condition. Patient's symptoms: Sore waist, occasional dizziness, red tongue, thin-yellow coating and a wiry-thready-rapid pulse. Because of the unsuccessful treatment experience of the right eye, the patient insisted on being treated with Chinese medicine instead of western medicine.

【Diagnosis】

TCM diagnosis: blurring vision

Western diagnosis: AMD.

【Pattern Differentiation】

Yin deficiency with yang hyperactivity and deficiency fire flaring upward, thus fire the injured ocular collateral and static blood blocked the eye.

【Treatment Principles】

Pacify the liver and subdue yang, cool the blood and stop bleeding.

【Prescription】

Tiān Má Gōu Téng Yǐn (Gastrodia and Uncaria Decoction, 天麻钩藤饮) adding *sān qī* (Radix et Rhizoma Notoginseng), *shēng pú huáng* (生蒲黄, Pollen Typhae) and *bái máo gēn* (Rhizoma Imperatae).

It was suggested that his blood pressure be treated and monitored regularly by his internist (MD).

【Follow-up】

After 14 doses of Chinese medicine, he felt the distorted vision was much better. Visual acuity was increased to 20/40. The fudus examination showed the retinal edema was alleviated, while hemorrhage spot was as the same. After continuing 21 doses of modified *Tiān Má Gōu Téng Yǐn,* he felt the distorted vision had vanished. The left eye fundus examination showed that the center of hemorrhage spot was absorbed with the periphery hemorrhage left in shape of half circularity. Central fovea could be seen and visual acuity was 20/30. No complaints with red tongue, thin coating, and deep-thready pulse. Thus the treatment principle was changed into supplementing the liver and kidney, and dissolving blood stasis. The recipe was *Qǐ Jú Dì Huáng Tāng* (Lycium Berry, Chrysanthemum and Rehmannia Decoction, 杞菊地黄汤) adding *xuè jié* (血竭, Sanguis Draconis) 1g. After 10 doses, the visual acuity was 20/25, retinal hemorrhage was totally absorbed in the left eye, only a few drusen and irregular pigmentation were in the local retina, light reflection of the central fovea could be seen. He was advised to take the Chinese patent drug *Qǐ Jú Dì Huáng Wán* (Lycium Berry, Chrysanthemum and Rehmannia Pill, 杞菊地黄丸) for three months afterward.

Question for Consideration

What Chinese medicinal would be added after pattern differentiation, when treating exudative AMD with retinal hemorrhage?

Section 7   Retinitis Pigmentosa

Retinitis pigmentosa (RP) is an inherited retinal dystrophy caused by the loss of photoreceptors and characterized by wax-yellow papillia, attenuate retinal vessels, and pigmentary deposits on the ambitus. Night blindness and peripheral vision loss (in the visual field) are the major clinical manifestations. The disease most often affects both eyes, and is a common genetic eye disease. RP is clinically divided for two types: typical RP and atypical RP. The disease occurs more in the offspring of blood-related parents. Some patients or relatives may accompany with high myopia, mental disorder, epilepsy, hypophrenia and deaf-mutism. Treatment methods of western medicine include symptomatic treatment, expanding blood vessels, tissue or cell transplantation and maintenance therapy. Up to now, there are no known effective treatments for RP.

The incidence of the disease ranges from about 5/1000 to 1/20,000 worldwide.

Traditional Chinese Medicine called the disease as *gāo fēng nèi zhàng* (高风内障), also known as *gāo fēng* Bird Eye (高风雀目) in the *Standards for Diagnosis and Treatment* (*Zhèng Zhì Zhǔn Shéng*, 证治准绳). The ancients considered that the cause was "debilitation of yang can not confront yin", due to a congenital jing deficiency, thin and astringent vessels and collaterals, and decadency of spirit light (Shen) It was an internal oculopathy disease which is characterized by night blindness, gradual vision loss and progressive narrowing of the visual field. There are many clinical treatment methods, but none are ideal. Chinese herbal medicine has some effect on systemic and eye symptoms. Some patients show different degrees of improvement in visual acuity, visual fields, and electrophysiological examinations. Generally, TCM treats RP with methods of supplementing yang and boosting qi, regulating blood and tonifying the kidney. TCM may stabilize symptoms and delay the occurrence of blindness if the patients with RP could stay in the treatment, but there are no known cure.

Clinical Manifestation

1. Night blindness, patients can not see in the twilight, in the dark or dimly lit places. There is a rise in the threshold for dark adaption (decrease in sensitivity).

2. Narrowed vision field in the early stage detection, ring dark spots can be seen in visual field examination, and gradually expands to the internal and external sides. In the late stages of RP, vision field may be constricted to a 10 degree tubular field. Central vision is normal or near normal in the early stages, but if/when the macula becomes affected, the loss of central vision can cause blindness.

3. Fundus examination shows consistency stenosis (hardening from plaque) of retinal vessels, significantly in the retinal arteries. In early stages, scattered bone-like pigments

appear in the equatorial parts. As the disease progresses, the papilla optica shows a yellow wax color. Pigments expand to the peripheral and posterior pole parts, cover in the retinal vessel. The retina often shows a blue gray color, and the choroidal vessels can be seen. Fluorescein angiography shows atrophy of choriocapillaris, snowflake-like high-fluorescence of fundus. Fluorescence leakage in the macula, posterior pole or peripheral parts can sometimes be seen as well.

4. ERG, the amplitude decreases and the peak time delays in a-wave, b-wave, even the waves disappear, which is called extinguished type.

Treatment

1. Pattern Differentiation and Treatment

(1) Insufficiency of Kidney Yang
【Syndrome Characteristics】
Night blindness, progressive constriction of visual field, fundus manifestation is the same as the above, systemic symptoms may include physical cold and cold limbs, limp aching lumbus and knees, pale tongue with thin white coating, a deep thready pulse.
【Treatment Principle】
Warm and supplement kidney yang.
【Representative Formula】
Yòu Guī Wán (Right-Restoring Pill, 右归丸)
【Prescription】

熟地	*shú dì*	20 g	Radix Rehmanniae Praeparata
山药	*shān yào*	15 g	Rhizoma Dioscoreae
山茱萸	*shān zhū yú*	10 g	Fructus Corni
枸杞子	*gǒu qǐ zǐ*	10 g	Fructus Lycii
菟丝子	*tù sī zǐ*	10 g	Semen Cuscutae
杜仲	*dù zhòng*	10 g	Cortex Eucommiae
当归	*dāng guī*	10 g	Radix Angelicae Sinensis
肉桂	*ròu guì*	5 g	Cortex Cinnamomi
制附子	*zhì fù zǐ*	10 g	Radix Aconiti Lateralis Praeparata

【Modifications】
➢ Add *hóng huā* (红花, Flos Carthami Safflower) 10g, *jī xuè téng* (鸡血藤, Caulis Spatholobi) 10g, *niú xī* (牛膝, Radix Achyranthis Bidentatae) 10g to enhance the effects of nourishing and invigorating blood.

(2) Liver-Kidney Yin Deficiency

【Syndrome Characteristics】

Night blindness, progressive constriction of visual field, fundus manifestation is the same as the above, dry eyes and uncomfortable. Systemic symptoms may include dizziness, tinnitus, deafness, insomnia and profuse dreams, red tongue with little coating, thready and rapid pulse.

【Treatment Principle】

Nourish the liver and kidney.

【Representative Formula】

Míng Mù Dì Huáng Tāng (Eye Brightener Rehmannia Decoction, 明目地黄汤)

【Prescription】

熟地	*shú dì*	15 g	Radix Rehmanniae Praeparata
生地	*shēng dì*	15 g	Radix Rehmanniae
山药	*shān yào*	10 g	Rhizoma Dioscoreae
山茱萸	*shān zhū yú*	10 g	Fructus Corni
泽泻	*zé xiè*	10 g	Rhizoma Alismatis
牡丹皮	*mǔ dān pí*	10 g	Cortex Moutan
柴胡	*chái hú*	10 g	Radix Bupleuri
茯苓	*fú líng*	10 g	Poria
当归	*dāng guī*	10 g	Radix Angelicae Sinensis
五味子	*wǔ wèi zǐ*	6 g	Fructus Schisandrae Chinensis

【Modifications】

➢ For cases with stasis macules on the tongue, thin retinal vessels, add *chuān xiōng* (川芎, Rhizoma Chuanxiong) 10g, *jī xuè téng* (鸡血藤, Caulis Spatholobi) 10g, *niú xī* (牛膝, Radix Achyranthis Bidentatae) 10g to strengthen the effect of quickening the blood and freeing the collaterals.

➢ For cases with dry mouth and constipation, add *zhī mǔ* (知母, Rhizoma Anemarrhenae) 10g, *huā fěn* (花粉, Radix Trichosanthis) 10g, *xuán shēn* (玄参, Radix Scrophulariae) 10g, *jué míng zǐ* (决明子, Semen Cassiae) 15g to eliminate heat by nourishing yin, and loosen bowel to relieve constipation.

(3) spleen qi deficiency

【Syndrome Characteristics】

Night blindness, progressive constriction of visual field, fundus manifest as upper shows. Systemic symptoms include white face and fatigued spirit, reduced eating and fatigue, pale tongue with white coating, a weak pulse.

【Treatment Principle】

Supplement the spleen and boost qi.

【 Representative Formula 】

Modified *Bǔ Zhōng Yì Qì Tāng* (Center-Supplementing and Qi-Boosting Decoction, 补中益气汤)

【 Prescription 】

黄芪	*huáng qí*	20 g	Radix Astragali
太子参	*tài zǐ shēn*	20 g	Radix Pseudostellariae
当归	*dāng guī*	15 g	Radix Angelicae Sinensis
白术	*bái zhú*	10 g	Rhizoma Atractylodis Macrocephalae
柴胡	*chái hú*	10 g	Radix Bupleuri
升麻	*shēng má*	6 g	Rhizoma Cimicifugae
陈皮	*chén pí*	10 g	Pericarpium Citri Reticulatae
甘草	*gān cǎo*	3 g	Radix et Rhizoma Glycyrrhizae

【 Modifications 】

➢ Add *chuān xiōng* (川芎, Rhizoma Chuanxiong) 10 g, *dān shēn* (丹参, Radix et Rhizoma Salviae Miltiorrhizae) 15 g, *jī xuè téng* (鸡血藤, Caulis Spatholobi) 10 g, *niú xī* (牛膝, Radix Achyranthis Bidentatae) 10 g to enhance the effects of nourishing and promoting blood.

2. Acupuncture

(1) Body needles

Mainly local acupoints are used, major acupoints include:

tài yáng (太阳)	BL 2 (*cuán zhú*)	ST 1 (*chéng qì*)
BL 1 (*jīng míng*)	GB 20 (*fēng chí*)	SJ 23 (*sī zhú kōng*)
GB 1 (*tóng zǐ liáo*)	*qiú hòu* (球后)	*yú yāo* (鱼腰)
GB 14 (*yáng bái*)		

Adjunct points include:

BL 23 (*shèn shù*)	BL 18 (*gān shù*)	GB 37 (*guāng míng*)
LI 4 (*hé gǔ*)	ST 36 (*zú sān lǐ*)	SP 6 (*sān yīn jiāo*)

For cases with congenital deficiency, debilitation of the *mìng mén* (life gate) fire, add RN 6 (*qì hǎi*), DU 4 (*mìng mén*), BL 23 (*shèn shù*). For cases with liver blood deficiency and deficiency of kidney-essence, add BL 17 (*gé shù*), BL 26 (*guān yuán shù*), RN 4 (*guān yuán*), KI 3 (*tài xī*).

For cases with spleen-stomach deficiency, insufficiency of essential qi, add BL 21 (*wèi shù*), RN 12 (*zhōng wǎn*), ST 36 (*zú sān lǐ*). Each time, select 2–3 local eye acupoints and

2 combination body acupoints.

For eye points acupuncture, use 30–32 guage, 1.5–2 *cun* needles, perpendicularly puncture and slowly insert the needle until an obvious qi sensation manifests, use the even supplementation and drainage method, DO NOT lift, thrust and rotate, retain the needles for 30 minutes, treat once every day. 10 sessions is a treatments course. Patients may take a rest for 3–5 days between two courses.

(2) Electroacupuncture Technique

Main points include *Xin Ming* I (located at the spot 5 fen anterior and superior to acupoint Yi Feng) and *qiú hòu* (球后). Combine points include *Xin Ming* II (located at the depression 1 *cun* above the external end of eyebrow and 5 *fen* lateral more), *yì míng* (翳明). All main points must be selected, but combine points are selected according to the condition.

Needle manipulation technique of *Xin Ming* I : After rapid insertion , slowly direct the needle to (outer) canthus. Needling may be performed differently from patient to patient. For example, someone may get a strong needle sensation when the needle inserted 1.5 centimeters, and someone else at 4.5 centimeters. Needle sensation may present with a local heat sensation in the temple and/or ocular muscle convulsion. Then lift and thrust, using rotate method with small amplitude for 1 minute, frequency of rotating is 160–180 times per minute, amplitude of lifting and thrusting is 1–2 millimeter.

Needle manipulation technique for *qiú hòu* (球后): Use 30–32 gauge, 2 *cun* needle , vertically insert the needle about 3–3.5 centimeters slowly until an obvious Qi-sensation manifests.

Needle manipulation technique for *yì míng* (翳明): Puncture vertically, other techniques are the same as *Xin Ming*.

Then connect electroacupuncture apparatus with bilateral *Xin Ming* II and *yì míng* (翳明). Patients should feel mild convulsion of the eyelids after turning on the apparatus, if not, adjust the direction of needlepoint. Continuous wave, frequency 200 times/min, the intensity should be adjusted to meet the patients pain threshold level. Stimulate for 15–30 minutes. Manipulate *Xin Ming* I and *Xin Ming* II acupoints again as mentioned above when withdrawing the needles. 2 times a week, 10 sessions is a treatment course.

3. Chinese Patent Medicines

(1) *Jīn Guì Shèn Qì Wán* (Golden Cabinet's Kidney Qi Pill, 金匮肾气丸)

Warm the kidney and invigorate yang, replenish essence and supplement the blood, applicable to RP caused by insufficiency of kidney yang, deficiency of kidney-essence.

(2) *Qǐ Jú Dì Huáng Wán* (Lycium Berry, Chrysanthemum and Rehmannia Pill, 杞菊地黄丸)

Enrich yin and supply the kidney, nourish the liver and brighten the eyes, applicable to RP caused by liver-kidney yin deficiency.

(3) *Shí Hú Yè Guāng Wán* (Dendrobium Night Vision Pill, 石斛夜光丸)

Enrich yin and supply the kidney, nourish the liver and brighten the eyes, applicable to RP caused by insufficiency of the liver and kidney, loss of essence and blood, yin deficiency and effulgent fire.

4) *Bǔ Zhōng Yì Qì Wán* (Center-Supplementing and Qi-Boosting Pill, 补中益气丸)
Supply the center and boost qi, upbearing yang and raising the fall, applicable to RP caused by spleen stomach qi deficiency, center qi fall.

4. Simple and proven recipes

Lóng Yǎn Sāng Shèn Gāo: *sāng shèn* (桑椹, Fructus Mori) 1000g, *lóng yǎn ròu* (龙眼肉, Arillus Longan) 500g, add appropriate amount water, stew slowly over heat until the decoction becomes thick, take orally 10g each time, two times a day to supplement the liver and kidney, nourish blood and brighten the eyes; applicable to RP caused by insufficiency of the liver and kidney, insufficiency of qi and blood.

5. External therapy

Acupuncture point injection:

(1) Acupoints: *tài yáng* (太阳); Drugs: Ligustrazine Hydrochloride Injection (*Chuān Xiōng Qín Zhù Shè Yè*, 川芎嗪注射液) or Astragalus Injection (*Huáng Qí Zhù Shè Yè*, 黄芪注射液);

Methods: Extract liquid 1 ml with a gauge 25# needle, after acupoints position and sterilization; insert the needle quickly with an angle of 30° between the needle-tip and the skin. After arriving of qi, inject slowly 0.3–0.5ml liquid into each point. After withdraw of the needle, press the acupoint with a dry and sterilized cotton balls for a moment. Once daily, 10 sessions is a treatment course. It is indicated to take 3-5 days as an interval between two treatment courses.

(2) Acupoints: BL 18 (*gān shù*), BL 23 (*shèn shù*). Drugs: *Fù Fāng Dān Shēn Zhù Shè Yè* (Compound Salviae Miltiorrhiza Injection, 复方丹参注射液), *Líng Zhī Zhù Shè Yè* (Mythic Fungus Injection, 灵芝注射液).

Method: 0.5 ml for each point, inject to bilateral BL 18 (*gān shù*) or BL 23 (*shèn shù*) alternatively, once a day or every other day, 10 sessions is a treatment course.

6. Treatment with Western Medicine

So far, there is no effective treatment for RP. If western medicine treatment needed, the patients might seek advice or treatment for eye doctors. Some recommendations are as follows: vasodilators, vitamin A and B_1, stem cell and tissue therapy and all kinds of growth factors.

7. Dietary Therapy and Preventive Care

(1) *Hé shŏu wū* (何首乌, Radix Polygoni Multiflori) porridge: *Hé shŏu wū* (何首乌, Radix Polygoni Multiflori) 60 g, *jīng mǐ* (粳米, Semen Oryza Sativa)200 g, *dà zăo* (大枣, Fructus Jujubae) 10 (enucleation). Method: Put *hé shŏu wū* in a cooking pot, add the right amount water, decoct for half an hour, then remove the dregs and keep the juice, add rice and Chinese date into the juice and heat it to make porridge. Eat in the morning and evening every day.

(2) *Gŏu qǐ* (枸杞, Fructus Lycii) porridge: *Gŏu qǐ zǐ* (枸杞子, Fructus Lycii) 30 g, *jīng mǐ* (粳米, Semen Oryza Sativa) 60 g, add the right amount water, heat it to make porridge in the usual way, eat in the morning and evening every day. It may supplement the kidney and nourish the liver, replenish vital essence to improve eye sight; applicable to RP caused by insufficiency of the liver and kidney.

(3) Pork Liver and Chinese Wolfberry Leaf Porridge

Pork liver 200 g, fresh Chinese wolfberry leaf 150 g. Method: Wash the pork liver clean and cut it into strips, then stew it with Chinese wolfberry leaf. Drink the soup and eat the liver slices with seasonings, two times everyday. It can supply the liver and boost essence; applicable to RP caused by insufficiency of the liver and kidney.

(4) Select suitable sunglasses to avoid the degeneration of outer segments of retinal cells. According to the lens color theory, sunglasses should use the reddish, purple or violet color. Patients may also select light gray on a cloudy day or when staying indoor, and use dark gray on a sunny day or in strong light. It is not suggested to wear blue-black or green color sunglasses for RP patients.

(5) Avoids mental and emotional stress. Under stress, blood catecholamines levels increase causing the choroid blood vessel to constrict, reducing blood flow and oxygen to the retina. This is one way the psychological stress can aggravate and accelerate the degeneration of retinal cells. Chinese qigong (static gong) can be used adjust the cerebral cortex and has a systemic relaxing effect on the organs of the body. By using one's intention, we can increase blood flow and qi to the eyes with qi gong exercise. If one willingly perseveres with qigong practice, it is possible to arrest the degenerative process.

(6) Prenatal and postnatal care, avoid inter-family marriages.

Case Studies

Pan, a 25-year-old male

[Chief Complaint]

Binocular night blindness for eight years. Before he came to our clinic, he was diagnosed with RP and told there was no treatment available.

【Examination】

Visual acuity: Binoculus 20/200; corrected 20/28, binocular visual fields showed concentric contract, within 15°, clear refracting media, wax yellow papilla, small optic disc with sharp rim, angiostegnosis, central fovea reflex of macula seen, bone cell-like pigmentation at retinal midperiphery, thready pulse, a reddish tongue with thin white coating.

【Diagnosis】

Retinitis pigmentosa.

【Pattern Differentiation】

Spleen deficiency and weak qi, insufficiency of liver blood.

【Treatment Principles】

Supply yang and boost qi, clear the liver and brighten the eyes.

【Prescription】

Modified *Rén Shēn Bǔ Wèi Tāng* (Ginseng supplement stomach Decoction, 人参补胃汤), for one doses everyday. At the same time, add *Huáng Lián Yáng Gān Wán* (Coptis and Goat's Liver Pill, 黄连羊肝丸), 1 pill everyday.

党参	dǎng shēn	12 g	Radix Codonopsis
炙黄芪	zhì huáng qí	15 g	Radix Astragali Praeparata cum Melle
黄柏	huáng bǎi	6 g	Cortex Phellodendri Chinensis
蔓荆子	màn jīng zǐ	10 g	Fructus Viticis
炒白芍	chǎo bái sháo	10 g	Radix Paeoniae Alba
炙甘草	zhì gān cǎo	5 g	Radix et Rhizoma Glycyrrhizae Praeparata cum Melle
夜明砂 (包煎)	yè míng shā (bāo jiān)	12 g	Faeces Vespertilionis (wrap)
谷精草	gǔ jīng cǎo	12 g	Flos Eriocauli

【Follow-up】

The patient visited our clinic six months later. He felt his vision improving, and night blindness obviously getting better. Examination: Visual acuity: binoculus 20/50; corrected 20/16, binocular near visual acuity was jegger1, visual fields extend to 25°, fundus was approximately the same as the previous. Previous representative formula was modified as follows: add *shí jué míng* (石决明, Concha Haliotidis) 25 g (decocted first), *yè míng shā* (夜明砂, bat feces) 15 g (wrap), *bái jí lí* (白蒺藜, caltrop fruit) 12 g, *wǔ wèi zǐ* (五味子, Fructus Schisandrae Chinensis) 3g, to strengthen the curative effect. The patient didn't return for treatment after this visit.

(*Wei Wen-gui Medical Cases Record*, 韦文贵医案)

Classic Quotes

隋·巢元方《诸病源候论》: "人有昼而睛明致瞑则不见物, 世谓之雀目。"

If a person could see clearly at the daylight, but not see at night, it is called bird eye (*què mù*, 雀目).

Treatise on the Origins and Manifestations of Various Diseases (*Zhū Bìng Yuán Hòu Lùn*, 诸病源候论), Sui Dynasty, Chao Yuan-fang

清·吴谦等《医宗金鉴》："高风内障为鸡盲，天晚不明天晓光，夜能上视难见下，损亏肝血肾精伤。"

Gāo fēng nèi zhàng (高风内障) is the same as chick blindness: one can see clearly in the daylight, but not at night, can see things upward clearly but not things at downward at night; caused by deficiency of liver blood and damage of kidney essence.

Golden Mirror of the Medical Tradition (*Yī Zōng Jīn Jiàn*, 医宗金鉴), Qing Dynasty, Wu Qian

Section 8　Retinal Detachment

Retinal detachment refers to the separation between the neuroepithelial and pigment epithelial layers. The disease is commonly seen among middle aged or elderly people, and in younger adults who are highly nearsighted (myopic). Retinal detachment may attack both eyes in succession. The risk factors of the disease include peripheral degeneration of the retina and liquefactive degeneration of the vitreous body, which are associated with age, genetic disposition and trauma. Based on the causes of the diseases, it can be classified into three types: rhegmatogenous, tractional and exudative retinal detachments. Exudative retinal detachment is secondary to severe ocular inflammation, circulation obstruction of the eye (and/or systemically) and the neoplasm of the choroid or orbit. Generally, there are no tears/holes in the retina of exudative retinal detachment cases, and the retina will reattach if the underlying causative factors are controlled. For rhegmatogenous retina detachment, an eye surgery is needed to reattach the retina as soon as possible. While for non- rhegmatogenous retina detachment, it is very important to treat the primary diseases which cause retinal detachment.

In Chinese medicine, retinal detachment is called *Shì Yī Tuō Lí* (视衣脱离). The causes and pathogenesis can be: (1) The spleen-qi deficiency with a collapse of clear yang causing the retina to have a weak attachment and eventually detaches; (2) Prolonged or chronic detachment of the retina results in gradual liver-kidney deficiency and the essence-qi insufficiency, which cause malnourishment of the eye. Integrated treatment between traditional Chinese and Western medicines is most effective. To treat a rhegmatogenous retinal detachment, Chinese medicine is best used post-operative, which can be quite helpful for a quick and more complete recovery. To treat non-rhegmatogenous retinal detachment, conventional medicine is also combined with Chinese medicine for best results.

Clinical Manifestations

Warning symptoms always occur before the detachment of retina which may include flashes of light that accompanies certain eye movements. When a partial retinal detachment happens, a cloudy shadow occurs in the contralateral visual field. Floaters may also be present which drift in the visual field due to vitreous opacity. Vision loss is identified by the location, the range, the degree of vitreous opacity and level of degeneration. If a macular detachment occurs, the central visual loss will be obvious. When a complete retinal detachment occurs, typically only light sensation remains or a complete visual loss results. Metamorphopsia may occur before visual loss. A shaky or "shivering image" may occur with specific eye movements. When a small surface detachment occurs, the intraocular pressure is usually normal or low. When the severity of retinal detachment increases surpassing a quadrant, the intraocular pressure decreases accordingly, and more severe if the detachment area is larger and the time is longer. However, if the retina is reattached and the subretinal fluid is absorbed, the intraocular pressure will typically revert back to a normal state.

To look for the degeneration region, breaks or local retinal detachment, you must dilate the patient's pupil thoroughly first. Examination of the periretinal region can be done by indirect ophthalmoscope along with a sclera buckle or slit lamp along with a three-mirror contact lens. The test can reveal the region where normal red light reflection has been lost and now presents with a gray or bluish gray, may be slight quivering with dark red vessels on the surface. The severe detached retina can cloud the optic disc and form folds. Without a careful examination, diagnosis of a flat retinal detachment can be easily missed. When macular region is involved, the macular center appears to be relatively dark red in color and somewhat transparent and is obviously different from the grayish-white presentation associated with a detached retina.

It is common to find holes or tears in retinal detachment. The key of the treatment of this disease is to find and seal the holes. A typical hole is normally red when compared, to the grayish-white color of the detached retina. This usually occurs in the superotemporal or subtermporal quadrant and is seldom seen in the nasal side. The holes in the ora serrata always show up in the subtemporal or the lower quadrant, however, they can also take place in the macular region or in areas where the retina is fully attached. The size and the number of the holes are typically not equal. The shapes of holes can vary. Some may appear round, u-shaped, barred, along the margin of ora serrata or irregular. The eminent detached retina may cover the holes. Therefore, when performing the examination, one can change the position of the patient's head or bind the two eyes, and let the patient lay in bed for 1 or 2 days, and then examine the fundus once the eminence of retina is reduced. In the cases with severe vitreous opacity, the back of the eye may be difficult to check. Ocular ultrasonic examination may be used to find out whether or not there is a retinal detachment.

Treatment

1. Pattern Differentiation and Treatment

(1) Spleen Qi Deficiency

【Syndrome Characteristics】

Blurred vision, vitreous opacity, retina detachment; or subretinal dropsy after the re-attachment; may be accompanied by fatigue, pale complexion, loose stool, anorexia; pale tongue body with teeth prints, white slippery coating, a thready or soft pulse.

【Treatment Principle】

Fortify the spleen and replenish the qi, ascend yang and restore the collapsed.

【Representative Formula】

Modified *Bǔ Zhōng Yì Qì Tāng* (Middle-Tonifying Qi-Replenishing Decoction, 补中益气汤) and *Sì Líng Sǎn* (Powder of Four Prescription with Poria, 四苓散)

【Prescription】

黄芪	*huáng qí*	20 g	Radix Astragali seu Hedysari
太子参	*tài zǐ shēn*	20 g	Radix Pseudostellariae
当归	*dāng guī*	15 g	Radix Angelicae Sinensis
白术	*bái zhú*	10 g	Rhizoma Atractylodis Macrocephalae
柴胡	*chái hú*	10 g	Radix Bupleuri
升麻	*shēng má*	6 g	Rhizoma Cimicifugae
陈皮	*chén pí*	10 g	Pericarpium Citri Reticulatae
泽泻	*zé xiè*	20 g	Rhizoma Alismatis
茯苓	*fú líng*	20 g	Poria
猪苓	*zhū líng*	20 g	Polyporus
甘草	*gān cǎo*	3 g	Radix et Rhizoma Glycyrrhizae

【Modifications】

➤ For cases with profuse dropsy, add *cāng zhú* (苍术, Rhizoma Atractylodis) 10 g, *chē qián zǐ* (车前子, Semen Plantaginis) 20 g (packed) and *yì yǐ rén* (薏苡仁, Semen Coicis) 10 g to promote urination and drain dampness.

(2) Stasis and Stagnation in the Vessels and Collaterals

【Syndrome Characteristics】

Retinal edema or subretinal dropsy after trauma or operation; could be accompanied by eye pain, headache; dark red tongue body with ecchymosis, a wiry and thready pulse.

【Treatment Principle】

Invigorate blood and resolve stasis, promote urination and relieve edema.

【 Representative Formula 】
Modified *Táo Hóng Sì Wù Tāng* (Peach Seed, Safflower and Four Prescription Decoction, 桃红四物汤)
【 Prescription 】

桃仁	*táo rén*	10 g	Semen Persicae
红花	*hóng huā*	10 g	Flos Carthami
生地	*shēng dì*	20 g	Radix Rehmanniae Recens
当归	*dāng guī*	10 g	Radix Angelicae Sinensis
赤芍	*chì sháo*	10 g	Radix Paeoniae Rubra
丹参	*dān shēn*	10 g	Radix Salviae Miltiorrhizae
防风	*fáng fēng*	10 g	Radix Saposhnikoviae
茯苓	*fú líng*	10 g	Poria
泽泻	*zé xiè*	10 g	Rhizoma Alismatis

【 Modifications 】
➢ For cases with eye pain, add *sū mù* (苏木, Lignum Sappan) 10 g and *zé lán* (泽兰, Herba Lycopi) 10 g to reinforce the action of resolving stasis, relieving pain and edema; for the cases with severe retinal edema accompanied by qi deficiency, add *shēng huáng qí* (生黄芪, Radix Astragali) 30 g and *chǎo bái zhú* (炒白术, dry-fried Rhizoma Atractylodis Macrocephalae) 15 g to replenish qi, dry dampness and relieve edema.

(3) liver and kidney yin deficiency
【 Syndrome Characteristics 】
Long term, chronic detachment of the retina, progressive retinal degeneration can be seen in the fundus of the eye or the post-operative improvement in vision is not satisfactory, dry eye; vertigo, tinnitus, aching lumbar and knee; pale tongue with little coating, a deep and thready pulse.
【 Treatment Principle 】
Nourish the liver and kidney.
【 Representative Formula 】
Modified *Bǔ Shèn Cí Shí Wán* (Tonify-kidney and Magnetite Pill, 补肾磁石丸)
【 Prescription 】

煅磁石	*duàn cí shí*	15 g	Calcined Magnetitum (decocted first)
菊花	*jú huā*	10 g	Flos Chrysanthemi
石决明	*shí jué míng*	20 g	Concha Haliotidis
肉苁蓉	*ròu cōng róng*	15 g	Herba Cistanches
菟丝子	*tù sī zǐ*	15 g	Semen Cuscutae
枸杞子	*gǒu qǐ zǐ*	15 g	Fructus Lycii

桑椹	*sāng shèn*	15 g	Fructus Mori
五味子	*wǔ wèi zǐ*	6 g	Fructus Schisandrae Chinensis
楮实子	*chǔ shí zǐ*	10 g	Fructus Broussonetiae
茺蔚子	*chōng wèi zǐ*	10 g	Fructus Leonuri

【Modifications】

➢ For cases with minimal or no eyesight improvement accompanied by insufficiency of qi and blood, add *mài dōng* (麦冬, Radix Ophiopogonis) 10 g, *tài zǐ shēn* (太子参, Radix Pseudostellariae) 20 g, *dāng guī* (当归, Radix Angelicae Sinensis) 10g, *chuān xiōng* (川芎, Rhizoma Chuanxiong) 10 g, *chì sháo* (赤芍, Radix Paeoniae Rubra) 10 g to replenish qi and nourish blood, nourish yin and brighten eyes.

2. Chinese Patent Medicines

(1) *Bǔ Zhōng Yì Qì Wán* (**Middle-Tonifying Qi-Replenishing Pill**, 补中益气丸)

Tonifying middle *jiao* and replenishing qi, ascending yang and relieving collapse. 9 g, twice a day, oral administration, applicable to the spleen qi deficiency and upward invasion of dampness-turbidity.

(2) *Jīn Guì Yì Qì Wán* (**Jingui Tonifying Qi Pill**, 金匮益气丸)

Warming kidney and strengthening yang, sufficing essence and tonifying blood. 9 g each time, twice a day, oral administration, applicable to spleen and kidney yang deficiency.

(3) *Shí Hú Yè Guāng Wán* (**Dendrobium and Night Light Pill**, 石斛夜光丸)

Nourishing yin and tonifying kidney, clearing liver and brightening eyes. 9 g, twice a day, oral administration; applicable to the insufficiency of the liver and kidney.

3. Treatment with Western Medicine

The chief treatment for retina detachment is an operation, which aims to seal retinal breaks, drain subretinal fluid and reattach retina. There are many surgical methods, such as the sclera buckle combined with cryotherapy or laser photocoagulation, and subretinal fluid drainage. In complicated cases, vitrectomy is necessary.

4. Dietary Therapy and Preventive Care

(1) Avoid eye strain and fatigue, as well as lifting heavy objects and violent exercise.

(2) Stay in bed before the eye surgery, wear stenopeic spectacles or cover both eyes; Avoid eye movement in order to prevent the exacerbating the existing retinal detachment condition.

(3) 1% atropine eye ointment is typically prescribed conventionally. It can fully

anaesthetize the ciliary and sphincter muscles of the pupil, thereby, hindering the pupil from contract during the operation.

Questions for Considerations

1. What is retinal detachment? How is it classified according to causes?

2. What is retinal detachment called in Chinese medicine, and what is the cause and pathogenesis?

Section 9   Ischemic Optic Neuropathy

Ischemic optic neuropathy is the most common acute optic neuropathy in people over the age of 50. Optic neuropathy is divided into two types based on the affected area of the optic nerve: anterior ischemic optic neuropathy and posterior ischemic optic neuropathy. The former is caused by ischemia of the short posterior ciliary arteries that supply the optic disc, resulting in hypoperfusion of anterior optic nerve. Presenting symptoms may include vision loss and papilloedema. The latter is acute ischemia of the optic nerve portion between cribriform plate and optic chiasm due to interruption of blood flow of arterial supply to the optic nerve. The cases present with vision impairment at the initial stages, and the fundus examination is always normal. The disease is also divided to two forms based on the causative factors: arteritic and non-arteritic. In clinic, non-arteritic anterior ischemic optic neuropathy (NAAION) is more common than the other type and occupies about 90% cases. According to the research carried out at the state of California in USA, the incidence occurs in (2.3–10.2)/100,000 in the people older than 50 years. The whole population incidence is 0.5/100,000, it also can be seen in the young people. Another statistic from 406 NAAION cases (done by Hayreh, USA) shows that the ages of onset range from 11 years old to 91 years old with average of (60 ± 14) years. The risk factors of ION mainly involve hypertension, arteriosclerosis, diabetes, hyperlipemia, hypotension due to blood loss and shock, abnormal blood flow and ocular hypertension.

In TCM, the disease is called *shì zhān hūn miǎo* (blurred vision, 视瞻昏渺) or *mù xì bào máng* (sudden blindness, 目系暴盲). The cause and pathogenesis can be associated with a diet high in fat, refined sugars, acrid and spicy food, drinking (alcohol) without continence. This results in internal phlegm and dampness, combined together with external wind pathogen obstructing the collaterals thus causing eye orifice blocked. Another causative factor is associated with yin damage due to prolonged illness or yin deficiency of the liver and kidney due to age. This pattern can result in yang hyperactivity harassing the eye collaterals. Another causative factor may be emotional rage which impairs the liver, causes counter flow of the qi dynamic and causes qi-fire to attack upward resulting in stasis and closure of eye collaterals. Besides yin and blood deficiency resulting from trauma, severe blood loss may also cause vacuity of the eye vessels and dystrophy of the ocular system.

In western medicine, most doctors insist on glucocorticoid therapy as well as vasodilation drugs that promote circulation, and nerve-nourishing supplements like Vitamin B_1 and Vitamin B_{12} in addition to treating the underlying cause. Some cases can also be treated with hyperbaric oxygen treatment to elevate aortic diastolic pressure, increase oxygen and blood flow of the common carotid artery, thus to improve the blood supply to the ophthalmic artery (OA). Improving blood flow to the OA will benefit and stabilize a patient's condition and improve overall visual acuity. In TCM, using individualized treatment method based on pattern differentiation may improve both the condition of the whole body and visual function.

Clinical Manifestations

1. Symptoms: Sudden vision loss or dark shadow in some area of the visual field which attacks one eye, often shortly upon awakening. Vision in the involved eye can range from almost normal to complete blindness. Usually, there is no pain, a few cases may complain transient vision blurred. The disease commonly attacks one eye, however, second eye involvement occurs in about 15%–30% of patients.

2. Signs: RAPD may be found in the affected eye. The optic disc or sectorial disk may be swollen, accompanied by small hemorrhages surrounding it. Some cases present with a smaller optic disc and a smaller or nonexistent cup. There may be segmental or a pale appearance to the optic nerve. The palor occurs after regression of edema, which is also known as optic atrophy. For patients with both eyes affected, edema may be present at one optic disc and optic atrophy in the other disk. The fundus examination is always normal in patients with posterior ischemic optic neuropathy during the initial stages. However, optic atrophy will occur as the condition progresses to the later stages.

3. Auxiliary examination: Auxiliary examination is very important for this condition, in order to help make the diagnosis and to help identify the causes and provide evidence to support a treatment plan.

(1) Perimetry: The classic finding in the AION patients is half visual field loss linked up with the physiological blind spot (either the upper or the lower). Fan-shaped or quadrant visual field defects may also be found. Some cases present with a perpendicular visual field loss, but it is not clearly defined. Patients may also present with bundle scotoma with normal central fixation, so the vision acuity may keep at 20/20–20/13.

(2) Visual Electrophysiology: Peak latency period of P100 may be delayed in pattern VEP or flash VEP examination, and amplitude may also be decreased.

(3) Fluorescence Fundus Angiography (FFA): In the early stage, fluorescence of the optic nerve may appear weak or delayed and uneven, during the later stages fluorescence leakage can be found.

(4) Transcranial Doppler Sonography (TCD) or Color Doppler Images (CDI): In some cases, the speed of blood flow in ophthalmic artery or posterior ciliary arteries may decrease or increase in the resistance index.

(5) Other examination: Blood glucose, blood pressure, blood fat, blood viscosity, erythrocyte sedimentation rate (ESR) and C reactive proteins (CRP) have been found useful in diagnosing.

4. If the patients are elderly and symptoms are accompanied by headache, tenderness of the scalp, fatigue, weight loss, marked elevated ESR, increased CRP and tenderness at temporal artery area, biopsy of temporal artery is highly recommended in order to find out if there is an arteritic anterior ischemic optic neuropathy present.

Treatment

1. Pattern Differentiation and Treatment

(1) Wind Phlegm Obstructing the Collaterals
〖 Syndrome Characteristics 〗
Acute vision loss, dizziness, dyspnea, phlegm in the throat, enlarged tongue with greasy coating, a wiry or slippery pulse.
〖 Treatment Principle 〗
Extinguish fire and transform phlegm, activate blood and dredge the collaterals.
〖 Representative Formula 〗
Modified *Dǎo Tán Tāng* (Phlegm-Expelling Decoction, 导痰汤)
〖 Prescription 〗

姜半夏	*jiāng bàn xià*	6 g	Rhizoma Pinelliae Praeparatum
枳实	*zhǐ shí*	6 g	Fructus Aurantii Immaturus
茯苓	*fú líng*	6 g	Poria
橘红	*jú hóng*	6 g	Exocarpium Citri Rubrum
甘草	*gān cǎo*	3 g	Radix et Rhizoma Glycyrrhizae
当归	*dāng guī*	6 g	Radix Angelicae Sinensis
丹参	*dān shēn*	6 g	Radix et Rhizoma Salviae Miltiorrhizae
枳壳	*zhǐ qiào*	10 g	Fructus Aurantii
胆南星	*dǎn nán xīng*	6 g	Arisaema cum Bile
生姜	*shēng jiāng*	10 pieces	Rhizoma Zingiberis Recens

〖 Modifications 〗
➢ For cases with marked heat syndromes add *huáng qín* (黄芩, Radix Scutellariae) 10 g, *zhú rú* (竹茹, Caulis Bambusae in Taenia) 6 g and *sāng yè* (桑叶, Folium Mori) 6 g to clear heat in the lung and the liver.

➤ For cases with constipation add *guā lóu* (瓜蒌, Fructus Trichosanthis) 6 g and *shú dà huáng* (熟大黄, Radix et Rhizoma Rhei Praeparata) 6 g to clear heat and relieve constipation.

(2) qi stagnation and blood stasis

【 Syndrome Characteristics 】

Acute vision loss, vexation and morosity, dull pain in the head and eyes, fullness in the chest and rib-side, dull purple tongue or stasis macule, a wiry and rapid pulse.

【 Treatment Principle 】

Move qi and invigorate blood.

【 Representative Formula 】

Xuè Fǔ Zhú Yū Tāng (Blood Stasis Expelling Decoction, 血府逐瘀汤)

【 Prescription 】

桃仁	*táo rén*	12 g	Semen Persicae
红花	*hóng huā*	9 g	Flos Carthami
生地	*shēng dì*	9 g	Radix Rehmanniae
川芎	*chuān xiōng*	5 g	Rhizoma Chuanxiong
赤芍	*chì sháo*	6 g	Radix Paeoniae Rubra
当归	*dāng guī*	9 g	Radix Angelicae Sinensis
牛膝	*niú xī*	9 g	Radix Achyranthis Bidentatae
桔梗	*jié gěng*	5 g	Radix Platycodonis
柴胡	*chái hú*	3 g	Radix Bupleuri
枳壳	*zhǐ qiào*	6 g	Fructus Aurantii
甘草	*gān cǎo*	3 g	Radix et Rhizoma Glycyrrhizae

【 Modifications 】

➤ For patients with lack of strength and no desire talk, add *huáng qí* (黄芪, Radix Astragali) 15 g and *dǎng shēn* (党参, Radix Codonopsis) 10 g to replenish qi and invigorate blood.

➤ For cases with marked vexation and qi stagnation add *fó shǒu* (佛手, Fructus Citri Sarcodactylis) 10 g and *mù xiāng* (木香, Radix Aucklandiae) 10 g to soothe the liver and regulate the spleen.

➤ For patients with hypertension add *zhēn zhū mǔ* (珍珠母, Concha Margaritiferae Usta) 20 g and *gōu téng* (钩藤, Ramulus Uncariae Cum Uncis) to calm the liver and release pressure.

(3) Yin deficiency and yang hyperactivity

【 Syndrome Characteristics 】

Acute vision loss or sudden dark shadow in front of the eye, dizziness and tinnitus, distending pain of the head and the eyes, impatience and irritability, low back and knee pain and/or weakness, insomnia and forgetfulness, red tongue with thin yellow coating, wiry and rapid pulse.

【 Treatment Principle 】

Calm the liver and extinguish the fire, nourish yin and activate the collaterals.

【 Representative Formula 】

Tiān Má Gōu Téng Yǐn (Gastrodia and Uncaria Decoction, 天麻钩藤饮)

【 Prescription 】

天麻	*tiān má*	10 g	Rhizoma Gastrodiae
钩藤	*gōu téng*	12 g	Ramulus Uncariae Cum Uncis
石决明 (先煎)	*shí jué míng (xiān jiān)*	18 g	Concha Haliotidis (wrap boiling and decocted first)
川牛膝	*chuān niú xī*	12 g	Radix Cyathulae
栀子	*zhī zǐ*	12 g	Fructus Gardeniae
黄芩	*huáng qín*	10 g	Radix Scutellariae
杜仲	*dù zhòng*	10 g	Cortex Eucommiae
益母草	*yì mǔ cǎo*	10 g	Herba Leonuri
桑寄生	*sāng jì shēng*	10 g	Herba Taxilli
茯神	*fú shén*	10 g	Sclerotium Poriae Pararadicis
夜交藤	*yè jiāo téng*	10 g	Caulis Polygoni Multiflori

【 Modifications 】

➢ For cases with emotional fluctuation or depression add *chái hú* (柴胡, Radix Bupleuri) 10 g and *yù jīn* (郁金, Radix Curcumae) 10 g to soothe the liver and regulate qi.

➢ For cases with normal or hypotension but marked stenosis of the retinal artery, remove *shí jué míng* (Concha Haliotidis) and add *tài zǐ shēn* (太子参, Radix Pseudostellariae) 20 g, *dǎng shēn* (党参, Radix Codonopsis) 10 g and *dì long* (地龙, Pheretima) 10 g to benefit qi, dredge collaterals and brighten the eyes.

➢ For cases with constipation add *jué míng zǐ* (决明子, Semen Cassiae) 15 g and *huǒ má rén* (火麻仁, Fructus Cannabis) to moisten the intestines to relieve constipation.

(4) Qi and Blood Deficiency

【 Syndrome Characteristics 】

Blurred vision, lack of energy, no desire to talk, pale complexion, palpitations and insomnia, pale tongue, weak and thready pulse.

【 Treatment Principle 】

Replenish qi and tonify blood, nourish the heart and tranquilize the mind.

【 Representative Formula 】

Modified *Guī Pí Tāng* (归脾汤, Spleen-Restoring Decoction)

【 Prescription 】

| 白术 | *bái zhú* | 15 g | Rhizoma Atractylodis Macrocephalae (dry-fried) |
| 黄芪 | *huáng qí* | 15 g | Radix Astragali |

茯苓	*fú líng*	15 g	Poria
人参	*rén shēn*	10 g	Radix et Rhizoma Ginseng
甘草	*gān cǎo*	6 g	Radix et Rhizoma Glycyrrhizae
木香	*mù xiāng*	10 g	Radix Aucklandiae
远志	*yuǎn zhì*	10 g	Radix Polygalae
酸枣仁	*suān zǎo rén*	15 g	Semen Ziziphi Spinosae
龙眼肉	*lóng yǎn ròu*	10 g	Arillus Longan
当归	*dāng guī*	10 g	Radix Angelicae Sinensis
枸杞子	*gǒu qǐ zǐ*	10 g	Fructus Lycii
楮实子	*chǔ shí zǐ*	10 g	Fructus Broussonetiae

【Modifications】

➢ For cases with marked symptoms of yin deficiency add *huáng qí* (Radix Astragali) to 30 g.

➢ For cases with marked symptoms of blood deficiency add *ē jiāo* (阿胶, Colla Corii Asini) 10 g and *zhì hé shǒu wū* (制何首乌, Radix Polygoni Multiflori Praeparata cum Succo Glycines Sotae) 10 g to nourish yin and tonify blood.

➢ For cases with marked syndrome of collaterals and vessels obstruction add *dān shēn* (丹参, Radix et Rhizoma Salviae Miltiorrhizae) 10 g, *dì lóng* (地龙, Pheretima) 10 g and *zhǐ qiào* (枳壳, Fructus Aurantii) 10g to dredge the collaterals and open the orifices.

2. Acupuncture

(1) Needling method

For cases with yin deficiency and yang hyperactivity, choose acupoints GB 20 (*fēng chí*), GB 43 (*xiá xī*), LR 2 (*xíng jiān*), GB 14 (*yáng bái*), GB 15 (*tóu lín qì*) and Bl 23 (*shèn shù*). For cases with qi stagnation and blood stasis choose acupoints LR 3 (*tài chōng*) LR 6 (*zhōng dū*), LR 5 (*lí gōu*), BL 18 (*gān shù*).

For cases with qi and blood deficiency choose acupoints ST 36 (*zú sān lǐ*), LI 4 (*hé gǔ*), SP 6 (*sān yīn jiāo*), BL 20 (*pí shù*) and RN 6 (*qì hǎi*). Choose 2–3 acupoints each time, mainly use supplementation method, however, for cases with qi stagnation and blood stasis mainly use the drainage method or even supplementation and drainage; treat daily or every other day, ten treatments equals one course of treatment.

(2) Electro-acupuncture: Choose the accurate acupoints (sample point prescription) and insert needles, turn on the electro-acupuncture device after arriving of qi, use continuous wave or sparse-dense wave with moderate stimulation, 20 minutes each time, 10 treatments equals one course.

(3) Scalp acupuncture: Choose optic area (originate 1 cm lateral to the midpoint of the occipital protuberance and runs for 4 cm parallel to the anterior-posterior line in an

anterior direction), puncture downwards symmetrically, one time each day or every other day, 10 sessions is a treatment course.

3. Chinese Patent Medicine

(1) *Xuè Fǔ Zhú Yū Jiāo Náng* (血府逐瘀胶囊 , **Blood Stasis Expelling Capsules**)

6 pills, two times a day. *Yín Xìng Yè Piàn* (银杏叶片, Ginggo Leaf Tablets), two tablets, three times a day. Both are useful as an adjunctive treatment for patterns of qi stagnation and blood stasis.

(2) *Huó Xuè Tōng Mài Piàn* (活血通脉片 , **Blood-Activating and Vessels-Freeing Tablets**)

4–5 tablets, 2–3 times a day. It is applicable to qi stagnation and blood stasis accompanied by qi deficiency.

(3) *Tiān Má Gōu Téng Kē Lì* (天麻钩藤颗粒 , **Gastrodia and Uncaria Granules**)

1 pouch (10 g), three times a day. *Zhèng Tiān Wán* (正天丸, Sky Righting Pill), 6 g, 2–3 times each day, 15 days is one course of treatment. These two drugs are more applicable to patterns of yin deficiency and yang hyperactivity accompanied by hypertension.

4. Dietary Therapy and Preventive Care

(1) Avoid fatty, sweet and heavy foods. Consume more fruits, vegetables and "white meat" like fish and shrimp. Drink enough water every day in order to keep hydrated, especially during the summer season. Alcohol should be limited and smoking should be prohibited.

(2) Lecithin, fish oils, blueberry and nuts are helpful for this condition.

(3) Get regular annual physical examinations after age 50, treat conditions of hypertension, diabetes and hyperlipidemia promptly.

(4) Get plenty of outdoor exercise every day, control emotion fluctuations and intemperance. Also, avoid mental overwork as this can exhaust the qi and blood.

Case Studies

Liao, male, 56 years old

First visit: August 6, 1989

【 Chief Complaint 】

The right eye vision loss for one month.

【 Medical History 】

The patient had a medical history of hypertension for 20 years, always suffered from dizziness and distending pain of head.

【 Examination 】

His visual acuity is 20/33 (corrected: 20/20) on the right and 20/600 (uncorrectable) on the left. The refractive media of both eyes was clear. Fundus examination: the right optic disc was normal, while the left disc presented obscure boundary with pale appearance at the temporal side, and there was a crossing sign of the artery and vein.

Visual field examination: It was normal on the right eye. There was a bundle-scotoma linked up with physiological blind spot on the left eye. In the P-VEP examination the peak latency period of P100 wave was delayed. There was no abnormal findings in brain CT test.

BP: 160/100 mmHg.

【Diagnosis】

Sudden blindness (ischemic optic atrophy)

【Pattern Differentiation】

Deficiency of the liver and the kidney, insufficiency of qi and blood.

【Treatment Principles】

Nourish blood and harmonize blood, supplement the liver and kidney.

【Prescription】

熟地黄	shú dì huáng	15 g	Radix Rehmanniae Praeparata
枸杞子	gǒu qǐ zǐ	15 g	Fructus Lycii
当归	dāng guī	10 g	Radix Angelicae Sinensis
女贞子	nǚ zhēn zǐ	10 g	Fructus Ligustri Lucidi
丝瓜络	sī guā luò	10 g	Retinervus Luffae Fructus
决明子	jué míng zǐ	10 g	Semen Cassiae
蔓荆子	màn jīng zǐ	10 g	Fructus Viticis
川芎	chuān xiōng	6 g	Rhizoma Chuanxiong

All medicinals decocted with water, one dose per day.

【Follow-up】

After 15 days treatment, the visual acuity of the left eye was increased to 20/40. There was no obvious change in anterior segment examination and fundus examination, but the bundle scotoma got smaller.

Classic Quotes

《秘传眼科龙木论》："此眼初患之时，眼朦昏暗，并无赤痛，内无翳膜"。

When attacked by this disease, vision will become blurred but there will be no pain, no redness and no nebula of the eye.

Longmu's Ophthalmology Secretly Handed Down (Mì Chuán Yǎn Kē Lóng Mù Lùn, 秘传眼科龙木论)

《灵枢·决气》："气脱者目不明"。

Those who are depleted of qi will lose their sight.

Magic Pivot – Understanding of Qi (Líng Shū – Jué Qì, 灵枢·决气)

Section 10   Optic Neuritis

Optic neuritis (ON) refers to inflammation of the optic nerve and is the most common optic nerve disorder seen in clinical practice. An epidemiology study from Minnesota, USA reported that most cases of ON are associated with demyelenation of the optic nerve, the annual incidence of acute optic neuritis caused by demyelenation is 5/100,000, with a prevalence estimated to be 115/100,000. ON typically affects young adults, 77 percent of patients are women. Up to 65% of patients present with symptoms of retrobulbar neuritis, which includes a sudden visual loss and central scotoma, while the fundus is normal during the acute episode. A small number of patients present with a swollen optic nerve head or/and exudates at the macular area, which are associated with papillitis optica and neuroretinitis respectively. Papillitis optica and neuroretinitis commonly afflict children and always attack binocularly.

The causes of ON are very complicated, in the past it was thought to be due to an infectious process of structures neighboring the optic nerve such as the accessory nasal cavity and/or gums. Now it is generally accepted that ON is an autoimmune demyelenating disease, clinically it appears as isolated and monosymptom optic neuritis, also called idiopathetic ON, or it may be the initial manifestation of multiple sclerosis, followed by other symptoms of the central nervous system in succession.

In traditional Chinese Medicine, ON pertains to the diseases of *bào máng* (sudden blindness, 暴盲) or *shì zhān hūn miǎo* (blurring vision, 视瞻昏渺). This disease process can be caused by exogenous pathogenic heat which attacks the *zang-fu* organs and promotes hyperactivity of liver fire that rises upwards and damages the eye(s). Another causative factor is the constraining of liver qi (caused by emotional depression) leading to stagnation of qi in the eye(s). Effulgent fire caused by yin deficiency or/and weakness due to prolonged disease flames upwards the eye can be another causative underlying pattern.

In western medicine, treatment with high dose corticosteroid such as intravenous methylprednisolone is commonly recommended for patients with severe vision damage at the acute episode. For those patients for whom steroids are unsuitable, or for those who do not respond to steroid therapy, or those who have serious adverse reaction to steroid therapy, TCM treatment will be necessary and highly effective with prompt treatment.

Clinical Manifestations

Manifestations of typical optic neuritis include one or more of the following:
- Usually, young adults aged 15–45 and typically attacked in one eye.
- Vision loss is acute or subacute with vision acuity dropping to light perception or even no light perception in several hours or several days. This can also happen as slow and

gradual onset with little or no symptoms.
- Pain may appear before vision loss occurs or during the process of vision loss. The pain may become worse when the patient move the eye.
- A relative afferent pupillary defect (RAPD) or Marcus Gunn pupil may be found in the affected eye. Direct pupillary light reaction will disappear if the affected eye has lost light perception.
- Central scotoma or paracentral scotoma.
- The optic head appears normal or slightly edema at acute episode and may become pale 2-8 weeks later.
- For most patients, majority of visual function will recover in several weeks or several months after onset.
- Some patients present with ambiopia, temporal limb anaesthesia, acratia, defecation or urinary disturbance, which indicate the possibility of multiple sclerosis.

Treatment

1. Pattern Differentiation and Treatment

(1) Excess Heat in the Liver Channel
【 Syndrome Characteristics 】
Sudden vision loss or blindness, distending pain in head and eye or ocular pain with eye movement, dysphoria and irritable, bitter taste in mouth and pain in hypochodrium, red tongue with yellow coating, a wiry and rapid pulse.
【 Treatment Principle 】
Clear the liver and reduce fire.
【 Representative Formula 】
Modified *Lóng Dǎn Xiè Gān Tāng* (Gentian Liver-Draining Decoction, 龙胆泻肝汤)
【 Prescription 】

龙胆草	*lóng dǎn cǎo*	10 g	Radix et Rhizoma Gentianae
黄芩	*huáng qí*	10 g	Radix Astragali
栀子	*zhī zǐ*	10 g	Fructus Gardeniae
车前子（包煎）	*chē qián zǐ (bāo jiān)*	15 g	Semen Plantaginis (wrap)
生地黄	*shēng dì huáng*	15 g	Radix Rehmanniae
当归	*dāng guī*	12 g	Radix Angelicae Sinensis
柴胡	*chái hú*	6 g	Radix Bupleuri
金银花	*jīn yín huā*	10 g	Flos Lonicerae Japonicae
连翘	*lián qiào*	10 g	Fructus Forsythiae
甘草	*gān cǎo*	6 g	Radix et Rhizoma Glycyrrhizae

【Modifications】

➢ For cases with severe distending pain in the head and eye, add *xià kū cǎo* (夏枯草, Spica Prunellae) 10 g and *jú huā* (菊花, Flos Chrysanthemi) 10 g to clear the head and eye thus relieving pain.

➢ For patients with dry mouth and tongue, and constipation add *tiān huā fěn* (天花粉, Radix Trichosanthis) 10 g and *jué míng zǐ* (决明子, Semen Cassiae) 10 g to nourish yin and engender liquid thus moistening the intestines to relieve constipation.

(2) Liver constraint and Qi Stagnation

【Syndrome Characteristics】

Severe vision loss, eye dull pain, emotional depression, chest stuffy pain or menstrual irregularities, red tongue with thin coating, a wiry pulse or wiry and rapid pulse.

【Treatment Principle】

Soothe the liver and relieve depression, cool the blood and dredge the collaterals.

【Representative Formula】

Modified *Dān Zhī Xiāo Yáo Sǎn* (Peony Bark and Gardenia Free Wanderer Powder, 丹栀逍遥散)

【Prescription】

柴胡	*chái hú*	15 g	Radix Bupleuri
栀子	*zhī zǐ*	10 g	Fructus Gardeniae
牡丹皮	*mǔ dān pí*	10 g	Cortex Moutan
当归	*dāng guī*	10 g	Radix Angelicae Sinensis
白芍	*bái sháo*	10 g	Radix Paeoniae Alba
茯苓	*fú líng*	10 g	Poria
蔓荆子	*màn jīng zǐ*	10 g	Fructus Viticis
石菖蒲	*shí chāng pú*	10 g	Rhizoma Acori Tatarinowii
薄荷 (后下)	*bò he (hòu xià)*	6 g	Herba Menthae (decocted later)
甘草	*gān cǎo*	10 g	Radix et Rhizoma Glycyrrhizae

【Modifications】

➢ For cases with stagnant heat obstructing collateral causing dull pain in head and eye, add *jué míng zǐ* (决明子, Semen Cassiae) 10 g and *dān shēn* (丹参, Radix et Rhizoma Salviae Miltiorrhizae) 10 g to clear heat, resolve stasis and relieve pain.

➢ For patients with emotional depression add *yù jīn* (郁金, Radix Curcumae) 10 g and *qīng pí* (青皮, Pericarpium Citri Reticulatae Viride) 10 g to regulate qi and relieve depression.

➢ For patients with severe chest stuffiness and pain in the rib-side add *chuān liàn zǐ* (川楝子, Fructus Toosendan) 10 g and *guā lóu* (瓜蒌, Fructus Trichosanthis) 10 g to soothe the emotions and move qi thus relieving pain.

(3) Yin Deficiency and Effulgent Fire

【Syndrome Characteristics】

Eye symptoms are the same as above accompanied by dizziness and tinnitus, vexing heat in chest, palms and soles, dry mouth and red cheeks, sore waist and dry stool.

【Treatment Principle】

Nourish yin and reduce fire.

【Representative Formula】

Modified *Zhī Bǎi Dì Huáng Tāng* (知柏地黄汤, Anemarrhena, Phellodendron and Rehmannia Decotion)

【Prescription】

生地黄	*shēng dì huáng*	15 g	Radix Rehmanniae
熟地黄	*shú dì huáng*	10 g	Radix Rehmanniae Praeparata
山茱萸	*shān zhū yú*	15 g	Fructus Corni
淮山药	*huái shān yào*	15 g	Rhizoma Dioscoreae
泽泻	*zé xiè*	10 g	Rhizoma Alismatis
牡丹皮	*mǔ dān pí*	10 g	Cortex Moutan
茯苓	*fú líng*	10 g	Poria
龟板	*guī bǎn*	15 g	Plastrum Testudinis
女贞子	*nǚ zhēn zǐ*	15 g	Fructus Ligustri Lucidi

【Modifications】

➢ For patients with dizziness and distending eye pain, add *shí jué míng* (石决明, Concha Haliotidis) 20 g (decocted first), and *gōu téng* (钩藤, Ramulus Uncariae Cum Uncis) 15 g to pacify the liver and subdue yang.

➢ For patients with vexing heat and thirst, add *shí gāo* (石膏, Gypsum Fibrosum) 10 g, *shí hú* (石斛, Caulis Dendrobii) 10 g and *lú gēn* (芦根, Rhizoma Phragmitis) 10 g to clear heat and promote fluid production thus quenching heat.

➢ For patients with constipation add *huǒ má rén* (火麻仁, Fructus Cannabis) and *jué míng zǐ* (决明子, Semen Cassiae) to moisten the intestines to relieve constipation.

(4) Deficiency of Qi and Blood

【Syndrome Characteristics】

This syndrome is always found in patients with prolonged disease or women during lactation. The symptoms include blurred vision, eye dull pain, mental fatigue and lack of strength, shortage of qi and reluctant to speech, pale complexion and lips, pale tongue, thready and weak pulse.

【Treatment Principle】

Tonify and replenish qi and blood.

【Representative Formula】

Modified *Bā Zhēn Tāng* (八珍汤, Eight Gem Decoction)

【 Prescription 】

熟地黄	*shú dì huáng*	10 g	Radix Rehmanniae Praeparata
当归	*dāng guī*	10 g	Radix Angelicae Sinensis
川芎	*chuān xiōng*	10 g	Rhizoma Chuanxiong
党参	*dǎng shēn*	12 g	Radix Codonopsis
白术	*bái zhú*	15 g	Rhizoma Atractylodis Macrocephalae
茯苓	*fú líng*	12 g	Poria
丹参	*dān shēn*	12 g	Radix et Rhizoma Salviae Miltiorrhizae
枳壳	*zhǐ qiào*	10 g	Fructus Aurantii
炙甘草	*zhì gān cǎo*	6 g	Radix et Rhizoma Glycyrrhizae Praeparata cum Melle

【 Modifications 】

➢ For patients with severe deficiency of qi, add *huáng qí* (黄芪, Radix Astragali) 10 g to replenish qi and nourish blood.

➢ For patients with palpitation and insomnia, add *suān zǎo rén* (酸枣仁, Semen Ziziphi Spinosae) 15 g, *bǎi zǐ rén* (柏子仁, Semen Platycladi) 10 g and *yè jiāo téng* (夜交藤, Caulis Polygoni Multiflori) to nourish heart and tranquilize the mind.

2. Acupuncture

(1) Acute stage

The main acupoints include:

qiú hòu (球后)	ST 1 (*chéng qì*)	BL 1 (*jīng míng*)
DU 23 (*shàng xīng*)		

Use even supplementation and drainage method and twirl in a gentle way. It's not advisable to lift and thrust the needle with amplitude.

Adjunct acupoints include:

GB 20 (*fēng chí*)	*tài yáng* (太阳)	DU 20 (*bǎi huì*)
LI 4 (*hé gǔ*)	LV 3 (*tài chōng*)	BL 18 (*gān shù*)

Use drainage method. Usually, choose 2–3 main acupoints and 2–4 combination acupoints each time, retain the needle for 30 minutes after the arrival of qi, treat once daily.

(2) Chronic or recurrence stage

BL 1 (*jīng míng*)	ST 1 (*chéng qì*)	GB 1 (*tóng zǐ liáo*)
ST 36 (*zú sān lǐ*)		

Use even supplementation and drainage with moderate stimulation, once a day or every other day.

3. Chinese Patent Medicines

(1) *Lóng Dǎn Xiè Gān Wán* (龙胆泻肝丸 , Gentian Liver-Draining Pill)
6 g each time, twice a day, applicable to patients with excess heat in liver Channel.

(2) *Qīng Kāi Líng Piàn* (清开灵片 , Heat-Removing Tablet) or *Qīng Kāi Líng Kǒu Fú Yè* (清开灵口服液 , Heat-Removing Oral Drink)
1–2 Tablets (or 10–20 ml) each time, twice or three times a day, applicable to patents with excess heat in the liver Channel or patients with acute onset.

(3) *Modified Xiāo Yáo Wán* (加味逍遥丸 , Modified Free Wanderer Pill) or *Modified Xiāo Yáo Kǒu Fú Yè* (加味逍遥口服液 , Modified Free Wanderer Oral Drink)
6 g or 10 ml each time, twice a day, applicable to liver constraint and qi stagnation.

(4) *Zhī Bǎi Dì Huáng Wán* (知柏地黄丸 , Anemarrhena, Phellodendron and Rehmannia Pill)
8–10 granules each time, twice a day, applicable to yin deficiency and effulgent fire.

(5) *Bā Zhēn Wán* (八珍丸 , Eight Gem Pill) or *Bā Zhēn Kē Lì* (八珍颗粒 , Eight Gem Granules)
6 g or one bag each time, twice a day, applicable for deficiency of qi and blood.

4. Simple and Proven Recipes

(1) *Jué Míng Gǒu Qǐ Tea* (决明枸杞茶, Cassia Seed and Chinese Wolfberry Fruit Tea): Take *jué míng zǐ* (决明子, Semen Cassiae) 30–50 g, *gǒu qǐ zǐ* (枸杞子, Fructus Lycii) 30–50 g, wash clean to remove impurity then add some water and boil it to make strong tea, filtrate the dregs, add some honey and sugar drink two to three times a day. The tea has the function of clearing the liver and brightening the eyes; applicable to patients with hyperactivity of liver yang, eye distending pain and constipation.

(2) *Jú Huā Chāng Pú Yǐn* (菊花菖蒲饮, Chrysanthemun Flower and Grassleaf Sweetflag Rhizome Drink): Take *jú huā* (菊花, Flos Chrysanthemi) 30 g, *shí chāng pú* (石菖蒲, Rhizoma Acori Tatarinowii) 15 g, *chē qián cǎo* (车前草, Herba Plantaginis) 30 g, soak the medicinals in 300–500 ml water for 15 minutes, then boil it for 30 minutes, filtrate dregs, take the decoction as tea, several times one day. The drink is applicable to acute patients with up-flaming liver fire.

5. Diet and Preventive Care

(1) In acute stage, avoid fishy food like fish and shrimp for it may aggravate the condition of ON. Spicy or deep fried food should be restrained too because it may induce pathogenic heat and fire. In recovery stage, the intake of cold and ice cold food should be prohibited to prevent the spleen and stomach damage due to accumulation of pathogenic cold, which will impede the recovery. Stimulants like coffee, tea, alcohol, nicotine, and refined sugar may also aggravate this condition.

(2) Wear more or less properly according to weather change in different seasons. Increase outdoor exercise to improve overall health and immune function.

(3) Prevent and cure infectious disease actively, treat eye infections, sinus infections, oral infections and ear infections promptly.

Case Study

Liu, a 21-year-old woman

First visit: April 4, 1994

【 Chief Complaint 】

With a 40-day history of acute vision loss.

【 Medical History 】

She had an argument with a colleague and became angry shortly before the disease onset. She had been diagnosed and treated as an optic neuritis case at another local hospital. She didn't respond well to the treatment and was still taking 40 mg of prednisone daily when she first came to us. Four examinations: Looking depressed, reluctant to speak, distending pain of the chest and hypochodrium, menstrual irregularities, red tongue with thin coating, a wiry pulse.

【 Examination 】

Her visual acuity was 20/333 (we need to change these to US eye chart equivalents) on the right and 20/16 on the left. A relative afferent pupillary defect (RAPD) was positive in the right eye where a 10 degree central scotoma was present. The optic disc appeared pale.

【 Diagnosis 】

Diagnosis of TCM: Sudden blindness

【 Pattern Differentiation 】

Liver constraint and qi stagnation.

【 Treatment Principles 】

Soothe the liver and relieve depression, clear the liver and brighten the eyes.

【 Prescription 】

Modified *Dān Zhī Xiāo Yáo Sǎn* (Peony Bark and Gardenia Free Wanderer Powder, 丹栀逍遥散) with removed *bò he* (薄荷, Herba Menthae) and *shēng jiāng* (生姜, Rhizoma Zingiberis Recens), added *xià kū cǎo* (夏枯草, Spica Prunellae) 10 g and *lián qiào* (连翘, Fructus Forsythiae) 10 g.

The second follow-up examination showed that visual acuity was 20/200 on the right eye. The dose of prednisolone had been reduced. Due to the effect, the primary formula was retained for a month. The third follow-up examination showed visual acuity of 20/33 on the right eye. Other signs and symptoms included mental fatigue, loose stool, no pleasure in eating, and a thin pulse. Based on the syndrome characteristics, a diagnosis was made of spleen and qi deficiency.

So the treatment principle was changed to invigorating spleen and regulating liver, activating blood and brightening eyes. Formula: *dǎng shēn* (党参, Radix codonopsis) 10 g, *fú líng* (茯苓, Poria) 10 g, *chǎo bái zhú* (炒白术, dry-fried Rhizoma Atractylodis Macrocephalae) 15 g, *zhì gān cǎo* (炙甘草, Radix et Rhizoma Glycyrrhizae Praeparata cum Melle), *dāng guī* (当归, Radix Angelicae Sinensis) 10 g, *chái hú* (柴胡, Radix Bupleuri) 10 g, *jú huā* (菊花, Flos Chrysanthemi) 10 g, *gǒu qǐ zǐ* (枸杞子, Fructus Lycii) 10 g, *chǎo gǔ yá* (炒谷芽, dry-fried Fructus Setariae Germinatus) 15 g, *chǎo mài yá* (炒麦芽, dry-fried Fructus Hordei Germinatus) 15 g. After having 15 doses, the right visual acuity increased to 20/20, the central scotoma was disappeared, and the other symptoms were obviously improved as well.

(*Ophthalmology Encyclopedia of Traditional Chinese Medicine*, 中医眼科全书)

Classical Quote

《证治准绳·杂病·七窍门》："平日素无他病，外不伤轮廓，内不损瞳神，倏然盲而不见也。"

The patient is otherwise healthy before they suddenly lose their vision. There is neither appearance of abnormal orbiculi and regins, nor any abnormalities of the pupil.

Standards for Diagnosis and Treatment–Miscellaneous Diseases-Seven Orifices (*Zhèng Zhì Zhǔn Shéng–Zá Bìng–Qī Qiào Mén*, 证治准绳·杂病·七窍门)

《审视瑶函》："其故有三：曰阴孤，曰阳寡，曰神离，乃闭塞关格之病。"

There are three causes for sudden blindness: yin deficiency, yang deficiency and vitality separated, hence yin-yang disharmony.

A Close Examination of the Precious Classic on Ophthalmology (*Shěn Shì Yáo Hán*, 审视瑶函)

Questions for Consideration

1. Which pattern is *Dān Zhī Xiāo Yáo Sǎn* (Peony Bark and Gardenia Free Wanderer Powder, 丹栀逍遥散) applicable to? Please write out the main syndrome characteristics of this pattern and prescription of the formula.

2. In the acute stage of optic neuritis, which acupoint(s) may be selected to treat it with acupuncture? What is the proper manipulation?

Section 11   Optic Atrophy

Optic atrophy can be defined as damage to the optic nerve which results in loss of visual function and discoloration (pallor) of the optic nerve. The disease is seen in every age group and may attack one eye or both eyes, and is commonly seen in clinic. In a normal eye, the optic nerve can transfer visual information to the brain via visual pathways. Under healthy circumstances, the eye can detect objects and colors within the visual field. If the optic nerve is damaged, it will cause severe visual dysfunction due to the death of ganglion cells and loss of function of the nerve fibers. Symptoms of optic atrophy can be a decrease in visual acuity, constriction of visual field, or defects of the visual field-even total blindness in severe cases.

There are many possible causes of optic atrophy, which include inflammation of the optic nerve and the retina, ischemia, trauma, degeneration, heredity, demyelinating diseases, malnutrition, and various kinds of toxicities (drugs, heavy metals, tobacco, and alcohol). In western medicine, it is accepted that optic atrophy is a pathology resulting from optic nerve damage, except for the treatment aimed directly at the causes, for example removing a brain tumor, there is no effective treatment, especially for the optic atrophy with no clear cause.

In TCM, optic atrophy is ascribed to *qīng máng* (bluish blindness, 青盲) some mild cases may be also called *shì zhān hūn miǎo* (blurred vision, 视瞻昏渺). TCM has treated this condition for centuries. In summary, the cause and pathogenesis of the disease is blocked sweat pore in the eyes, therefore, qi and blood can not nourish the optic nerve which results in visual dysfunction. The specific causes include insufficiency of native endowment wind pathogen and toxin attacking fetus, improper diet, exhaustion of blood, excessive use of eyesight, internal damage by the excessive seven emotions, trauma of brain and eyes, oncothlipsis, etc. It may be also associated with retinitis pigmentosa, glaucoma and retinal arterial obstruction. TCM has exact curative effect on optic atrophy by treatment with medicinals combined with acupuncture. However, it is also very important to ascertain the underlying causes, such as the brain tumor, if it is not detected and removed as soon as possible, the treatment by TCM is not only in vain, but may delay the chance of proper treatment and aggravate patients' condition. Based on the literature report and our clinical experiences, TCM treatment (including medicinals and acupuncture) will be highly effective at improving visual function, in some cases it can even cure the disease. For some chronic or severe condition, TCM treatment can stabilize the visual acuity and prevent the deterioration of visual function.

Clinical Manifestation

1. Severe vision loss, no light perception in some cases.

2. Color vision can be affected at different levels, especially red and green.

3. A relative afferent pupillary defect (RAPD) may be found in unilaterally affected cases, which is also called Macus-Gunn pupil. Direct pupillary reaction will delay or disappear according to the condition in bilaterally affected patients.

4. The disc is discolored or may be totally pale. Based on the signs of fundus, optic

atrophy is classified into primary optic atrophy and secondary optic atrophy. In conditions of primary optic atrophy, the disc is white and sharply demarcated, the retina and the vessels are normal. The causes are associated with the damage to retrobulbar portion of optic nerve or intracalvarium. In conditions of secondary optic atrophy, besides that the disc is discolored, the vessels of retina may get thinner or surrounded by white sheaths, hyperpigmented spot, large area atrophy or proliferation lesion may also be found too.

5. Auxiliary Examination:

(1) Visual field: Most cases present with concentric contraction of visual field. Other visual field defects include central scotoma, paracentral scotoma, fan-shaped defect, bitemporal hemianopia or homonymous hemianopia.

(2) Visual electrophysiology: The latency period of P-VEP or F-VEP will increase, and the amplitude will decrease obviously, or the wave may totally disappear.

(3) FFA: There is nothing abnormal in the early stages. In the later stages, low fluorescence of disc is commonly seen in FFA examination.

Treatment

1. Pattern Differentiation and Treatment

(1) liver qi depression

【Syndrome Characteristics】

Blurred vision, central visual field defect, or shadow in a certain quadrant visual field, vexation and depression, bitter taste in mouth and hypochondriac pain, red tongue with thin white coating, rapid and thready pulse.

【Treatment Principle】

Soothe the liver and relieve the depression

【Representative Formula】

Modified *Dān Zhī Xiāo Yáo Sǎn* (Peony Bark and Gardenia Free Wanderer Powder, 丹栀逍遥散)

【Prescription】

牡丹皮	*mǔ dān pí*	10 g	Cortex Moutan
栀子	*zhī zǐ*	10 g	Fructus Gardeniae
柴胡	*chái hú*	8 g	Radix Bupleuri
茯苓	*fú líng*	10 g	Poria
白术	*bái zhú*	10 g	Rhizoma Atractylodis Macrocephalae
当归	*dāng guī*	10 g	Radix Angelicae Sinensis
甘草	*gān cǎo*	3 g	Radix et Rhizoma Glycyrrhizae
薄荷 (后下)	*bò he (hòu xià)*	3 g	Herba Menthae (decocted later)
生姜	*shēng jiāng*	2 pieces	Rhizoma Zingiberis Recens

【 Modifications 】

➢ For cases with long time depression and dullness in the chest and rib-side, add *zhǐ qiào* (枳壳, Fructus Aurantii) 10 g, *yù jīn* (郁金, Radix Curcumae) 10 g and *chuān liàn zǐ* (川楝子, Fructus Toosendan) 10 g to regulate qi, resolve depression and stop pain.

➢ For cases with long time depression causing qi stagnation and marked blood stasis, add *dān shēn* (丹参, Radix et Rhizoma Salviae Miltiorrhizae) 10 g, *hóng huā* (红花, Flos Carthami) 10 g and *chuān xiōng* (川芎, Rhizoma Chuanxiong) 10 g to enhance the function of moving blood and activating blood.

➢ For cases with the liver constraint and blood deficiency, add *zhì hé shǒu wū* (制何首乌, Radix Polygoni Multiflori Praeparata cum Succo Glycines Sotae) to benefit qi and nourish blood.

➢ For cases with tinnitus, hearing loss and vexation add *shí chāng pú* (石菖蒲, Rhizoma Acori Tatarinowii) 10 g and *yuǎn zhì* (远志, Radix Polygalae) 10 g to sharpen the hearing, open the orifices, brighten the eyes, quite the heart and tranquilize mind.

(2) qi stagnation and blood stasis

【 Syndrome Characteristics 】

Visual decease or loss, headache, poor memory and forgetfulness, insomnia and profuse dreams, dusky red tongue or with stasis maculae, thin white coating, thin rough pulse or knotted and intermittent pulse.

【 Treatment Principle 】

Move qi and invigorate blood, regulate qi and dredge collaterals.

【 Representative Formula 】

Modified *Táo Hóng Sì Wù Tāng* (Peach Kernel and Carthamus Four Substances Decoction, 桃红四物汤)

【 Prescription 】

桃仁	*táo rén*	10 g	Semen Persicae
红花	*hóng huā*	6 g	Flos Carthami
当归	*dāng guī*	10 g	Radix Angelicae Sinensis
川芎	*chuān xiōng*	10 g	Rhizoma Chuanxiong
白芍	*bái sháo*	10 g	Radix Paeoniae Alba
熟地黄	*shú dì huáng*	10 g	Radix Rehmanniae Praeparata
柴胡	*chái hú*	10 g	Radix Bupleuri
枳壳	*zhǐ qiào*	10 g	Fructus Aurantii
党参	*dǎng shēn*	12 g	Radix Codonopsis
路路通	*lù lù tōng*	10 g	Fructus Liquidambaris

【 Modifications 】

➢ For cases with marked qi deficiency, add *huáng qí* (黄芪, Radix Astragali) 10 g and *bái zhú* (白术, Rhizoma Atractylodis Macrocephalae) 10 g to benefit qi and nourish blood.

➢ For cases with pale disk and narrow vessels add *jī xuè téng* (鸡血藤, Caulis Spatholobi) 10 g, *sī guā luò* (丝瓜络, Retinervus Luffae Fructus) 10 g and *ē jiāo* (阿胶, Colla Corii Asini) 10 g to enhance the function of nourishing blood and dredging collaterals.

(3) yin deficiency of the liver and kidney

【 Syndrome Characteristics 】

Prolonged blurred vision and get worse gradually, dryness of the eyes and mouth, dizzy and tinnitus, sore waist and limb legs, vexation heat and night sweat, emission, dry stool, red tongue with thin white coating, thready pulse.

【 Treatment Principle 】

Supplement the liver and the kidney.

【 Representative Formula 】

Modified *Míng Mù Dì Huáng Wán* (Eye Brightener Rehmannia Pill, 明目地黄丸)

【 Prescription 】

生地	*shēng dì*	15 g	Radix Rehmanniae
熟地黄	*shú dì huáng*	15 g	Radix Rehmanniae Praeparata
山茱萸	*shān zhū yú*	10 g	Fructus Corni
干山药	*gān shān yào*	15 g	Rhizoma Dioscoreae
泽泻	*zé xiè*	10 g	Rhizoma Alismatis
茯苓	*fú líng*	10 g	Poria
柴胡	*chái hú*	10 g	Radix Bupleuri
当归	*dāng guī*	10 g	Radix Angelicae Sinensis
五味子	*wǔ wèi zǐ*	6 g	Fructus Schisandrae Chinensis
枸杞子	*gǒu qǐ zǐ*	10 g	Fructus Lycii
丹参	*dān shēn*	10 g	Radix et Rhizoma Salviae Miltiorrhizae
川芎	*chuān xiōng*	10 g	Rhizoma Chuanxiong

【 Modifications 】

➢ For cases accompanied by yang deficiency, add *tù sī zǐ* (菟丝子, Semen Cuscutae) 10 g and *ròu cōng róng* (肉苁蓉, Herba Cistanches) 10 g to supplement yang and strengthen the kidney.

➢ For cases with vexing heat in the five heart, add *zhī mǔ* (知母, Rhizoma Anemarrhenae) 10 g, *huáng bǎi* (黄柏, Cortex Phellodendri Chinensis) 10 g and *dàn zhú yè* (淡竹叶, Herba Lophatheri) 10 g to clear heat, resolve vexation and tranquilize the mind.

➢ For cases with sore waist and limb legs, add *gǒu jǐ* (狗脊, Rhizoma Cibotii) 10 g and *dù zhòng* (杜仲, Cortex Eucommiae) 10 g to tonify the kidney and strengthen the waist.

(4) qi and blood deficiency

【Syndrome Characteristics】

Gradual vision loss to total blindness, lusterless complexion, pale lips and nails, lassitude spirit and lack of strength, laziness to speak and reluctant to talk, palpitation and short of breath, pale tongue with thin white coating, thready and weak pulse.

【Treatment Principle】

Benefit qi and nourish blood.

【Representative Formula】

Bā Zhēn Tāng (Eight Gem Decoction, 八珍汤)

【Prescription】

党参	*dǎng shēn*	15 g	Radix Codonopsis
黄芪	*huáng qí*	20 g	Radix Astragali
白术	*bái zhú*	10 g	Rhizoma Atractylodis Macrocephalae
茯苓	*fú líng*	10 g	Poria
熟地黄	*shú dì huáng*	15 g	Radix Rehmanniae Praeparata
当归	*dāng guī*	10 g	Radix Angelicae Sinensis
白芍	*bái sháo*	10 g	Radix Paeoniae Alba
川芎	*chuān xiōng*	10 g	Rhizoma Chuanxiong
丹参	*dān shēn*	10 g	Radix et Rhizoma Salviae Miltiorrhizae
石菖蒲	*shí chāng pú*	10 g	Rhizoma Acori Tatarinowii
枳壳	*zhǐ qiào*	10 g	Fructus Aurantii
炙甘草	*zhì gān cǎo*	5 g	Radix et Rhizoma Glycyrrhizae Praeparata cum Melle

【Modifications】

➢ For cases with marked blood deficiency, add *zhì hé shǒu wū* (制何首乌, Radix Polygoni Multiflori Praeparata cum Succo Glycines Sotae) 10 g and *lóng yǎn ròu* (龙眼肉, Arillus Longan) 10 g to nourish blood and brighten the eyes.

➢ For cases with obvious qi deficiency, add more *huáng qí* (黄芪, Radix Astragali) to 30–40 g. For cases with qi stagnation and depressed emotion, add *chái hú* (柴胡, Radix Bupleuri) 10 g and *xiāng fù* (香附, Rhizoma Cyperi) 10 g.

➢ For cases accompanied by blood stasis with thin rough pulse, add *hóng huā* (红花, Flos Carthami) 10 g and *jī xuè téng* (鸡血藤, Caulis Spatholobi) 10 g to nourish the blood and invigorate the blood.

2. Acupuncture

(1) Body Acupuncture Therapy

Choose acupoints guided by the principle of pattern differentiation and treatment. Commonly used acupoints include:

① Local acupoints around the eye:

ST 1 (*chéng qì*)	BL 1 (*jīng míng*)	BL 2 (*cuán zhú*)
yú yāo (鱼腰)	*qiú hòu* (球后)	GB 1 (*tóng zǐ liáo*)
SJ 23 (*sī zhú kōng*)	*shàng míng* (EX-HN19)	

② Acupoits at the head area:

GB 14 (*yáng bái*)	*tài yáng* (太阳)	ST 2 (*sì bái*)
DU 24 (*shén tíng*)	BL 3 (*méi chōng*)	DU 20 (*bǎi huì*)
ST 8 (*tóu wéi*)	*sì shén cōng* (四神聪)	GB 20 (*fēng chí*)
yì míng (翳明)	GB 16 (*mù chuāng*)	

③ Body acupoints:

ST 36 (*zú sān lǐ*)	SP 6 (*sān yīn jiāo*)	GB 34 (*yáng líng quán*)
GB 37 (*guāng míng*)	LR 2 (*xíng jiān*)	LR 3 (*tài chōng*)
GB 42 (*dì wǔ huì*)	BL 60 (*kūn lún*)	LI 4 (*hé gǔ*)
BL 18 (*gān shù*)	Bl 23 (*shèn shù*)	

Choose 2–3 acupoints around the eye, 2–4 head acupoints and 2–4 body acupoints, treat each day, use even supplementation method, ten treatments is one course of treatment. For chronic or prolonged cases, or cases that do not respond well to conventional or other treatments, or for those cases who have lost most or all of their eyesight, it is suggested to choose ST 1 (*chéng qì*), BL 1 (*jīng míng*), *shàng míng* (EX-HN19) – 0.5 *cun* below *Yú yāo*), which is also called "eye tri-acupoints", and puncture appropriately with in-situ gently twisting. Do not lift and thrust the needle. In recent years, we use "tri-acupoints combining nine needles method" to treat severe optic atrophy and get better therapeutic effect than before. In detail, we puncture SJ 23 (*sī zhú kōng*) joined to *yú yāo* (EX-HN 4), *tài yáng* (EX-HN5) joined to GB 1 (*tóng zǐ liáo*), and GB 14 (*yáng bái*) joined to BL 2 (*cuán zhú*) besides the "tri-acupoints" as above. And also choose body acupoints like ST 36 (*zú sān lǐ*), SP 6 (*sān yīn jiāo*), GB 37 (*guāng míng*) and LI 4 (*hé gǔ*) guided by the principle of pattern differentiation and treatment.

(2) Scalp Acupuncture

Choose optic area (originate 1 cm lateral to the midpoint of the occipital protuberance and runs for 4 cm parallel to the anterior-posterior line in an anterior direction), puncture downwards symmetrically, one time each day or every other day, 10 sessions is a treatment course.

(3) Electro-Acupuncture

Electro-acupuncture enhances the treatment effect by combining the effects of both filiform needle puncture and electric stimulation. The acupoints could be the same as the above. One time each day, 20 minutes every time, 10 sessions is treatment course. Be cautious that the electric circuits should be paired as far as possible, and choose acupoints of neighborhood to pair.

(4) Medicinal Iontophoresis by Direct Current

Use the effect of a direct current field, put the (medicinal) at the same electropolarity. This is based on the theory of repulsion by same electropolarity and attraction by opposite eletropolarity, introduce medicinal ions into the eyes without the help of the blood circulation. The commonly used Chinese medicinals include: *dān shēn* (Radix et Rhizoma Salviae Miltiorrhizae), *chuān xiōng* (Rhizoma Chuanxiong) and *jué míng zǐ* (Semen Cassiae), the treatment course is the same as the electro-acupuncture therapy.

(5) Acupoint Injection

The Chinese medicinals that have the function of activating blood and resolving stasis are commonly used for acupoint injection, including *Fù Fāng Dān Shēn Zhù Shè Yè* (Compound Salviae Miltiorrhiza Injection, 复方丹参注射液), *Fù Fāng Zhāng Liǔ Jiǎn Zhù Shè Yè* (Compound Anisodine Hydrobromide Injection, 复方樟柳碱注射液), etc. This method has the double effect of both drug and acupoints stimulation, however, the acupoints close to the eyeball such as ST 1 (*chéng qì*), BL 1 (*jīng míng*), *qiú hòu* (球后) and *Shàng míng* (EX-HN19) are not suggested for injection.

3. Chinese Patent Medicines

The available Patent Medicines include *Míng Mù Dì Huáng Wán* (Brighten Eye and Rehmannia Root Pill, 明目地黄丸), *Qǐ Jú Dì Huáng Wán* (Lycium Berry, Chrysanthemum and Rehmannia Pill, 杞菊地黄丸), *Shí Hú Yè Guāng Wán* (Dendrobium Night Vision Pill, 石斛夜光丸), *Bǔ Zhōng Yì Qì Wán* (Center-Supplementing and Qi-Boosting Pill, 补中益气丸), *Shēng Mài Sǎn Kǒu Fú Yè* (Pulse-Engendering Oral Liquid, 生脉口服液) and *Xiāo Yáo Wán* (Free Wanderer Pill,逍遥丸). Choose the appropriate formula based on the pattern differentiation. Because the disease course has been very long, for cases that need long-term treatment, it is suggested to take decoction and pills alternatively every other day. *Shí Hú Yè Guāng Wán* (Dendrobium Night Vision Pill, 石斛夜光丸) is composed by 25 medicinals, thus it is not advisable for long time use due to the complicated prescription and cool flavor.

4. Simple and Proven Recipes

(1) *Huáng qí* (黄芪, Radix Astragali) 30 g, *dǎng shēn* (党参, Radix Codonopsis) 15 g and *yì yǐ rén* (薏苡仁, Semen Coicis) 20 g, one dose every day, decocted with water and taken twice each day. It is applicable to cases with qi deficiency of spleen.

(2) *Lóng yǎn ròu* (龙眼肉, Arillus Longan) 30 g, *bǎi hé* (百合, Bulbus Lilii) 20 g and *dāng guī* (当归, Radix Angelicae Sinensis) 15 g, decocted with water and taken twice

each day, one dose every day. It is applicable for cases with blood deficiency of the heart and restless of heart spirit.

(3) *Gǒu qǐ zǐ* (枸杞子, Fructus Lycii) 30 g, *nǚ zhēn zǐ* (女贞子, Fructus Ligustri Lucidi) 15 g, decocted with water and taken twice each day, one dose every day. It is applicable for cases with yin deficiency of the liver and the kidney.

5. Dietary Therapy and Preventative Health Care

Dietary Therapy is helpful to stabilize the visual acuity, thus it can even reduce the course of treatment depending on the patients' condition.

(1) Chinese angelica-hoantchy root Chicken soup: Put one hen, *dāng guī* (当归, Radix Angelicae Sinensis) 15 g and *huáng qí* (黄芪, Radix Astragali) 20 g into water and braise it for two hours, get the soup and take it twice every week. It is applicable to cases with deficiency of qi and blood.

(2) Lamb liver gruel: Put 100 g lamb liver slices and 120 g rice into water and boil it into gruel, take once every day. It is helpful to reinforce the spleen and brighten the eyes.

(3) Dried Longan gruel: Put 15 g dried longan, 10 pieces common jujube and rice 100 g into appropriate water, boil it into gruel. Take it in the morning and in the evening for weeks. It is useful to nourish the heart, tonify blood and strengthen the spleen and applicable for patients with heart blood deficiency.

(4) Dwarf yellow daylily and finger citron fruit Drink: Dwarf yellow daylily 30 g, finger citron fruit 30 g, make soup and sauce it with salt or sugar, take once or two times a day for two weeks, which can soothe the liver and regulate qi. It is applicable for cases with liver qi depression.

Preventative health care is also very important for all patients with optic atrophy. Pay attention to nourishing yin and tranquilizing the mind, avoid excessive stress, upset, outrage, impatience and anxiety. Live a regular life, avoid too much sexual indulgence with ejaculation (for men), stay warm, restrain from drinking alcohol, and quit smoking. Diet should be abundant in nutrients that are easily digested, consume more fresh fruits and vegetables, juicing is an option. Increase outdoor exercise appropriately in order to strengthen your overall constitution condition. This will help to stabilize the patient's condition.

Case Studies

Case 1#

Zhu, a 21-year-old female
[Chief Complaint]
Vision loss of the nine months.

【 Medical History 】

She was diagnosed with Optic Atrophy and had no form of treatments.

The patient had irregular menstrual periods for a long time, once every two years. The other symptoms included vexation and insomnia, dusky tongue with thin white coating, deep-thready and rapid pulse.

【 Examination 】

Her visual acuities were 20/50 on both eyes, uncorrectable. The fundus examination showed that both discs were discolored and pale at the temporal side, and the retinal arteries were thin, nothing else was abnormal of the fundus examination. The visual field presented with concentric contraction (right 12°, left 12°).

【 Diagnosis 】

Blurred vision (the liver constraint and qi stagnation).

【 Pattern Differentiation 】

Essence and blood can not nourish the eyes due to ascent-descent disorder of qi.

【 Treatment Principles 】

Soothe the liver and relieve the depression, nourish and invigorate blood, and in combination with some medicinals that have the function of nourishing yin, clearing the liver and brightening the eyes.

【 Prescription 】

当归	dāng guī	10 g	Radix Angelicae Sinensis
白芍	bái sháo	10 g	Radix Paeoniae Alba
桑叶	sāng yè	10 g	Folium Mori
枸杞子	gǒu qǐ zǐ	10 g	Fructus Lycii
焦白术	jiāo bái zhú	6 g	Rhizoma Atractylodis Macrocephalae (stir-fried)
柴胡	chái hú	6 g	Radix Bupleuri
牡丹皮	mǔ dān pí	6 g	Cortex Moutan
栀子	zhī zǐ	6 g	Fructus Gardeniae (prepared)
白菊花	bái jú huā	6 g	Flos Chrysanthemi Indici
茯苓	fú líng	12 g	Poria
生地	shēng dì	15 g	Radix Rehmanniae
熟地黄	shú dì huáng	15 g	Radix Rehmanniae Praeparata
川芎	chuān xiōng	3 g	Rhizoma Chuanxiong
甘草	gān cǎo	3 g	Radix et Rhizoma Glycyrrhizae

One dose every day or every other day, 90 doses in total.

【 Follow-up 】

At the second follow-up visit, her visual acuities were 20/33, and her menstrual period was normal. She complained of dizziness. Her pulse was thready and weak, accompanied by red tongue with less fluid.

Pattern differentiation: Hyper activity of the liver due to yin deficiency.

Treatment principle: Nourish and tonify the liver and the kidney, assistant with pacifying the liver and brightening the eyes.

Formula: Modified *Qǐ Jú Dì Huáng Wán* (Lycium Berry, Chrysanthemum and Rehmannia Pill, 杞菊地黄丸). At her third and forth following-up visit, she was administered with modified *Míng Mù Dì Huáng Wán* (Eye Brightener Rehmannia Pill, 明目地黄丸) and *Yì Qì Cōng Míng Tāng* (Qi-Boosting Intelligence Decoction, 益气聪明汤) based on the pattern differentiation. At her last visit, the visual acuities were 20/20 on the right eye and 20/16 on the left eye, and the visual field was almost recovered to normal though there was not much change of fundus examination. The patient complained of nothing uncomfortable, thus the treatment was stopped.

Case 2#

Ma, a 53-year-old male

【Chief Complaint】

Vision loss for the three years with a diagnosis of optic atrophy.

【Medical History】

Besides many western drugs, he had been treated with methods of optic nerve massage and burying catgut, but none had helped him.

【Examination】

The visual acuities were 20/100 on the right eye and 20/290 on the life eye. The fudus examination showed a pale discs and thin vessels. His visual field presented with concentric contraction. The pulses of both sides were soft and weak, more obvious on the right side.

【Diagnosis】

Bluish blindness (optic atrophy)

【Pattern Differentiation】

Deficiency of kidney yang and debilitation of blood and essence.

【Treatment Principles】

Supplement the kidney and benefit yang, nourish blood and brighten the eyes.

【Prescription】

肉苁蓉	*ròu cōng róng*	90 g	Herba Cistanches
熟地黄	*shú dì huáng*	180 g	Radix Rehmanniae Praeparata
补骨脂	*bǔ gǔ zhī*	120 g	Fructus Psoraleae
菟丝子	*tù sī zǐ*	120 g	Semen Cuscutae
当归	*dāng guī*	120 g	Radix Angelicae Sinensis
党参	*dǎng shēn*	120 g	Radix Codonopsis
枸杞子	*gǒu qǐ zǐ*	120 g	Fructus Lycii
茯苓	*fú líng*	120 g	Poria

All the medicinals of the above were ground up and made into pills by mixing with honey, 9 g each day.

At the second visit (after 6 months), all the symptoms improved but the visual acuity. He was administered the same formula added with *chǔ shí zǐ* (楮实子, Fructus Broussonetiae) 90 g and *chái hú* (柴胡, Radix Bupleuri) 30 g. All the medicinals were made into pills and taken as the above. When he had his third visit six months later, the visual acuities were 20/50 on the right eye and 20/500 on the left eye. There was no change in the fundus examination. He was administered the same formula but the patient stopped treatment. We did the follow-up visit his visual acuity on the right eye was stable at 20/500, while the visual filed was still very small. The visual acuity on the left eye decreased from 20/500 to light perception.

Case 3#

A 60-year-old female patient

【 Chief Complaint 】

Severe vision loss, she had pituitary surgery 13 years ago.

【 Examination 】

Visual acuities were no light perception on the right eye and 20/400 on the left. Nothing abnormal was found in the outer eye examination. The right eye fundus examination showed that the disc was pale and the retinal arteries and veins got thinner, moreover, the color of the retina were dirty gray. For the left eye fundus, except that the disc of the left was light white and the arteries became thinner, there was no other abnormal findings in the examination.

【 Prescription 】

Chinese medicinals combined with acupuncture.

Yǎng Mù Wán (Eye-Nourishing Pills, 养目丸) with the function of nourishing the kidney and the liver as well as activating blood and removing stasis.

Acupuncture: Selected points include GB 20 (*fēng chí*), GB 12 (*wán gǔ*), BL 10 (*tiān zhù*), *shàng jīng míng*, BL 1 (*jīng míng*), *qiú hòu* (球后), ST 1 (*chéng qì*), ST 2 (*sì bái*), *tài yáng* (太阳), DU 20 (*bǎi huì*), LI 4 (*hé gǔ*), BL 18 (*gān shù*), Bl 23 (*shèn shù*), and etc.

Chosen 4–6 points alternatively every day, and acupunctured one time daily. After 20 days of treatment, the visual acuity on the left eye was increased to 20/30. Continued the same treatment for two months (an additional 60 treatments) and then reduced the acupuncture frequency to 3 times one week.

Classic Quotes

《目经大成·青盲篇》: "青盲不似暴盲奇, 暴盲来速青盲迟。"

Bluish blindness doesn't like sudden blindness, it happens slowly.

The Great Compendium of Classics on Ophthalmology–Bluish Blindness Chapter (目经大成 · 青盲篇, *Mù Jīng Dà Chéng–Qīng Máng Piān*)

《证治准绳 · 杂病 · 七窍门》"青盲者，瞳神不大不小，无缺无损，仔细观之，瞳神内并无别样色气，俨然与好人一般，只是自看不见，方为此证，若有何气色，即是内障，非青盲也。"

In bluish blindness case, the pupil is not big or small, incomplete or damaged, it looks like the normal one, just the patient can not see. If there is some qi and colors behind the pupil other than normality, it is internal blindness but bluish blindness.

Standards for Diagnosis and Treatment – Miscellaneous Diseases–Seven Orifices Sect (*Zhèng Zhì Zhǔn Shéng–Zá Bìng–Qī Qiào Mén*, 证治准绳 · 杂病 · 七窍门)

Questions for Consideration

1. In the opinion of western medicine, what is the cause of optic atrophy? What is the classification based on the characteristic of the fundus change?

2. What are the common patterns of optic atrophy? Write out the relative treatment principle and representative formula.

Section 12   Stargardt's Disease

Stargardt macular dystrophy, also named as Stargardt's disease, is the most common form of inherited juvenile macular dystrophies. The inheritance is usually autosomal recessive with only occasional cases resulting from autosomal dominant mode. It is considered that Stargardt and fundus flavimaculatus are two variants of one disease. Stargardt's disease typically begins with a visual loss at age 6 to 20, while may also be noticed until age 30 to 40 with vision problems. Central vision loss is the main symptom and no gender difference is related to the incidence. In traditional Chinese medicine, the disease is belonged to *shì zhān hūn miǎo* (blurring vision, 视瞻昏渺), which is caused by yin deficiency in the liver and kidney, or local qi stagnation and blood stasis.

Clinical Manifestation

1. Gradually central vision loss is bilateral with no pain.

2. At early stage only nonspecific speckles could be seen in the central fovea. Because of inconspicuous ocular fundus signs, patients might be considered as malingery.

3. In fundus examination, the typical lesion is in the shape of oval about the size of 1.5 times of optic disc bilaterally, appears as "snail mucus" or forged bronze. Yellow-white flecks encircle the macular lesion in a few cases.

4. Diagnosis could be made by fundus fluorescein angiography, electroretinography, electro-oculography and optical coherence tomography.

5. The disease progresses slowly, but the visual prognosis is severe. Once the vision falls down to 20/40, it will rapidly drops to and stabilizes around 20/200 to 20/400.

Treatment

1. Pattern Differentiation and Treatment

There are no effective drugs in western medicine. In Chinese medicine, hereditary macular diseases are belonged to congenital "jing" insufficiency. The kidney is the congenital foundation, stores essence of life; the liver stores blood, thus the liver and kidney have a common source in essence and blood. Eyes could see things if the qi of liver and kidney is sufficient, otherwise eyes would become dim with vertigo. The treatment principle in Chinese medicine of this kind of disease is to supplement the liver and kidney with regulating qi and activating blood to smooth flow of blood and enhance local nourishment. If acupuncture is added, the therapeutic effect would be better. We have treated 8 patients who suffered from Stargardt's disease, after the treatment, the vision in 4 patients was steady around 20/100 to 20/66, the vision was improved to 20/50 to 20/40 in the other two patients. The treatment was as follows:

【Treatment Principle】
Supplement the liver and kidney, regulate qi and activate blood.

【Representative Formula】
Modified *Qǐ Jú Dì Huáng Tāng* (Lycium Berry, Chrysanthemum and Rehmannia Decoction, 杞菊地黄汤)

【Prescription】

枸杞子	*gǒu qǐ zǐ*	10 g	Fructus Lycii
菊花	*jú huā*	6 g	Flos Chrysanthemi
熟地黄	*shú dì huáng*	6 g	Radix Rehmanniae Praeparata
淮山药	*huái shān yào*	6 g	Rhizoma Dioscoreae
山茱萸	*shān zhū yú*	6 g	Fructus Corni
茯苓	*fú líng*	6 g	Poria
泽泻	*zé xiè*	6 g	Rhizoma Alismatis
牡丹皮	*mǔ dān pí*	6 g	Cortex Moutan
柴胡	*chái hú*	6 g	Radix Bupleuri
当归	*dāng guī*	6 g	Radix Angelicae Sinensis
红花	*hóng huā*	6 g	Flos Carthami

【 Modifications 】
➢ For cases with poor appetite, abdominal distention and loose stool in Children, add *dǎng shēn* (党参, Radix Codonopsis) 6 g, *chǎo bái zhú* (炒白术, dry-fried Rhizoma Atractylodis Macrocephalae) 6 g and *jī nèi jīn* (鸡内金, Endothelium Corneum Gigeriae Galli) 6 g to invigorate the spleen, promote digestion and remove stagnation.

2. Acupuncture

GB 14 (*yáng bái*)	ST 2 (*sì bái*)	ST 1 (*chéng qì*)
SJ 23 (*sī zhú kōng*)	LI 4 (*hé gǔ*)	ST 36 (*zú sān lǐ*)
SP 6 (*sān yīn jiāo*)	BL 18 (*gān shù*)	BL 23 (*shèn shù*)
BL 20 (*pí shù*)		

10 to 14 days is a course of treatment, 2 to 4 courses are needed (20 – 40 treatments).

Questions for Consideration

1. Based on the theory of TCM, what is the cause and pathogenesis of Stargardt's Disease?

2. Give the treatment principle and representative formula.

Chapter 15
Other Eye Diseases

Section 1　Amblyopia

Amblyopia is an eye disease involving one or both eyes in which the best possible corrected visual acuity is lower than the normal corrected level. There are no organic changes corresponding to the hypopsia. Usually, it is caused by the insufficient stimulations to the visual cells during the critical period of visual development. It has four types: strabismic, anisometropic, refractive and form-deprivation and occlusion amblyopia. Statistics shows that the incidence of the disease among juveniles is 2%–5%.

In Chinese medicine, amblyopia was attributed to strabismus (*tōng jīng*, 通睛), anisometropia (*néng jìn qiè yuǎn*, 能近怯远) and congenital cataract (*tāi huàn nèi zhàng*, 胎患内障). The best corrected visual acuity for amblyopia can be reversed by proper treatment. So, in addition to the western conventional treatment for amblyopia, the treatment of Chinese medicine, acupuncture and massage can effectively shorten the treatment course, and raise the therapeutic effect. The etiology and pathogenesis of the disease is most often attributed to congenital insufficiency, a genuine essence deficiency or spleen-stomach deficiency, which result in the shortage of source for the production of qi and blood that fail to transports essence to the eyes.

Classification according to visual acuity:

Mild amblyopia: Best corrected visual acuity: 20/33–20/25.

Medium amblyopia: Best corrected visual acuity: 20/100–20/40.

Serious amblyopia: Best corrected visual acuity: ≤20/200.

Clinical Manifestation

1. Subjective Symptoms

Blurred vision. Parents typically bring their kids to see the eye doctor when they notice their child squinting.

2. Visual Function

The best corrected visual acuity is lower than normal level and can be improved after treatment. The ability to distinguish the visual targets in a line is more difficult than identifying a single visual target, referred to as the "crowding phenomenon". The patient may suffer poor spatial acuity without a structural pathologies. This is a functional problem.

3. Paracentral Fixation

In severe cases, the child may suffer abnormal fixation. Examination by funduscope shows that the reflection focal point of central fovea of macula is not centrally located.

4. Synoptophore Examination

The exam is used to assess binocular vision and measures both the property and level of ocular deviation.

5. Visual Evoked Potential (VEP)

VEP diagram shows that P100 wave latency (WL) is delayed and amplitude is reduced.

Treatment

1. Pattern Differentiation and Treatment

(1) congenital deficiency
〖 Syndrome Characteristics 〗
Blurred vision or strabismus caused by congenital ametropia or after the operation for congenital cataract; night terror, bed wetting, even delayed growth. Light pale tongue with thin coating, weak pulse.
〖 Treatment Principle 〗
Supplement the liver and kidney.
〖 Representative Formula 〗
Modified *Sì Wù Wǔ Zǐ Wán* (Four Ingredients and Five Seeds Pill, 四物五子丸)
〖 Prescription 〗

熟地黄	*shú dì huáng*	10 g	Radix Rehmanniae Preparata
当归	*dāng guī*	10 g	Radix Angelicae Sinensis
地肤子	*dì fū zǐ*	10 g	Fructus Kochiae

白芍	bái sháo	10 g	Radix Paeoniae Alba
菟丝子	tù sī zǐ	10 g	Semen Cuscutae
川芎	chuān xiōng	10 g	Rhizoma Ligustici Chuanxiong
覆盆子	fù pén zǐ	10 g	Fructus Rubi
枸杞子	gǒu qǐ zǐ	10 g	Fructus Lycii
车前子 (包煎)	chē qián zǐ (bāo jiān)	10 g	Semen Plantaginis (wrapped)

【Modifications】

➢ For the cases with cold body and extremities, add *bǔ gǔ zhī* (补骨脂, Fructus Psoraleae) 15 g and *ròu cōng róng* (肉苁蓉, Herba Cistanches) 10 g to tonify kidney and warm yang; for the cases with aching lumber and knee, and tinnitus, add *chǔ shí zǐ* (楮实子, Fructus Broussonetiae) 10g and *sāng shèn* (桑椹, Fructus Mori) 10 g to tonify the kidney and brighten the eyes.

(2) spleen and stomach deficiency

【Syndrome Characteristics】

Blurred vision, feeling fatigue to lift eyelids; poor appetite, food preference, sallow complexion, dizziness, weariness, loose stool. Light moist tongue body, white thin coating, and weak thready or moderate pulse.

【Treatment Principle】

replenishing qi and fortifying spleen.

【Representative Formula】

Modified *Shēn Líng Bái Zhú Sǎn* (Ginseng, Poria and White Atractylodes Powder, 参苓白术散)

【Prescription】

太子参	tài zǐ shēn	15 g	Radix Pseudostellariae
白术	bái zhú	15 g	Rhizoma Atractylodis Macrocephalae
山药	shān yào	15 g	Rhizoma Dioscoreae
白扁豆	bái biǎn dòu	10 g	Semen Dolichoris Album
砂仁	shā rén	10 g	Fructus Amomi Villosi
薏苡仁	yì yǐ rén	15 g	Semen Coicis
茯苓	fú líng	15 g	Poria
陈皮	chén pí	10 g	Pericarpium Citri Reticulatae
当归	dāng guī	10 g	Radix Angelicae Sinensis
白芍	bái sháo	10 g	Radix Paeoniae Alba
桃仁	táo rén	10 g	Semen Persicae
川芎	chuān xiōng	10 g	Rhizoma Chuanxiong
桂枝	guì zhī	10 g	Ramulus Cinnamomi

【 Modifications 】

➢ For the cases with food stagnation, add *jiāo sān xiān* (Tres Immortales Usti, 焦三仙) 10 g and *jī nèi jīn* (鸡内金, Endothelium Corneum Gigeriae Galli) 10 g to promote digestion and resolve stagnation.

2. Acupuncture

(1) Body acupuncture

BL 1 (*jīng míng*)	BL 2 (*cuán zhú*)	ST 1 (*chéng qì*)
GB 37 (*guāng míng*)	GB 20 (*fēng chí*)	*qiú hòu* (EX-HN 7)

Modification: For cases with liver and kidney insufficiency, add ST 2 (*sì bái*), SP 6 (*sān yīn jiāo*), BL 18 (*gān shù*), BL 23 (*shèn shù*). For the cases with spleen and stomach deficiency, add CV 4 (*guān yuán*), BL 20 (*pí shù*), BL 21 (*wèi shù*), ST 36 (*zú sān lǐ*).

Manipulations: Mainly use even supplementation and drainage method, BL 18 (*gān shù*), BL 23 (*shèn shù*) and ST 36 (*zú sān lǐ*) can be applied supplementation method. Retain the needle for 30 minutes, once a day, 10 sessions is a treatment course.

(2) Ear acupuncture: Choose the points eye (LO5), liver (CO12), spleen (CO13), kidney (CO10), heart (CO15). Retain the needle for 30–60 minutes, use intermittent manipulation.

(3) Acupressure with ear seeds: Choose the same points as that in the above ear acupuncture; stimulate the points by pressing the plaster-fixed Semen Vaccariae, several times a day.

3. Chinese Patent Medicines

(1) *Míng Mù Dì Huáng Kē Lì* **(Brighten Eye and Rehmannia Root Granule, 明目地黄颗粒)**

6 g, twice a day. For the child younger than 4 years old, reduce the dose to 3 g. The medicine is suitable for the patient with congenital deficiency.

(2) *Huà Jī Kǒu Fú Yè* **(Resolving Food Stagnation Oral Liquid, 化积口服液)**

10 ml, twice a day. Or *Shān Zhā Wán* (Hawthorn Fruit Pill, 山楂丸), 1 pill, 3 times a day. The medicine is suitable for patients with spleen and stomach deficiency.

4. Simple and Proven Recipes

(1) *Huā Shēng Mì Yǐn* (Peanut and Honey Decoction, 花生蜜饮): Milk 200 g, peanut 50 g, honey 15 g, 1 egg. Stir up the egg and add it into boiled milk, heat it to boil again, then add peanut and honey, and mix the ingredients up. Take it once a day for breakfast.

(2) *Yáng Gān Huáng Qí Gēng* (Lamb Liver and Astragalus Soup, 羊肝黄芪羹):

Lamb liver 40 g, *huáng qí* (黄芪, Radix Astragali) 15 g. Slice the liver and stew it with Astragalus. Drink the soup and eat the liver slices with seasonings, once a day.

5. Treatment with Western Medicine

(1) Remove etiology: Remove the factors which cause form deprivation and correct squint and ametropia with corrective lenses.

(2) Amblyopia training: The training includes occlusion therapy (eye patch), pleoptics, penalization, episcotister stimulation therapy, Haidinger brush therapy and the training for stereoscopic vision etc. A vision therapist/vision educator or optometrist may choose the trainings according to the specific eye condition of the patient.

6. Preventive Care

(1) The critical period of visual development of a child is from 0-3 years old. Visual acuity testing is necessary during the period. Once the abnormal visual acuity was found, one should go to see an eye doctor as soon as possible. Early detection and early treatment can greatly increase the chance of successful treatment and long-term cure. Successful treatment can also be easily reached in mild cases. If the treatment started before 8 years old, good therapeutic effect can be achieved; and typically if the child is over 12 years old, the chances for successful treatment will decrease. However, persistence in long-term treatment will sometimes bring good results.

(2) Amblyopia is a developmental eye disease; the treatment course is designed to promote vision development and is a relatively long process, whereas the treatment may take several months or even a few years. In cases where young children lack self-control and refuse to wear glasses and follow the treatment regiment, the parents need to be patient, persistent and supportive.

(3) Once the therapeutic effect has been achieved, after treatment must be insisting on to stabilize the effect. Regular follow-up evaluations are necessary.

(4) Creating and maintaining good dietary habits with balanced nutrition is imperative, avoid junk-food and processed foods.

Question for Consideration

Briefly describe the main syndrome characteristics of amblyopia caused by congenital deficiency. Give the treatment principle and representative formula.

Section 2   Acquired Paralytic Strabismus

Acquired paralytic strabismus is an eye disease characterized by a sudden deviation of eyeball, limited eye movement and diplopia. This disease is the result of pathological changes of nucleus, neural stem or ocular muscles most often caused by trauma, inflammation, vascular disease, tumor and metabolic diseases. In Chinese medical ophthalmology, the term used is *fēng qiān piān shì* (paralytic strabismus, 风牵偏视) or *mù piān shì* (strabismus, 目偏视). The cause and pathogenesis is associated with qi and blood deficiency, thus coupled with pathogen wind invading the channels and collaterals, causing muscle and tendon flaccidity; or the condition may also be due to a spleen-stomach disharmony causing a failure of body fluids to distribute, resulting in collecting dampness and engendering sputum, combined with an external attack of pathogen wind. The wind-phlegm stagnates the collaterals causing an extra ocular muscle disorder. Another cause may be due to consumption of yin caused by febrile disease, yin-deficiency producing wind. The wind and phlegm flare upwards, disturbing the eyes. Vessel or collateral damage due to trauma in the head and face or oncothlipsis compression may be yet another causative factor.

Clinical Manifestation

The disease occurs with a sudden onset presenting with double vision, often accompanied by blurred vision, dizziness, nausea, instability of gait and so on. The eye squints to the opposite direction of the paralytic muscle with limited movement. If the abducent muscle group is attacked, the eye will bias to the nasal side and cause direct diplopia. While, if the abductor group is attacked, the eye will bias to the temporal side and result in crossed diplopia. Generally, the head will lean to the side of palsy muscle. Some cases may also have mydriasis and vision loss. The laboratory and special examinations include:

Arc perimeter strabismometry: Second angle of strabismus is bigger than the first angle of strabismus, which means when the palsy eye fixes at the target, the deviation of the healthy eye is more obvious.

Synoptophore examination: It can be used to determine the angle of strabismus. Imaging examination: Take orbit X-ray, cerebral CT or MRI examination to exclude fracture of the orbit, cerebral hemorrhage and occupying lesion.

Treatment

1. Pattern Differentiation and Treatment

(1) Wind Striking the Channel
【 Syndrome Characteristics 】
Acute onset, squinting, motor eye disorder, tilting the head back to see better, blurred vision, double vision, dizziness and instability of gait, pale tongue, rapid pulse.

【 Treatment Principle 】
Dispel wind and dissipate pathogen, invigorate blood to remove and dredge the collaterals.

【 Representative Formula 】
Modified *Qiāng Huó Shèng Fēng Tāng* (Notopterygium Wind-Eliminating Decoction, 羌活胜风汤) and *Qiān Zhèng Sǎn* (Symmetry-Correcting Powder, 牵正散)

【 Prescription 】

柴胡	*chái hú*	10 g	Radix Bupleuri
黄芩	*huáng qín*	10 g	Radix Scutellariae
荆芥	*jīng jiè*	10 g	Fructus Aurantii
枳壳	*zhǐ qiào*	10 g	Fructus Arctii
川芎	*chuān xiōng*	10 g	Rhizoma Chuanxiong
防风	*fáng fēng*	10 g	Radix Saposhnikoviae
羌活	*qiāng huó*	10 g	Rhizoma et Radix Notopterygii
独活	*dú huó*	10 g	Radix Angelicae Pubescentis
前胡	*qián hú*	10 g	Radix Peucedani
薄荷	*bò he*	10 g	Herba Menthae
桔梗	*jié gěng*	10 g	Radix Platycodonis
白芷	*bái zhǐ*	10 g	Radix Angelicae Dahuricae
甘草	*gān cǎo*	3 g	Radix et Rhizoma Glycyrrhizae
白附子	*bái fù zǐ*	6 g	Rhizoma Typhonii
僵蚕	*jiāng cán*	10 g	Bombyx Batryticatus
全蝎	*quán xiē*	3 g	Scorpio

【 Modifications 】
➢ For cases with liver deficiency and lack of blood, add *dāng guī* (当归, Radix Angelicae Sinensis) 10 g, *bái sháo* (白芍, Radix Paeoniae Alba) 10 g, and *shú dì huáng* (熟地黄, Radix Rehmanniae Praeparata) 10 g to tonify and nourish blood.

➢ For cases with dizziness, add *dāng guī* (当归, Radix Angelicae Sinensis) 10 g, *bái sháo* (白芍, Radix Paeoniae Alba) 10 g, *tiān má* (天麻, Rhizoma Gastrodiae) 10 g, and *jú huā* (菊花, Flos Chrysanthemi) 10 g to nourish blood, dispel wind and dredge the collaterals.

(2) wind-phlegm blocking the collaterals

【 Syndrome Characteristics 】

Eye syndromes is similar to the above condition, may be accompanied by dyspnea, nausea and vomiting, poor appetite, vomiting sputum, white-greasy coating, wiry-slippery pulse.

【 Treatment Principle 】

Dispel wind and eliminate dampness, resolve phlegm and dredge collaterals.

【 Representative Formula 】

Modified *Zhèng Róng Tāng* (Face-Restoring Decoction, 正容汤)

【 Prescription 】

羌活	*qiāng huó*	10 g	Rhizoma et Radix Notopterygii
白附子	*bái fù zǐ*	10 g	Rhizoma Typhonii
防风	*fáng fēng*	10 g	Radix Saposhnikoviae
秦艽	*qín jiāo*	10 g	Radix Gentianae Macrophyllae
胆南星	*dǎn nán xīng*	10 g	Arisaema cum Bile
半夏	*bàn xià*	10 g	Rhizoma Pinelliae
僵蚕	*jiāng cán*	10 g	Bombyx Batryticatus
木瓜	*mù guā*	10 g	Fructus Chaenomelis
甘草	*gān cǎo*	3 g	Radix et Rhizoma Glycyrrhizae
黄松节	*huáng sōng jié*	3 g	Lignum Pini Nodi
生姜	*shēng jiāng*	3 g	Rhizoma Zingiberis Recens

【 Modifications 】

For cases with nausea and vomiting, add *zhú rú* (竹茹, Caulis Bambusae in Taenia) 10 g to clear up phlegm and arrest vomiting. For cases with severe syndrome of phlegm-dampness pattern, add *yì yǐ rén* (薏苡仁, Semen Coicis) 15 g, *shí chāng pú* (石菖蒲, Rhizoma Acori Tatarinowii) 10 g, *pèi lán* (佩兰, Herba Eupatorii) 10 g to eliminate wetness-pathogenic with drugs of fragrant flavor, remove dampness and dispel phlegm.

(3) Stasis and Obstruction of the Channels and Collaterals

【 Syndrome Characteristics 】

Most of the causes are associated with head and face direct trauma, direct injury to the eye or stroke. The symptoms and signs include double vision, dark red tongue with ecchymosis, thin white coating, wiry-rapid or astringent pulse.

【 Treatment Principle 】

Invigorate blood and move qi, resolve stasis and dredge collaterals.

【Representative Formula】

Modified *Táo Hóng Sì Wù Tāng* (Peach Kernel and Carthamus Four Substances Decoction, 桃红四物汤)

【Prescription】

桃仁	*táo rén*	10 g	Semen Persicae
红花	*hóng huā*	10 g	Flos Carthami
当归	*dāng guī*	10 g	Radix Angelicae Sinensis
熟地黄	*shú dì huáng*	10 g	Radix Rehmanniae Praeparata
白芍	*bái sháo*	10 g	Radix Paeoniae Alba
川芎	*chuān xiōng*	10 g	Rhizoma Chuanxiong

【Modifications】

➢ For cases in the initial stage, add *fáng fēng* (防风, Radix Saposhnikoviae) 10 g, *jīng jiè* (荆芥, Herba Schizonepetae) 10 g, *bái fù zǐ* (白附子, Rhizoma Typhonii) 10 g, *jiāng cán* (僵蚕, Bombyx Batryticatus) 10 g, *quán xiē* (全蝎, Scorpio) 3 g to enhance the function of dispelling wind and eliminating pathogen. For case in late stage, add *dǎng shēn* (党参, Radix Codonopsis) 10 g and *huáng qí* (黄芪, Radix Astragali) 15 g to benefit qi and support healthy qi.

(4) Yin-Deficiency With Yang Hyperactivity

【Syndrome Characteristics】

Chronic, gradual onset, often presents with a history of hypertension, dizziness, squint, eye movement disorder, double vision, red tongue with thin coating, thready-rapid pulse.

【Treatment Principle】

Nourish yin and subdue yang, calm the liver and extinguish wind.

【Representative Formula】

Modified *Yù Yīn Qiǎn Yáng Xī Fēng Tāng* (Yin-Fostering, Yang-Subduing and Wind-Extinguishing Decoction, 育阴潜阳息风汤)

【Prescription】

生地	*shēng dì*	15 g	Radix Rehmanniae
白芍	*bái sháo*	12 g	Radix Paeoniae Alba
枸杞子	*gǒu qǐ zǐ*	12 g	Fructus Lycii
麦冬	*mài dōng*	10 g	Radix Ophiopogonis
天冬	*tiān dōng*	10 g	Radix Asparagi
盐知母	*yán zhī mǔ*	10 g	Rhizoma Anemarrhenae (salt-prepared)
盐黄柏	*yán huáng bǎi*	10 g	Cortex Phellodendri Chinensis (salt-fried)
石决明	*shí jué míng*	15 g	Concha Haliotidis
龙骨	*lóng gǔ*	10 g	Os Draconis

牡蛎	*mǔ lì*	10 g	Concha Ostreae
怀牛膝	*huái niú xī*	10 g	Radix Achyranthis Bidentatae
钩藤	*gōu téng*	10 g	Ramulus Uncariae Cum Uncis
全蝎	*quán xiē*	10 g	Scorpio
菊花	*jú huā*	10 g	Flos Chrysanthemi
黄芩	*huáng qín*	10 g	Radix Scutellariae

【Modifications】

➢ For cases with constipation, add *fān xiè yè* (番泻叶, Folium Sennae) 10 g.

➢ For cases with dyspnea, palpitation and knotted pulse, remove *shí jué míng* (石决明, Concha Haliotidis), *lóng gǔ* (龙骨, Os Draconis), *mǔ lì* (牡蛎, Concha Ostreae, oyster shell), and add *zǐ sū zǐ* (紫苏子, Fructus Perillae) 10 g, *dǎng shēn* (党参, Radix Codonopsis) 10 g, *yuǎn zhì* (远志, Radix Polygalae) 10 g, and *suān zǎo rén* (酸枣仁, Semen Ziziphi Spinosae) 10 g.

2. Acupuncture

| *Tòu Méi* ("joining eyebrow", joining SJ 23 to BL 2) | BL 1 (*jīng míng*) | ST 1 (*chéng qì*) |
| *qiú hòu* (球后) | *tài yáng* (太阳) | GB 20 (*fēng chí*) |

Manipulation: Insert the needle for 3–5 *fen* when puncturing at *tài yáng* (太阳) and GB 20 points, and 1 *cun* for the other acupuncture points.

If the eye deviates inward, select "joining eyebrow", *qiú hòu* (球后), *tài yáng* (太阳), and GB 20. If outward, select "joining eyebrow", *jīng míng* (睛明, BL1), *tài yáng* (太阳), and GB 20. If the eye deviates upward, select "joining eyebrow", ST 1 (*chéng qì*), *tài yáng* (太阳), and GB 20.

If downward, select "joining eyebrow", *tài yáng* (太阳), and GB 20. Use even supplementation and drainage methods, retain the needles for 30–45 minutes after arrival of qi, treat once every day or every other day. 12 treatments equals one course, 20–40 courses may be needed.

Main points: BL 1, ST 1, BL 2, *yú yāo*, GB 14, GB 20. Use 1–*cun* needle, retain the needles for 30–45 minutes, treat once every day or every other day, 12 sessions is a treatment course.

3. Massage

First, arrange the patient in supine position, then massage the acupoints DU 20 (*bǎi huì*), BL1 (*jīng míng*), BL 2 (*cuán zhú*), *yú yāo* (鱼腰), *tài yáng* (太阳), GB 1 (*tóng zǐ liáo*), SJ 23 (*sī zhú kōng*), GB 20 (*fēng chí*) with manipulation of finger-pressing, pressing and rubbing alternatively for about 30 minutes. After that, arrange the patient in sitting position, massage the points of BL 18 (*gān shù*), BL19 (*dǎn shù*), BL 20 (*pí shù*), LI 4 (*hé gǔ*), and GB 37 (*guāng míng*) with manipulations of finger-pressing, pressing, kneading and pinching, for 5 minutes, once a day, 10 sessions is a treatment course.

4. Chinese Patent Medicines

(1) *Sàn fēng Huó Luò Wán* (散风活络丸, Wind-Dissipating and Collateral-Activating Pill)
Take orally, 6 g (1 tablet), two times a day, applicable to wind phlegm obstructing the collaterals.
(2) *ZhèngTiān Wán* (正天丸, Sky-Righting Pill)
Take orally, 2 tablets, three times a day, applicable to yin deficiency with yang hyperactivity.
(3) *Nǎo Xīn Tōng Jiāo Náng* (脑心通胶囊, Troxerutin and Diprophylline Capsules)
Take orally, 2–4 tablets, three times a day, applicable to qi deficiency and blood stasis and phlegm obstructing meridian collaterals.

5. External Treatment

Point application therapy
Fù Fāng Qiān Zhèng Gāo (复方牵正膏, Compound Symmetry-Correcting Paste): Apply to *tài yáng* (太阳), ST 7 (*xià guān*), ST 6 (*jiá chē*) on the affected side, one point every time, 7–10 days interval between two points' application, it is applicable to patterns of wind-phlegm obstructing the collaterals.

6. Treatment with Western Medicine

Take oral supplementation of vitamin B1, B2 and Inosine tablets. If the course of the disease has existed for more than 10 days and if the condition is stable, surgery may be advised to correct the position of the eye.

7. Dietary Therapy and Preventive Care

Cover the paralytic eye to eliminate diplopia. Avoid fatty, sweet and greasy-fried foods in order to prevent production of dampness and sputum/mucous, which may aggravate the disease. Live a regular life and stay warm to prevent the disease or alleviate the symptoms.

Case Study 1

Wu, female, 28-year-old

【Chief Complaint】

Diplopia for one month.

【Examination】

The vision was 20/20 on the right eye and 20/25 on the left eye. Movement of the left eye was limited at directions of lateral, supra-outside and infra-outside, and diplopia is present even when the left eye moves slightly outwards. There was nothing abnormal with the right eye. The fundus of both eyes was normal. Blood pressure: 90/55 mmHg. The patient also presented with red tongue with slight yellow-greasy coating, wiry-rapid pulse.

【Diagnosis】

Squinting of the left eye, seeing one thing as two.

【Pattern Differentiation】

Liver constraint and qi stagnation causing obstruction of the vessel, and pathogens wind invading the underlying deficiency.

【Treatment Principles】

Calm the liver and clear heat, extinguish wind and resolve spasms.

【Prescription】

Modified *Bǔ Gān Sǎn* (Liver-Tonifying Powder, 补肝散)

车前子（包煎）	*chē qián zǐ (bāo jiān)*	9 g	Semen Plantaginis (wrap)
细辛	*xì xīn*	2 g	Radix et Rhizoma Asari
茯苓	*fú líng*	12 g	Poria
防风	*fáng fēng*	5 g	Radix Scrophulariae
玄参	*xuán shēn*	9 g	Radix Paeoniae Rubra
黄芩	*huáng qín*	5 g	Radix Scutellariae
羌活	*qiāng huó*	5 g	Rhizoma et Radix Notopterygii
党参	*dǎng shēn*	12 g	Radix Codonopsis
石决明	*shí jué míng*	24 g	Concha Haliotidis
钩藤	*gōu téng*	5 g	Ramulus Uncariae Cum Uncis
五味子	*wǔ wèi zǐ*	9 g	Fructus Schisandrae Chinensis
僵蚕	*jiāng cán*	6 g	Bombyx Batryticatus
白附子	*bái fù zǐ*	2 g	Rhizoma Typhonii

All the medicinals were decocted with water and 1 dose was administered each day. Besides the decoction, the patient was also administered a Chinese patent drug *Cí Zhū Wán* (磁朱丸, Loadstones and Cinnabar Pill), 6 g per day, pounded into pieces and taken with warm boiled water.

【Follow-up】

After taking 27 doses, she visited our clinic again. Her diplopia disappeared when seeing things within one foot, and the patient reported that the symptoms occurred occasionally when looking laterally - outwards. She now complained of insomnia and mildly low blood pressure. The position of the left eye was normal and the eye could move upwards, downwards, rightwards and leftwards without limit. The fundus of both eyes was normal. She presented with a deep-thready pulse, pale tongue with white coating. The muscle and tendon spasm was resolved after treatment so that the squinting disappeared. However, the prolonged course had damaged qi and caused deficiency of the spleen and stomach, thus the eye connector was still not as flexible as before, and there was still a degree of minor eye movement disorder that remained. So as to secure root and bank up original qi thus cure the disease completely, the treatment principle was changed to replenish qi and elevate yang, quiet the heart and calm mind. Formula: Modified *Bǔ Zhōng Yì Qì Tāng* (Center-Supplementing and Qi-Boosting Decoction, 补中益气汤). Prescription as the following:

炙黄芪	*zhì huáng qí*	15 g	Radix Astragali Praeparata cum Melle
炒白术	*chǎo bái zhú*	10 g	Rhizoma Atractylodis Macrocephalae (dry-fried)
陈皮	*chén pí*	6 g	Pericarpium Citri Reticulatae
升麻	*shēng má*	6 g	Rhizoma Cimicifugae
柴胡	*chái hú*	6 g	Radix Bupleuri
党参	*dǎng shēn*	10 g	Radix Codonopsis
炙甘草	*zhì gān cǎo*	10 g	Radix et Rhizoma Glycyrrhizae Praeparata cum Melle
丹参	*dān shēn*	10 g	Radix et Rhizoma Salviae Miltiorrhizae
炒枣仁	*chǎo zǎo rén*	15 g	Semen Ziziphi Spinosae (dry-fried)
夜交藤	*yè jiāo téng*	15 g	Caulis Polygoni Multiflori
五味子	*wǔ wèi zǐ*	6 g	Fructus Schisandrae Chinensis

The patient was administered 14 doses to strengthen the effect.

Case Study 2

A 27-year-old female
【Chief Complaint】
Double vision for the last seven days
【Medical History】
The patient stated that she has been working with computer more than ten hours everyday. Seven days ago after a common cold, she suddenly found she saw one thing as two, and also felt slightly sick.

【Examination】

The corrected vision is 20/20 on both eyes, the anterior segment and fundus was normal. The right eye movement was limited when turning outwards, it was full range of motion in all other directions.

Diplopia image examination: Horizontal homonymous, the deviation was most obvious with a lateral eye movement, and the peripheral one of the two images was seen by the right eye.

【Diagnosis】

Paralytic strabismus (right abducens nerve palsy). Due to the fact that the patient had nothing abnormal of tongue and pulse, he was treated only with acupuncture.

Point selection:

GB 20 (*fēng chí*)	GB 12 (*wán gǔ*)	BL 10 (*tiān zhù*)
ST 1 (*chéng qì*)	GB 1 (*tóng zǐ liáo*)	*qiú hòu* (球后)
tài yáng (太阳)	DU 20 (*bǎi huì*)	SJ 5 (*wài guān*)
LI 4 (*hé gǔ*)		

Treatment was administered once a day.

【Follow-up】

After seven days of acupuncture, her diplopia disappeared. To strengthen the effectiveness, the same treatment was given 5 more times.

Section 3   Thyroid-Associated Opthalmopathy

Thyroid-associated opthalmopathy is the most common orbital disease. It is considered to be an autoimmune action and is closely related with the endorine function. It is also called Graves' disease, mostly accompanied by hyperthyoidism. If the patient has no past or present history of hyperthyroidism and only present with eye symptoms, it is called ocular Graves' disease. Clinically thyroid-associated ophthalmopathy may present with different degrees of proptosis regardless of thyroid function, patients maybe hyperthyroid, normal or hypothyroid function. In severe cases, irreversible vision loss maybe occurs if the enlarged extraocular muscles compress and damages the optic nerve. Therefore, it is important to diagnose and treat promptly in the early stages of the disease. In Traditional Chinese Medicine, the disease is called *tū qǐ jīng gāo* (sudden bulging of the eyes, 突起睛高), or *hú yǎn níng jīng* (dove-like fixed eye, 鹘眼凝睛). Another name is *yú jīng bū yè* (nightless fish eyes) from *Mù Jīng Dà Chéng* (The Great Compendium of Classics on Ophthalmology, 目经大成) because proptosis eyes look like unclosed fish eyes. The cause and mechanism of the disease patterns is heat toxin of five viscera congesting in the upper body, causing internal wind-heat of brain attacking the eye. The other possible causative factors include yin deficiency and yang hyperactivity, which may be due to constitutional yin deficiency, or excess heart stress resulting in the heart yin deficiency and liver yin damage. When western medicine is unsuitable or ineffective for these patients, Traditional Chinese Medicine can be quite effective, even for some intractable cases. TCM therapeutic methods may relieve symptoms and decrease complications which may result in permanent vision loss.

Incidence rate

Statistics from England indicate that this disease is more common in women aged 40–50 years old. The female to male ratio is 8:1. In China, a study was done in 3,406 cases of orbital diseases from 1976 to 1995, it showed Grave's disease presented itself in 622 cases (about 18.26%) and occurred in all ages; the majority occurring in women aged 20–40 years.

Clinical manifestation

The disease may manifest in one or several symptoms and signs as seen below.

1. Diplopia: Binocular horizontal or vertical diplopia may occur when extraocular muscles are involved.

2. Eyelid retraction: Retraction may occur in both upper and lower eyelids. The patients often describe it as "the eyes open wider" or "gazing". It's called Von Graefe sign when superior eyelids lag upon downward gaze and expose more of the sclera.

3. Proptosis: Exposure keratitis may occur in some severe cases.

4. Other symptoms: Other symptoms include restricted eyeball movement, discomfort or pain in retrobulb (back of the eye) and periorbit (around the eye), vision loss, intraocular pressure elevation and so on. When swelling of inner orbital tissues and raise of intraocular pressure, it can bring out compression of optic nerve and optic neuropathy. The patients will complain of loss of visual acuity, constriction of visual field or pathological scotoma. Manifestations of fundus oculi include papilledema, retinal exudation and edema, tortuosity and extension of the retinal vein. Severe conditions may lead to optic atrophy which results in serious impaired vision and pallor papillae.

Patients with hyperthyroidism may have some systemic symptoms, such as rash and impatient nature, emaciation, increased appetite, hand tremor, pulse speeding up and basic metabolic rate increasing.

Treatment

When the function of thyroid is abnormal, it is important to seek help from endocrine doctors. If there is severe swelling of orbital tissues and obvious ophthalmological symptoms, western medicine mainly uses glucocorticoids or radiotherapy. When drug treatment is ineffective for high pressure of the orbital cavity, orbital decompression surgery may be an option.

1. Pattern Differentiation and Treatment

(1) Heat Toxin Congestion in the Upper Body
【Syndrome Characteristics】
Binocular progressive proptosis, hard swelling of the eyelid, limitation of eye movement, red face and generalized heat, constipation and reddish urine, red tongue with yellow greasy coating, rapid pulse.
【Treatment Principle】
Clear heat and remove toxin, invigorate blood and free the collaterals.
【Representative Formula】
Xiè Nǎo Tāng (Brain-Draining Decoction, 泻脑汤)
【Prescription】

车前子	*chē qián zǐ*	10 g	Semen Plantaginis (wrap)
木通	*mù tōng*	10 g	Caulis Akebiae
茯苓	*fú líng*	10 g	Poria
熟大黄	*Shú dà huáng*	10 g	Rhei Radix et Rhizoma Conquiti
玄明粉	*xuán míng fěn*	10 g	Natrii Sulfas Exsiccatus (add at end)
黄芩	*huáng qín*	10 g	Radix Scutellariae
茺蔚子	*chōng wèi zǐ*	10 g	Fructus Leonuri
防风	*fáng fēng*	10 g	Radix Saposhnikoviae
桔梗	*jié gěng*	10 g	Radix Platycodonis
玄参	*xuán shēn*	10 g	Radix Scrophulariae

【Modifications】
➢ For cases with proptosis accompanying with pain caused by heat scorching, add *mǔ dān pí* (牡丹皮 Cortex Moutan) 10 g, *chì sháo* (赤芍 Radix Paeoniae Rubra) 10 g and *xià kū cǎo* (夏枯草, Spica Prunellae) 10 g to cool blood and dissipate blood stasis, dissipate mass and stop pain;
➢ For cases with headache and stiff nape, add *shí jué míng* (石决明, Concha Haliotidis) 15 g, *qīng xiāng zǐ* (青葙子, Semen Celosiae) 10 g and *bái jí lí* (白蒺藜, Fructus Tribuli) 10 g to clear the liver and drain fire, calm the liver and relieve pain.

(2) yin deficiency and yang hyperactivity
【Syndrome Characteristics】
Proptosis, staring and not easy movement, dizzy and eye distention, dysphoria,

insomnia and profuse sweating, few tongue coating, rapid and thready pulse.

【 Treatment Principle 】

Nourish yin and subdue yang.

【 Representative Formula 】

Tiān Má Gōu Téng Yǐn (Gastrodia and Uncaria Decoction, 天麻钩藤饮)

【 Prescription 】

天麻	*tiān má*	10 g	Rhizoma Gastrodiae
钩藤	*gōu téng*	12 g	Ramulus Uncariae Cum Uncis
生石决明	*Shēng shí jué míng*	20 g	Concha Haliotidis
栀子	*zhī zǐ*	10 g	Fructus Gardeniae
黄芩	*huáng qín*	10 g	Radix Scutellariae
川牛膝	*chuān niú xī*	12 g	Radix Cyathulae
杜仲	*dù zhòng*	10 g	Cortex Eucommiae
益母草	*yì mǔ cǎo*	10 g	Herba Leonuri
桑寄生	*sāng jì shēng*	10 g	Herba Taxilli
夜交藤	*yè jiāo téng*	10 g	Caulis Polygoni Multiflori
朱茯神	*zhū fú shén*	15 g	Sclerotium Poriae Pararadicis

【 Modifications 】

➢ For cases with dry mouth and constipation, add *shēng dì* (生地, Radix Rehmanniae) 15 g, *xuán shēn* (玄参, Radix Scrophulariae) 10 g, and *huǒ má rén* (火麻仁, Fructus Cannabis) 10 g to enrich yin, moisten dryness and free the stool.

➢ For cases with yin deficiency and heat accumulation, proptosis and congestion, add *chì sháo* (赤芍, Radix Paeoniae Rubra) 10 g, *zǐ cǎo* (紫草, Radix Arnebiae) 10 g, and *lián qiào* (连翘, Fructus Forsythiae) 10 g to cool blood, dissipate stasis, and resolve swelling.

➢ For cases with difficult-to-treat proptosis, add *zhè bèi mǔ* (浙贝母, Bulbus Fritillariae Thunbergii) 15 g, *shēng mǔ lì* (生牡蛎, Ostreae Concha Cruda) 15 g, and *kūn bù* (昆布, Thallus Laminariae) 10 g to enhance the effect of breaking stasis and dissipating masses.

2. Acupuncture

Acupoints of body needles selected include GB 20 (*fēng chí*), *tài yáng* (太阳), GB 14 (*yáng bái*), ST 2 (*sì bái*), ST 1 (*chéng qì*), LI 4 (*hé gǔ*), SJ 5 (*wài guān*), SI 3 (*hòu xī*), LV 2 (*xíng jiān*), GB 42 (*dì wǔ huì*), and so on.

Choose 3–4 eye aupoints and 2-3 body acupoints every time, use even supplementation and drainage method, retain the needle for 30 minutes, once every day. For the cases with severe heat syndrome, prick LI 20 (*yíng xiāng*), *tài yáng* (太阳), and DU 23 (*shàng xīng*) using three edged needle to open astringent and abduct stagnation, drain the superabundance and free the stasis.

3. Chinese Patent Medicines

(1) *Xià Kū Cǎo Jiāo Náng* (Spica Prunellae Capsules, 夏枯草胶囊)

0.7g each time, two times a day, applicable to clear fire, dissipate binds, disperse swelling.

(2) *Zhī Bǎi Dì Huáng Wán* (Anemarrhena, Phellodendron and Rehmannia Pill, 知柏地黄丸)

8 pills (concentrated pill) each time, two times a day, applicable to nourish yin and reduce fire, clear heat and eliminate vexation.

4. External Treatment

黄芪	*huáng qí*	30 g	Radix Astragali
细辛	*xì xīn*	10 g	Radix et Rhizoma Asari
当归	*dāng guī*	30 g	Radix Angelicae Sinensis
杏仁	*xìng rén*	30 g	Semen Armeniacae Amarum
防风	*fáng fēng*	30 g	Radix Saposhnikoviae
松脂	*sōng zhī*	30 g	Pini Resina
黄蜡	*huáng là*	30 g	Wax
白芷	*bái zhǐ*	120 g	Radix Angelicae Dahuricae
小麻油	*xiǎo má yóu*	120 g	Oleum Ricini

Usage: Grind all the medicinals into powder and then decoct it to make paste. Put the paste onto *tài yáng* (太阳), two times a day. It is applicable to invigorate blood, free the collaterals and disperse swelling. However, it is used with care for the cases of skin hypersensitivity.

5. Dietary Therapy and Preventive Care

(1) For the cases with obvious proptosis or hypophasis during sleep, drop artificial tears several times a day, apply antibiotics eye ointment to moisten eyelids before sleep.

(2) Take bland diet, do not eat fried, fatty foods, and inhibit the consumption of lamb meet, rooster meat and seafood.

(3) Dredge psychology and adjust spirit, build up the idea of insisting on treatment for long time.

Classic Quotes

《秘传眼科龙木论》:"此疾皆因五脏热壅冲上，脑中风热入眼所致。"

The disease was caused by heat toxin of five viscera congesting in the upper body, wind heat of brain going into the eyes.

The Secret Transmission of Long-mu's Ophthalmology (*Mì Chuán Yǎn Kē Lóng Mù Lùn*, 秘传眼科龙木论)

《银海精微》谓:"突起睛高，险峻厉害之症也……皆因五脏毒风所蕴，热极充眼者……"

"Sudden proptosis is a severe disease......caused by toxin wind congesting in the five *zang* and extreme heat filling the eyes....."

Essentials from the Silver Sea (*Yín Hǎi Jīng Wēi*, 银海精微)

Section 4   Myopia

Myopia is, by definition an ocular refraction problem. The occurrence of myopia is related with heredity, growth & development, diet, environment and so on, but the exact cause is still unclear. In recent years, myopia tends to affect children early on, and the incidence increases from elementary school, up through middle school.

TCM realized the disease of myopia a long time ago and named it *mù bù néng yuǎn shì* (nearsightedness, 目不能远视) or *néng jìn qiè yuǎn zhèng* (nearsightedness, 能近怯远症). It is also called *jìn qū* (近觑) or *qū qū yǎn* (squinting eye, 觑觑眼) if it is a congenital myopia with a high diopter. The cause and pathogenesis of the disease is associated with excessive use of eyes for reading, computer and close work during young ages. These results in the damage of qi and blood and deficiency of heart yang, therefore the eye can not see distant objects clearly. Another associated pattern is that of prenatal essence deficiency causing deficiency of the liver and kidney, essence and blood, which results in the weakness of sight.

Classification

Based on the degree of diopter, myopia is divided into three grades:

Low myopia: the diopter is 3.0 or less than 3.0

Medium myopia: the diopter is between 3.0 and 6.0

High myopia: the diopter is higher than 6.0

Based on the cause of refraction, myopia is divided into two types: axial myopia and refractive myopia.

Axial myopia: the axis of the eye is quite long, but the refractive power is normal.

Refreactive myopia: the axis is normal but the refractive power increases.

Based on the clinical characteristics of myopia, it is divided to simple myopia and pathological myopia. The main differences are listed below:

Classification	Simple myopia	Pathological myopia
Incidence	High	Low
Age	Juvenile	At birth or early stage of childhood
Development	Stabilize when growth process completed	Progress fast, the diopter increases following the age
Axis length	< 28mm	>28mm, accompanied by scleral posterior staphyloma
Corrected visual acuity	≥20/20	<20/20
Final diopter	Always less than -12.0D	Always higher than -12.0D
Fundus	Few complications in the retina and macula	Lattice degeneration in the peripheral retina, retinochoroidal atrophy spot, hemorrhage, degeneration, Fuchs spot and lacquer cracks in the macula area
Pathogenesis	Acquired	Polygene hereditary

Clinical Manifestation

1. Symptoms

Blurred vision when trying to see distant objects, but the individual can see near objects relatively clearly. The patient will typically squint in order to see distant objects from far away. Patients with high myopia may report flashing sensations, floaters, shadow-like shapes in the field of vision, low vision in dim environment, visual fatigue and so on.

2. Visual acuity

Far vision decreases, near vision remains normal. Those patients with high myopia or pathologic myopia may have blurred vision for both near sight and distant sight.

3. Ophthalmic examination

Those patients with high myopia may present with axial proptosis, exotropia or exophoria. The fundus is often normal in people with simple myopia, though some cases present with myopic crescent and atrophic change like leopard-spot. Besides the fundus change of the above, the pathologic myopia patients may also present with vitreous liquefaction, posterior vitreous detachment, and posterior scleral staphyloma at young ages. Lazy eye may occur in the pre-school children with medium or high myopia if their vision is not corrected through wearing proper glasses.

Treatment

1. Pattern Differentiation and Treatment

(1) Insufficiency of Heart Yang

【 Syndrome Characteristics 】

Nearby objects seen clearly but distant objects appear blurred. No obvious complaints, and may be accompanied by palpitations and mental fatigue, and forgetfulness, pale complexion, pale tongue with thin coating, thready and weak pulse.

【 Treatment Principle 】

Supplement the heart and replenish qi, quiet the spirit and stabilize the mind.

【 Representative Formula 】

Modified *Dìng Zhì Wán* (Spirit-Quieting Pill, 定志丸)

【 Prescription 】

远志	*yuǎn zhì*	10 g	Radix Polygalae
石菖蒲	*shí chāng pú*	10 g	Rhizoma Acori Tatarinowii
党参	*dǎng shēn*	10 g	Radix Codonopsis
茯苓	*fú líng*	10 g	Poria
朱砂	*zhū shā*	3 g	Cinnabaris

【 Modifications 】

➢ For cases with eye distending pain and fatigue, add *mù guā* (木瓜, Fructus Chaenomelis) 10 g and *bái sháo* (白芍, Radix Paeoniae Alba) 10 g to nourish blood and activate collaterals.

➢ For cases with dull pain in the head and eye, add *dān shēn* (丹参, Radix et Rhizoma Salviae Miltiorrhizae) 10g and *gé gēn* (葛根, Radix Puerariae Lobatae) 10 g to activate blood and dredge collaterals.

➢ For cases with eyebrow bone pain, add *màn jīng zǐ* (蔓荆子, Fructus Viticis) 10 g, *quán xiē* (全蝎, Scorpio) 3 g and *bái zhǐ* (白芷, Radix Angelicae Dahuricae) 10 g to stop wind and dredge collaterals.

(2) Deficiency of Both Liver and Kidney

【 Syndrome Characteristics 】

See nearby objects clearly but distant objects appear to be blurred, floaters in the visual filed are common, may accompanied by vitreous liquefaction and turbid, dizziness and tinnitus, insomnia profuse dreaming, limp aching lumbus and knees, dribbling urination, pale tongue with thin coating, thready pulse or wiry and thready pulse.

【 Treatment Principle 】

Supplement the liver and the kidney, nourish essence and blood.

【 Representative Formula 】

Modified *Zhù Jǐng Wán* (Long Vistas Pill, 驻景丸)

【 Prescription 】

熟地黄	*shú dì huáng*	10 g	Radix Rehmanniae Praeparata
菟丝子	*tù sī zǐ*	20 g	Semen Cuscutae
楮实子	*chǔ shí zǐ*	10 g	Fructus Broussonetiae
枸杞子	*gǒu qǐ zǐ*	10 g	Fructus Lycii
车前子	*chē qián zǐ*	10 g	Semen Plantaginis
五味子	*wǔ wèi zǐ*	10 g	Fructus Schisandrae Chinensis
当归	*dāng guī*	10 g	Radix Angelicae Sinensis
花椒	*huā jiāo*	10 g	Pericarpium Zanthoxyli

【 Modifications 】

➢ For cases accompanied by qi deficiency syndromes like shortage of breath and reluctancy to speak , add *dǎng shēn* (党参, Radix Codonopsis) 15 g and *huáng qí* (黄芪, Radix Astragali) 15 g to strengthen the effect of replenishing qi.

➢ For cases with spleen-stomach disharmony, add *jiāo sān xiān* (焦三仙,Tres Immortales Usti) and *chén pí* (陈皮, Pericarpium Citri Reticulatae) 10 g to invigorate the spleen and promote digestion.

2. Acupuncture

(1) Dermal Needle:

Choose one of the five acupoint groups:

Group 1 includes ST 1 (*chéng qì*) and *yì míng* (翳明),

Group 2 includes ST 2 (*sì bái*) and SI 15 (*jiān zhōng shù*),

Group 3 includes ST 8 (*tóu wéi*) and *qiú hòu* (球后)

Group 4 includes BL 1 (*jīng míng*) and GB 37 (*guāng míng*),

Group 5 includes SJ 23 (*sī zhú kōng*), LV 3 (*tài chōng*), and KI 6 (*zhào hǎi*).

Choose one group each day with alternation, mainly use supplementation method, 10 sessions for a treatment course.

(2) Embedding Seeds at Ear Points

Wáng bù liú xíng (王不留行, Vaccariae Semen) seeds on sticky fabric to make ear seed , choose auricular acupuncture points spirit gate (*shén mén*, HT7), liver (*gān*), spleen (*pí*), kidney (*shèn*, CO10), and ear apex (*ěr jiān*, HX6), stick the ear seed on the points, press and kneed the points 2–3 times each day, one treatment course includes 15 days. The ear bean is suggested to be changed 1–2 times every week to keep clean and working effectively.

(3) Chinese Massage / Acupressure

Choose the point 3 fen below BL 2 (*cuán zhú*) as the "main myopia acupoint", and BL 2 (*cuán zhú*), *yú yāo* (鱼腰), SJ 23 (*sī zhú kōng*), ST 2 (*sì bái*), BL 1 (*jīng míng*) as the combination acupoints, press and knead the main myopia acupoint first using the forefinger and then the combination acupoints, 10 minutes each time. One treatment course includes 30 times.

3. Simple and Proven Recipes for Improving Eye Sight

(1) Spiney date seed conjee

Take *suān zǎo rén* (酸枣仁, Semen Ziziphi Spinosae) 30 g and rice 50 g, pound the spine date seeds into pieces and wrap it with a gauze cloth, put it into 500 ml water together with rice and boil it until the rice turns mushy, then remove the gauze bag, add some brown sugar, tighten the cover and keep it close for 5 minutes. Warm and take 1 hour before bedtime every night. This method is applicable to patients with syndrome of deficiency of heart yang.

(2) Cooked Chinese Wolfberry Fruit and Pork Liver

Take Chinese wolfberry fruit 50 g and pork liver 250 g, use lard, salt, cooking wine, monosodium glutamate as sauces. First, dip the Chinese wolfberry fruit in boiled water for two hours and then dry it in air, cut the pork liver into slices, mix it well with the salt and cooking wine, then cook the liver slices with lard until it is medium done, add the Chinese wolfberry fruit and cook together until the liver slices is well done, at last add some monosodium glutamate. It can be taken with rice and bread and suggested to those with syndrome of insufficiency of both liver and kidney.

(3) Tremella and Chinese Wolfberry Fruit Eye-Brightening Decoction

Yín ěr (银耳, Tremella) 20g, Chinese wolfberry fruit 20 g, jasmine 10 g, decocted with water one dose per day and taken as tea for days. It's applicable to patients with deficiency of both the live and kidney.

4. Treatment with Western Medicine

Corrective eyeglasses is the main treatment for myopia. Laser refractive surgery has been developed in recent years and is another possible alternative treatment for nearsightedness in adults older than 18 years old with high diopters. The final decision of whether laser surgery is a suitable option should be made after the comprehensive examination has been performed by an optometrist.

5. Prevention and Health Care

(1) Develop good habits for eye health, it is suggested to read under proper lighting and sit in a correct posture when reading.

(2) Youths should limit their consumption of sweet foods like chocolate and ice-cream. The diet should be comprehensive and arranged well with coarse and processed flour, supplemented with calcium, magnesium, phosphorus and zinc daily.

(3) Exercise regularly to improve and maintain your overall health.

(4) Have regular ophthalmic examination so that nearsightedness can be found early and treated early.

(5) Do eye care massage daily.

Classic Quotes

《诸病源候论·目病诸候》:"劳伤肝腑，肝气不足，兼受风邪，使精华之气衰弱，故不能远视。"

Overstrain may damage the liver and result in liver qi deficiency. If re-attacked by wind pathogen, the essential qi will be destroyed badly, thus the eyes can not see objects in distance clearly for lack of nutrients.

Treatise on the Origins and Manifestations of Various Diseases – Eye Disease (*Zhū Bìng Yuán Hòu Lùn–Mù Bìng Zhū Hòu*, 诸病源候论·目病诸候)

《审视瑶函·内障》:"怯远症，肝经不足肾经病，光华咫尺视模糊，莫待精衰盲已定" 及 "阳不足，病于火少者也。无火，是以光华不能发越于远。"

One with nearsightedness can not see objects in distance even in very young ages. It is caused by deficiency of both the liver and kidney. It may also be seen in the patients with yang deficiency syndrome,for the eyes can not be warmed by yang, thus the vision brilliance can not reach distance.

Jade Case of Perspicacity – Internal Visual Obstruction (*Shěn Shì Yáo Hán–Nèi Zhàng*, 审视瑶函·内障)

Questions for Consideration

1.What is the cause and pathogenesis of myopia?

2. Briefly describe the embedding of seeds at ear points.

Section 5   Visual Fatigue

Visual fatigue is characterized by distending eye pain, dizziness, heavy eyelids, blurred vision, headache, pain around the eyebrow bone, and in some cases, nausea. The symptoms occur after extensive reading and will typically disappear with rest. In modern medicine, the disease is classified into retinal visual fatigue, muscular visual fatigue and accommodative visual fatigue and etc. In Chinese ophthalmology, visual fatigue is ascribed to *gān láo* (肝劳, liver taxation). The causative factors are associated with qi deficiency or yang deficiency, thus yang qi cannot bear upward to the eyes resulting in eye fatigue. Other causative factors are associated with blood deficiency or yin deficiency, thus yin blood fails to nourish the eyes causing fatigue. Deficiency of the kidney essence may be another causative factor. The pathogenesis is due to lack of source for blood nourishment or closing of the pores, thus the eyes cannot get enough nutrients.

Clinical Manifestation

The patients feel dryness and discomfort of the eyes, distending pain, dizziness, vexation and nausea after extensive work at close distances (reading, computer work, etc.). Symptoms may resolve with rest. There are no obvious abnormities in the visual acuity or upon eye examination. Some patients may present with myopia and presbyopia.

Treatment

1. Pattern Differentiation and Treatment

(1) Deficiency of Both the Liver and the Kidney

Main syndrome characteristics: Blurred vision after extensive use of the eyes, distending eye pain, dryness. Some patients may have refractive errors like myopia, hyperopia or presbytia. The other body symptoms include dizziness, tinnitus, aching lumbus and limp knees, pale tongue with few coating, theady pulse.

Treatment principle: Nourish the kidney and the liver, enrich essence and brighten the eyes.

Representative formula: Modified *Qǐ Jú Dì Huáng Wán* (Lycium Berry, Chrysanthemum and Rehmannia Pill, 杞菊地黄丸) combined with *Chái Gé Jiě Jī Tāng* (Bupleurum and Pueraria Muscle-Resolving Decoction, 柴葛解肌汤)

【 Prescription 】

熟地黄	*shú dì huáng*	10 g	Radix Rehmanniae Praeparata
山茱萸	*shān zhū yú*	10 g	Fructus Corni

干山药	gān shān yào	10 g	Rhizoma Dioscoreae
泽泻	zé xiè	10 g	Rhizoma Alismatis
茯苓	fú líng	10 g	Poria
牡丹皮	mǔ dān pí	10 g	Cortex Moutan
枸杞子	gǒu qǐ zǐ	10 g	Fructus Lycii
菊花	jú huā	10 g	Flos Chrysanthemi
柴胡	chái hú	10 g	Radix Bupleuri
葛根	gé gēn	10 g	Radix Puerariae Lobatae
甘草	gān cǎo	3 g	Radix et Rhizoma Glycyrrhizae
黄芩	huáng qín	10 g	Radix Scutellariae
赤芍	chì sháo	10 g	Radix Paeoniae Rubra
知母	zhī mǔ	10 g	Rhizoma Anemarrhenae
贝母	bèi mǔ	10 g	Bulbus Fritillaria
牡丹皮	mǔ dān pí	10 g	Cortex Moutan

【Modifications】

➢ For cases with severe eye dryness, add *běi shā shēn* (北沙参, Radix Glehniae) 10 g and *mài dōng* (麦冬, Radix Ophiopogonis) 10 g to benefit the qi and nourish the yin.

(2) Spleen Qi Deficiency

【Syndrome Characteristics】

Eye distending pain or eye pain, heavy eyelids, vision blurred after extensive reading or computer use. Pale complexion, reduced eating, powerless limbs, loose stools, pale tongue, thready pulse.

【Treatment Principle】

Benefit qi and raise yang, dispel wind and stop pain

【Representative Formula】

Modified *Zhù Yáng Huó Xuè Tāng* (Yang-Helping and Blood-Activating Decoction, 助阳活血汤)

【Prescription】

黄芪	huáng qí	20 g	Radix Astragali
白芷	bái zhǐ	10 g	Radix Angelicae Dahuricae
防风	fáng fēng	10 g	Radix Saposhnikoviae
当归	dāng guī	10 g	Radix Angelicae Sinensis
升麻	shēng má	10 g	Rhizoma Cimicifugae
柴胡	chái hú	10 g	Radix Bupleuri
炙甘草	zhì gān cǎo	10 g	Radix et Rhizoma Glycyrrhizae Praeparata cum Melle
蔓荆子	màn jīng zǐ	10 g	Fructus Viticis

【Modifications】

➢ For cases with light loose stool, add *chǎo bái zhú* (炒白术, dry-fried Rhizoma Atractylodis Macrocephalae) 15 g, roasted ginger 3 g to strengthen the spleen, warm the middle and dissipate cold.

➢ For cases with severe eye pain at night, add *xià kū cǎo* (夏枯草, Spica Prunellae) 10 g.

(3) Qi and Blood Deficiency

【Syndrome Characteristics】

Pain of eyeball and supra-orbital bone, being unable to see for a long time. The other symptoms may include pale complexion and pale lips, mental fatigue and lack of strength, forgetful and profuse dreams, pale white tongue, thready and weak pulse.

【Treatment Principle】

Benefit qi and nourish blood, dispel wind and stop pain.

【Representative Formula】

Modified *Dāng Guī Yǎng Róng Tāng* (Chinese Angelica Qi-Nourishing Decoction, 当归养荣汤)

【Prescription】

当归	*dāng guī*	10 g	Radix Angelicae Sinensis
川芎	*chuān xiōng*	6 g	Rhizoma Chuanxiong
白芍	*bái sháo*	10 g	Radix Paeoniae Alba
熟地黄	*shú dì huáng*	10 g	Radix Rehmanniae Praeparata
羌活	*qiāng huó*	6 g	Radix et Rhizoma Notopterygii
防风	*fáng fēng*	6 g	Radix Saposhnikoviae
白芷	*bái zhǐ*	6 g	Radix Angelicae Dahuricae
党参	*dǎng shēn*	15 g	Radix Codonopsis

【Modifications】

➢ For cases with marked syndromes of qi deficiency add *zhì huáng qí* (炙黄芪, Radix Astragali Praeparata cum) 20 g to tonify lung and spleen qi. For cases with severe syndromes of blood deficiency, add *zhì hé shǒu wū* (制何首乌, Radix Polygoni Multiflori Praeparata cum Succo Glycines Sotae) 10 g and *lóng yǎn ròu* (龙眼肉, Arillus Longan) 10 g to nourish blood and tranquilize spirit. For cases with serious supra-orbital bone pain, add *mù guā* (木瓜, Fructus Chaenomelis) 10 g and *gōu téng* (钩藤, Ramulus Uncariae Cum Uncis) 10 g to subdue wind and stop pain.

(4) Liver Constraint and Blood deficiency

【Syndrome Characteristics】

Being unable to read for an extensive period of time, complaining of blurred vision, headache, eye distending pain after long time reading, or tightness sensation of the forehead, heavy eyelids, or sore and dryness of the eye. Usually there is no obvious systemic symptom. Pale tongue with white coating, deep wiry and thready rapid pulse or deep and weak, forceless pulse.

【Treatment Principle】

Enrich yin and nourish blood, clear the liver and harmonize.

【Representative Formula】

Zī Yīn Yǎng Xuè Hé Jiě Tāng (Yin-enriching, blood-nourishing and harmonizing decoction, 滋阴养血和解汤)

【Prescription】

熟地黄	*shú dì huáng*	30 g	Radix Rehmanniae Praeparata
枸杞子	*gǒu qǐ zǐ*	12 g	Fructus Lycii
麦冬	*mài dōng*	10 g	Radix Ophiopogonis
沙参	*shā shēn*	10 g	Radix Adenophorae
当归	*dāng guī*	5 g	Radix Angelicae Sinensis
白芍	*bái sháo*	5 g	Radix Paeoniae Alba
黄芩	*huáng qín*	10 g	Radix Scutellariae
半夏	*bàn xià*	10 g	Rhizoma Pinelliae
银柴胡	*yín chái hú*	10 g	Radix Stellariae
荆芥	*jīng jiè*	10 g	Herba Schizonepetae
防风	*fáng fēng*	10 g	Radix Saposhnikoviae
香附	*xiāng fù*	10 g	Rhizoma Cyperi
夏枯草	*xià kū cǎo*	15 g	Spica Prunellae
甘草	*gān cǎo*	3 g	Radix et Rhizoma Glycyrrhizae

【Modifications】

➢ For cases with dry stool, add *fān xiè yè* (番泻叶, Folium Sennae) 10 g.

➢ For cases with loose stool and acid swallowing, remove *shú dì huáng* (熟地黄, Radix Rehmanniae Praeparata), add *bái zhú* (白术, Rhizoma Atractylodis Macrocephalae) 10 g, *cāng zhú* (苍术, Rhizoma Atractylodis) 10 g, and *wú zhū yú* (吴茱萸, Fructus Evodiae) 10 g.

2. Acupuncture

(1) Body Acupuncture Therapy

ST 1 (*chéng qì*)	BL 2 (*cuán zhú*)	*tài yáng* (太阳)
GB 20 (*fēng chí*)	*yú yāo* (鱼腰)	SJ 23 (*sī zhú kōng*)
qiú hòu (球后)	LI 4 (*hé gǔ*)	

Choose 4–6 points using 1 inch filiform needles, retain the needle for 30–45 minutes

after the arrival of qi, treat one time each day, 12 treatments is one course of treatment.

(2) **Massage**

Choose acupoints around the eye like

ST 1 (*chéng qì*)	BL 2 (*cuán zhú*)	BL 1 (*jīng míng*)
SJ 23 (*sī zhú kōng*)	GB 14 (*yang bái*)	*yú yāo* (鱼腰)

Massage the points with fingers in combination with gentle acupressure, for 10 minutes, 3 times a day.

3. Chinese Patent Medicines

(1) *Rén Shēn Guī Pí Wán* (人参归脾丸 , **Ginseng Spleen-Restoring Pill**)

1 pill (6g), twice a day. It is applicable to spleen qi deficiency.

(2) *Bā Zhēn Kē Lì* (八珍颗粒冲剂 , **Eight Gem Granules**)

One bag (6 g), twice a day, applicable to deficiency of qi and blood.

(3) *Qǐ Jú Dì Huáng Wán* (**Lycium Berry, Chrysanthemum and Rehmannia Pill,** 杞菊地黄丸)

1 pill, twice a day, applicable to liver-kidney yin deficiency.

4. Simple and Proven Recipes

(1) *Jú huā* (菊花, Flos Chrysanthemi) 30 g, *jué míng zǐ* (决明子, Semen Cassiae) 30 g, *mài dōng* (麦冬, Radix Ophiopogonis) 30 g, *gǒu qǐ zǐ* (枸杞子, Fructus Lycii) 30 g, wrap the medicinals individually, take 1 g of each every time, put in a teapot and add some boiled water to make medicinal tea, take 6–9 times each day.

(2) *Jú huā* (菊花, Flos Chrysanthemi) 30 g, *mài dōng* (麦冬, Radix Ophiopogonis) 30 g, *pàng dà hǎi* (胖大海, Semen Sterculiae Lychnophorae) 30 g, *shān zhā* (山楂, Fructus Crataegi) 30 g, wrap the medicinals individually, take 1 g of each, put in a teapot and add some boiled water to make medicinal tea, take 6-9 times each day.

5. External Treatment

Slice Chinese waxgourd and soak the slices into cool water for 15 minutes, close the eyes, put the slice on the skin of eyelid, 10 minutes each time, three times a day.

6. Western Medicine

(1) *Guǒ Wéi Kāng Piàn* (果维康片, Vitamin C Buccal Tablets), take orally, 1 tablet, once a day.

(2) Vitamin C, take orally, 20 mg, three times a day.

(3) Vitamin B$_1$, take orally, 20 mg, three times a day.

7. Dietary Therapy and Preventative Health Care

Do not stay up late (past 11pm), eat more vegetables and fruits, rest the eyes for 15 minutes after every 1 hour of reading, eat green plants frequently, do not watch TV, view computer, and play visual games infrequently.

Consume gruel/congee made of rice or millet with black bean, soybean, red bean, walnut, and sesame, peanut and red dates in the morning and again in the evening.

Case Study

Huang, a 26-year-old female

〖 Chief Complaint 〗

Presented to our clinic with chief complaints of distending eye pain and soreness of the eyebrow bone for the last two weeks.

〖 Medical History 〗

She had been in good overall health. She had moderate bleeding at her first labor. She didn't pay attention to rest and taking care of herself after giving birth. She had read three novels successively and weaved a sweater. A month later she felt a distending pain in her eyes and soreness of her eyebrow bones, the pain became unbearable after 15 minutes of reading. She also experienced headaches and nausea, felt flustered and a lack of composure. It was suspected that she may have glaucoma before she came to our clinic.

〖 Examination 〗

Vision, intraocular pressure and the fundus examination is normal. The systemic symptoms and signs include pale complexion, mental fatigue and lack of power, pale tongue, deep and thready pulse.

〖 Diagnosis 〗

Visual fatigue (blood deficiency and wind attack).

〖 Treatment Principles 〗

Nourish blood and dispel wind.

〖 Prescription 〗

Formula: Modified *Dāng Guī Yǎng Róng Tāng* (Chinese Angelica Qi-Nourishing Decoction, 当归养荣汤)

当归	*dāng guī*	10 g	Radix Angelicae Sinensis
川芎	*chuān xiōng*	10 g	Rhizoma Chuanxiong
白芍	*bái sháo*	10 g	Radix Paeoniae Alba

熟地黄	*shú dì huáng*	10 g	Radix Rehmanniae Praeparata
羌活	*qiāng huó*	10 g	Rhizoma et Radix Notopterygii
防风	*fáng fēng*	10 g	Radix Saposhnikoviae
白芷	*bái zhǐ*	10 g	Radix Angelicae Dahuricae
蔓荆子	*màn jīng zǐ*	10 g	Fructus Viticis

One dose per day, decocted with water, 14 doses in total. At her second visit, all of her symptoms completely disappeared.

Classic Quotes

It says in the Introduction to Medicine - Miscellaneous Disease – The Eye (*Yī Xué Rù Mén – Zá Bìng Fēn Lèi –Yǎn*, 医学入门 · 杂病分类 · 眼): "Eye pain caused by excessive reading and embroidering is called *Gān Láo* (肝劳, liver taxation), one needs to close the eyes and take a rest.

Section 6   Lyme Disease

Lyme disease, also called Borreliosis, is caused by the genus Borrelia Burgdorferi. This is a kind of spirochetal infection originated from a tick bite. The typical rash of the disease is called erythema chronicum migrans, and may appear in the groin, thigh or armpit. Several days or several weeks later, the pathological changes may affect the whole body including the central nervous system. If the eyes are effected, it may cause retinitis or orbital optic neuritis, which is named as Lyme disease-induced optic neuritis.

The disease can be seen all over the world, most frequently in spring and summer, and without gender differences. The incidence rate is higher in Northeastern United States. Wisconsin is another endemic area for Lyme disease.

Clinical Manifestation

Lyme disease may result in pathological changes in ocular and neuro-optic system. The typical clinical manifestation can be divided into three stages.

Stage 1: 60%–80% of patients have a rash presenting with expanding erythema chronicum migrans, sometimes accompanied by fever, regional lymph and slight general malaise. If the eyes are involved, it may present as conjunctivitis, photophobia, periorbital edema, diffuse choroiditis, exudative detachment of retina and iridocyclitis.

Stage 2: The infection may spread through bloodstream or lymphatic system, which leads to symptoms on the skin, nervous system or musculoskeletal system, like annulare erythema on the cheek, joint pain, myocarditis, lymphadenopathy, splenomegalia, hepatitis, haematuria, albuminuria, malaise and fatigue. The eye infection may include symptoms of keratitis, panophthalmitis, papilloedema (similar to pseudotumor cerebri syndrome), granuloma iritis, hyalitis and orbital myositis etc. About two thirds of the patients develop ocular complications and central nervous system problems, of which the most common disorders are facial paralysis, optic neuritis, meningitis and radiculopathy.

Stage 3: The symptoms at later stages are caused by persistent infection, typically includes arthritis and skin lesion similar to dermatosclerosis. Keratitis and nervous system disorders like encephalomyelitis, spastic paraparesis, ataxia gait, paraphora and chronic radiculopathy are very common too. Symptoms of the nervous system and the relative radiation examination have similar characteristics of multiple sclerosis.

The diagnosis of Lyme disease is mainly made by a specialist of infectious diseases. Serological tests by means of enzyme-linked immunosorbent assay (ELISA) is suggested for the patient when the disease is suspected by clinical manifestation. Lyme disease spirochetes antibody-positive of cerebrospinal fluid is the sensitive indicator for nervous system disorders. PCR and specific immune complex detection assay can improve the sensitivity and accuracy of the diagnosis for nervous system and other patterns Lyme disease. The patients who have a typical rash after a tick bite in the endemic area should be highly suspected, for up to 80% of those are diagnosed with Lyme disease.

Treatment

Treatment of Lyme disease should be administered by an infectious disease specialist due to different stages and systems involved. However, intravenous ceftriaxone antibiotic is effective at the early stage. In TCM, the eye disorders of Lyme disease can be treated with medicinals and acupuncture, detailed therapies referred to treatments for keratitis, iritis, optic neuritis.

Summary

Chinese medicine was discovered thousands of years ago to prevent and treat many eye diseases. Every person is born with inherent strengths and weaknesses that affect the eyes. Trauma, stress, emotions, infections, exercise, diet, habits, and lifestyle all affect vision. When we learn to manage our weaknesses and maximize our strengths, good health and optimal vision endure.

There are many factors that cause degenerative vision loss, including genetic predisposition, metabolic diseases, poor circulation, overuse, etc. Chinese medicine may lead you to fully understand your constitutional strengths and weaknesses, showing you how to safeguard your health and vision.

Personal accountability and responsibility for one's own state of health is the hallmark of Chinese Medicine. Many cultures have become dependent on pharmaceuticals and conventional medical intervention. Medical treatments can be extremely beneficial and are primarily geared towards acute care, and relief of symptoms - rather than identifying and correcting the true underlying causes of disease.

Modern medicine is highly effective in managing acute trauma and emergency cases, but generally is a poor system for managing chronic illness, especially ophthalmic conditions. Conventional treatment for many of the leading chronic eye conditions may greatly benefit from an integrative strategy. These include macular degeneration, retinitis pigmentosa, glaucoma, ushers syndrome, uveitis, optic atrophy, optic neuritis, etc.

Cataract surgery often works very well. Glaucoma meds and trabulectomies, implants may control intra-ocular pressure, but people with glaucoma are still going blind. Avastin/ Lucentis injections and/or laser treatment for cases retinal bleeding may be helpful. In cases like wet macular degeneration, macula edema, and diabetic retinopathy, laser and injections may work short-term to control bleeding; however extensive laser procedures and frequent injections may weaken the blood vessels in the eye resulting in a possible higher rate of recurrence. It may be that the best strategy for most chronic cases of eye disease would be to incorporate both Eastern and Western medicine.

In China, many hospitals and eye clinics integrate modern medicine with acupuncture and Chinese Medicine. In most other countries, like the United States, there is virtually no integration. Most seek medical treatment for their eye diseases, unaware of the benefits that Chinese Medicine may provide. Acupuncture, herbs and adjunctive therapies are generally "dismissed" by Western medicine (especially in the US) because there is little or no medical research supporting its efficacy. We believe that once conventional medicinal community becomes more open to Chinese Medicine, we can then begin evidence-based research which will increase acceptance and integration. Incorporating both Western and Eastern medical treatment strategies for eye disease may ultimately prove to be most beneficial approach.

In addition to being a practical clinical manual for practitioners of Chinese medicine in the treatment of ophthalmic conditions, we hope that the field of TCM ophthalmology grows internationally so as to aid in providing the absolute best possible care for our eye patients.

We thank you for considering our ideas and hope you find the information in this text useful.

Appendix

Glossary

five orbiculi	*wǔ lún*, 五轮
flesh orbiculus; eyelid	*ròu lún*, 肉轮
blood orbiculus; canthus	*xuè lún*, 血轮
qi orbiculus; white of the eye	*qì lún*, 气轮
wind orbiculus; the black of the eye	*fēng lún*, 风轮
water orbiculus; pupil	*shuǐ lún*, 水轮
inner canthus	*mù nèi zì*, 目内眦
outer canthus	*mù wài zì*, 目外眦
the white of the eye	*bái jīng*, 白睛
the black of the eye	*hēi jīng*, 黑睛
pupil	*tóng shén*, 瞳神
spirit water (aqueous humor; tear)	*shén shuǐ*, 神水
petaloid nebula with a sunken center (ulcerative keratitis)	*huā yì bái xiàn*, 花翳白陷
wind-orbiculus red bean (fascicular keratitis)	*fēng lún chì dòu*, 风轮赤豆
sparrow vision (night blindness)	*què mù*, 雀目
contracted pupil (iridocyclitis)	*tóng shén jǐn xiǎo*, 瞳神紧小
pupillary metamorphosis (posterior synechia)	*tóng rén gān quē*, 瞳人干缺
green glaucoma (acute angle-closure glaucoma)	*lǜ fēng nèi zhàng*, 绿风内障
bluish wind glaucoma (primary open angle glaucoma)	*qīng fēng nèi zhàng*, 青风内障
round nebula cataract (senile cataract)	*yuán yì nèi zhàng*, 圆翳内障
fog moving before eye (vitreous opacity)	*yún wù yí jīng*, 云雾移睛
bluish blindness (optic atrophy)	*qīng máng*, 青盲
high-wind internal visual obstruction (retinitis pigmentosa)	*gāo fēng nèi zhàng*, 高风内障

blurring vision	*shì zhān hūn miǎo*, 视瞻昏渺
paralytic strabismus	*fēng qiān piān shì*, 风牵偏视
stye	*zhēn yǎn*, 针眼
phlegm node in eyelid (chalazion)	*bāo shēng tán hé*, 胞生痰核
drooping of upper eyelid (blepharoptosis)	*shàng bāo xià chuí*, 上胞下垂
epidemic red eye (acute contagious conjunctivitis)	*tiān xíng chì yǎn*, 天行赤眼
fulminant wind and invading fever (acute contagious conjunctivitis)	*bào fēng kè rè*, 暴风客热
clustered stars nebula (herpes simplex keratitis)	*jù xīng zhàng*, 聚星障
seasonal eye itching	*shí fù mù yǎng*, 时复目痒
wind red sore (herpes zoster of the eye lid)	*fēng chì chuāng yí*, 风赤疮痍
red ulceration of the palpebral margin	*jiǎn xián chì làn*, 睑弦赤烂
wind wheel red bean (phlyctenular keratoconjunctivitis)	*fēng lún chì dòu*, 风轮赤豆
twitching eyelid (blepharospasm)	*bāo lún zhèn tiào*, 胞轮振跳
fire gan (scleritis)	*huǒ gān*, 火疳
tinted vision (central serous chorioretinopathy)	*shì zhān yǒu sè*, 视瞻有色
seeing straight things as crooked (central serous chorioretinopathy)	*shì zhí rú qū*, 视直如曲
seeing small things as big (central serous chorioretinopathy)	*shì xiǎo wéi dà*, 视小为大
sudden bulging of the eyes (hyroid-associated opthalmopathy)	*tū qǐ jīng gāo*, 突起睛高
strabismus	*tōng jīng*, 通睛
hyphema	bleeding into the anterior chamber of the eye
goniosynechia	adhesion of the iris to the posterior surface of the cornea in the angle of the anterior chamber of the eye

图书在版编目（CIP）数据

中医眼科学：英文 / 韦企平，（美）安迪·罗森法
尔布，梁丽娜主编 . —2 版 . —北京：人民卫生出版社，
2018

国际标准化英文版中医教材

ISBN 978–7–117–27737–2

I. ①中… II. ①韦… ②安… ③梁… III. ①中医五
官科学 – 眼科学 – 教材 – 英文　IV. ①R276.7

中国版本图书馆 CIP 数据核字（2018）第 261314 号

人卫智网	www.ipmph.com	医学教育、学术、考试、健康， 购书智慧智能综合服务平台
人卫官网	www.pmph.com	人卫官方资讯发布平台

国际标准化英文版中医教材

中医眼科学

第 2 版

主　　编：韦企平　（美）安迪·罗森法尔布　梁丽娜
出版发行：人民卫生出版社（中继线 010-59780011）
地　　址：北京市朝阳区潘家园南里 19 号
邮　　编：100021
E - mail：pmph @ pmph.com
购书热线：010-59787592　010-59787584　010-65264830
印　　刷：北京虎彩文化传播有限公司
经　　销：新华书店
开　　本：787×1092　1/16　　印张：26
字　　数：633 千字
版　　次：2011 年 5 月第 1 版　　2018 年 12 月第 2 版
　　　　　2019 年 12 月第 2 版第 2 次印刷（总第 3 次印刷）
标准书号：ISBN 978-7-117-27737-2
定　　价（含光盘）：480.00 元
打击盗版举报电话：010-59787491　E-mail：WQ @ pmph.com
（凡属印装质量问题请与本社市场营销中心联系退换）